Comments for Priceless

"With his head for the practical and his heart for the disadvantaged, John Goodman has long been the clearest and most insightful healthcare thinker we have. Now that our perverse, accidental 'insurance' system has reached its inevitable crisis, it's time we acted on his common sense, fact-based wisdom in *Priceless*."

—**Mitch E. Daniels**, Governor of Indiana

"John Goodman's book *Priceless* provides more good thinking from the person who taught us that incentives matter."

—**Michael O. Leavitt**, former Governor of Utah; former Secretary, US Department of Health and Human Services; former Administrator, US Environmental Protection Agency

"*Priceless* is an important contribution to a market-friendly approach to reforming healthcare."

—**Martin S. Feldstein**, George F. Baker Professor of Economics, Harvard University; President Emeritus, National Bureau of Economic Research

"If liberal commentators wish to sharpen their claws, there is no better stone on which to do it than John Goodman's book *Priceless*."

—**Uwe E. Reinhardt**, James Madison Professor of Political Economy and Professor of Economics and Public Affairs, Princeton University; former Commissioner, Physician Payment Review Commission

"John Goodman, widely known as the father of health savings accounts, is as provocative and controversial as ever in his new book, *Priceless*. His prescription for fixing what ails American healthcare is to free American consumers to seek the healthcare that best suits their needs and to free physicians and hospital administrators to provide the best, lowest cost care they can by getting rid of the constraints and disincentives provided by insurance companies and public payers. An interesting read for all who have been frustrated in their search for a workable solution to our healthcare woes."

—**Gail R. Wilensky**, Senior Fellow, Project HOPE; former Administrator, Centers for Medicare and Medicaid Services

"There's no question that today's healthcare system is littered with distorted incentives and what John Goodman calls dysfunctionality. This book is a call to arms to do something about it. Even if you don't agree with all of Goodman's ideas—and there are plenty I disagree with—you should read this book if you want to be an informed participant in the debate over the future of healthcare in this country."

—**Peter R. Orszag**, former Director, Congressional Budget Office; Vice Chairman, Global Banking, *Citigroup*, Inc.

"*Priceless* is unique in that it combines a general discussion of the issues in health; access, cost and quality, with specific implications of the Patient Protection and Affordable Act of 2009 on these same issues. The book is provocative and instructive, a combination that is difficult to pull off but done here in John Goodman's style of combining humor with fact. This book should be on the reading list for everyone interested in healthcare reform."

—**Thomas R. Saving**, Jeff Montgomery Professor of Economics and Director of Private Enterprise Research Center, Texas A&M University

"John Goodman is a highly influential health policy analyst, organization leader, and entrepreneur whose ideas are always provocative and simply can't be ignored. You may not agree with every proposal he makes, but he is right on target when he notes that future solutions to unsustainable health-cost growth must convince consumers and patients that they gain from those reforms."

—**C. Eugene Steuerle,** MD, Institute Fellow and Richard B. Fisher Chair, Urban Institute

"In *Priceless*, Goodman argues that doctors are trapped in a dysfunctional system and they need to be liberated. He's right. Restore liberty. End coercion."

—**Donald J. Palmisano**, former President, American Medical Association

"In *Priceless: Curing the Healthcare Crisis*, John Goodman explains why so many Americans—the sick, the healthy, consumers, employers, medical professionals and insurers—feel trapped by the US healthcare system. Thankfully, he demonstrates that there *are* ways to escape the health-care traps, and his solutions deserve serious attention, regardless of one's political persuasions."

—**John Engler**, President, Business Roundtable; former Governor of Michigan

"John Goodman's terrific book *Priceless* is indeed priceless. It offers a breath of fresh air in a tired healthcare debate that demonstrates once again that markets enjoy their greatest advantage in complex settings that call for imaginative solutions that no government-driven system can deliver. Critics may carp that healthcare markets are never perfectly competitive. Goodman offers chapter and verse to explain why market innovation beats top-down schemes by a mile—ACA especially included."

—**Richard A. Epstein**, Laurence A. Tisch Professor of Law,
New York University

"In *Priceless*, John Goodman provides a much needed perspective on healthcare issues—he is the leading proponent of using market-based reforms to solve health policy problems."

—**Kevin M. Murphy**, George J. Stigler Distinguished Service
Professor of Economics, University of Chicago

"John Goodman's analysis is incisive and compelling. The insight and innovative thinking in *Priceless* will be invaluable in avoiding the harms of government-run healthcare."

—**Steve Forbes**, Chairman and Editor-in-Chief, *Forbes* Media

"John Goodman is always interesting, always provocative. His ideas are not to be ignored."

—**Jim Cooper**, US Congressman (D-TN)

"John Goodman's timely and important book *Priceless* has much to like. The presentation of healthcare economics is clear as is the discussion of the perverse incentives in healthcare. Good writing and clear explanations have always been hallmarks of Goodman's writing. I particularly like three aspects of this book: the consideration of the role of time prices and the surprising winners and losers that emerge from the healthcare reform legislation; the analysis of the political economy of healthcare systems and Goodman's explanation of why European systems look and act so differently from ours; and the policy prescriptions to reform health insurance, Medicare and Medicaid. Anyone seriously interested in understanding healthcare reform should look carefully at the proposals offered here."

—**Michael A. Morrisey**, Professor of Health Economics and Health
Insurance and Director of the Lister Hill Center for Health Policy,
University of Alabama at Birmingham

"In the sea of perplexity and inefficiency that characterizes health policy, John Goodman's new book, *Priceless,* provides fresh and original insights to help steer us into a system that harnesses individual choice, aligns price and quality, and more effectively utilizes financing to achieve these ends."

—**June E. O'Neill**, Wollman Distinguished Professor of Economics and Director of the Center for the Study of Business and Government, Baruch College; former Director, Congressional Budget Office

"I have not agreed with Goodman's emphasis on high-deductible health insurance in healthcare.... But no one who is serious about health reform can afford to ignore the ideas in *Priceless*."

—**Alain C. Enthoven,** Eccles Professor of Public and Private Management Emeritus, Stanford University

"In *Priceless,* John Goodman's challenge to the conventional wisdom of a healthcare system broken because of excessive freedom can not be more timely. As we stand on the brink of hyper-regulating our system further, Goodman cogently argues that our answer is to free our system from the traps policymakers, insurers and providers have built over the decades."

—**Stephen T. Parente,** Professor of Finance and Director of the Medical Industry Leadership Institute, University of Minnesota

"*Priceless* illustrates the importance of market-based solutions to drive affordability, access, and higher quality experience for today's empowered healthcare consumers."

—**Angela F. Braly,** Chair, President, and Chief Executive Officer, WellPoint, Inc.

"Everyone who wants to understand the mess Washington has made of health policy should read John Goodman's incisive book, *Priceless*. Generations of health reformers have tried to engineer a new system based on regulation and centralized control, only to find higher cost for healthcare that too often fails to provide value to patients. Goodman has a better idea: replace the perverse economic incentives of first dollar coverage and top-down regulation with real insurance, and let competition work."

—**Joseph R. Antos,** Wilson H. Taylor Scholar in Healthcare and Retirement Policy, American Enterprise Institute

"Too many American health economists have looked to government to solve healthcare problems, without realizing that government is the fundamental cause of these problems. John Goodman is the welcome exception and his innovative work has been influential in his creation of health savings accounts. His book *Priceless* is now full of equally useful ideas for restoring healthcare to the market, and when ACA disappears this book will provide the framework for truly reforming healthcare for all."

—**Paul H. Rubin**, Samuel Candler Dobbs Professor of Economics, Emory University

"John Goodman has been developing innovative ideas on how to create a better health system, a less expensive health system, a health system with more access for well over two decades. He really was the creator of the health-savings-account model and developed that entire initiative to try to give people increased resources and increased control over their health."

—**Newt Gingrich**, 58th Speaker of the US House of Representatives

"I have been following John Goodman's health policy ideas for as long as I've been on Capitol Hill. John's latest effort, *Priceless: Curing the Health Care Crisis*, makes it abundantly clear why he is a source of wisdom, insight, and innovative thinking."

—**Paul Ryan**, US Congressman (R-WI)

"While many people discuss the problems within our healthcare system, few propose real solutions. John Goodman has written a book that not only accurately describes what is happening with healthcare in our nation, it provides key solutions and answers to a problem that so desperately needs to be corrected."

—**Jeb Bush**, former Governor of Florida

"In a health policy world dominated by old tarnished ideas recycled under new acronyms, it is a pleasure to read *Priceless* that goes back to first principles, defies pigeonholing, and ends up with imaginative yet eminently practical proposals for reform."

—**Mark V. Pauly**, Bendheim Professor, Professor of Health Care Management, and Professor of Business and Public Policy, Wharton School, University of Pennsylvania; former Commissioner, Physician Payment Review Commission

"John Goodman is one of the nation's top thinkers in healthcare policy. His new book, *Priceless*, will be an important resource for policy makers in Washington and around the country."

—**Kay Bailey Hutchison**, US Senator (R-TX)

"*Priceless* makes a very persuasive case that liberating people is the key to health reform. When we free the patients and the healthcare professionals from payer and government shackles, we will drive quality up and price down and eliminate an enormous amount of waste."

—**Stephen B. Bonner**, President and Chief Executive Officer, Cancer Treatment Centers of America

"America is in perilous times. In *Priceless: Curing the Healthcare Crisis* John Goodman deftly explains how to jettison the overgrown dysfunctional gridlock that prevents reform of healthcare and healthcare entitlements."

—**Earl L. Grinols**, Distinguished Professor of Economics and Director of Doctoral Programs Development, Robbins Institute for Health Policy and Leadership, Baylor University

"John Goodman explains in *Priceless* why the health sector is so dysfunctional and why problems cannot be solved by adding even more layers of government bureaucracy, regulation, and price distortion. Goodman brings his clear thinking as an economist to explain how we could employ market forces in health care to realign incentives so patients, doctors, and all of the players in the health care marketplace are seeking greater efficiency, higher quality, and better value."

—**Grace-Marie Turner**, President, Galen Institute

"From the author of *Patient Power*, *Priceless* is a new book about why we need to empower doctors as well as patients."

—**Daniel H. Johnson, Jr.**, MD, former President, American Medical Association; former President, World Medical Association

"With *Priceless*, John Goodman has written a path-breaking book that everyone should read."

—**William A. Archer, Jr.**, former US Congressman and Chairman, House Ways and Means Committee

PRICELESS

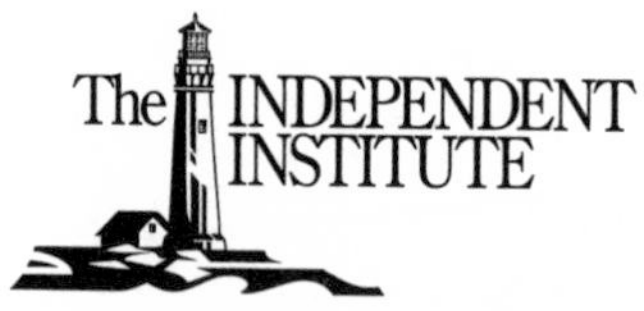

THE INDEPENDENT INSTITUTE is a non-profit, non-partisan, scholarly research and educational organization that sponsors comprehensive studies in political economy. Our mission is to boldly advance peaceful, prosperous, and free societies, grounded in a commitment to human worth and dignity.

Politicized decision-making in society has confined public debate to a narrow reconsideration of existing policies. Given the prevailing influence of partisan interests, little social innovation has occurred. In order to understand both the nature of and possible solutions to major public issues, the Independent Institute adheres to the highest standards of independent inquiry, regardless of political or social biases and conventions. The resulting studies are widely distributed as books and other publications, and are debated in numerous conference and media programs. Through this uncommon depth and clarity, the Independent Institute is redefining public debate and fostering new and effective directions for government reform.

100 Swan Way, Oakland, California 94621-1428, USA
Telephone: 510-632-1366 • Facsimile: 510-568-6040 • Email: info@independent.org • www.independent.org

JOHN C. GOODMAN

PRICELESS

CURING THE HEALTHCARE CRISIS

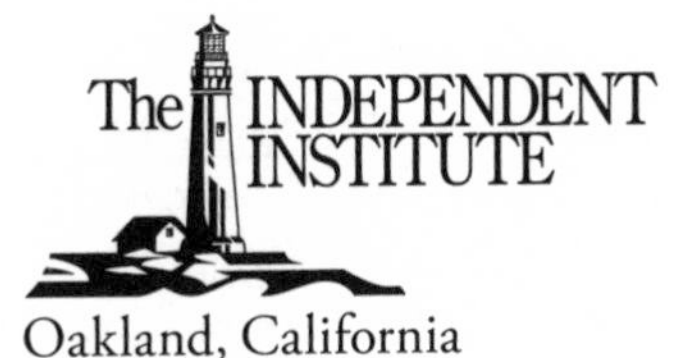

Oakland, California

The Independent Institute 100 Swan Way, Oakland, CA 94621-1428
Telephone: 510-632-1366 Fax: 510-568-6040 Email: info@independent.org
Website: www.independent.org

Cover Design: Keith Criss
Cover Image: © Jamie Grill/Getty
Interior Design and Composition by Leigh McLellan Design

Library of Congress Cataloging-in-Publication Data

Goodman, John C.
Priceless : curing our healthcare crisis / John C. Goodman.
p. cm.
ISBN 978-1-59813-083-6 (hardcover : alk. paper)
1. Medical care—United States. 2. Medical policy—United States.
3. Medical care, Cost of—United States. 4. Health care reform—United States. I. Title.
RA395.A3G657 2012
362.10973—dc23 2012008379

16 15 14 13 12 5 4 3 2

Contents

Preface

An Intellectual Odyssey

WHEN GERALD MUSGRAVE and I wrote *Patient Power*[1] two decades ago, we had no idea we were starting a revolution in thinking about health policy. At the time, just about everybody in the field was advocating managed care and managed competition. And I really mean *everybody*. The large insurance companies, the employer trade groups, the medical organizations, even the American Medical Association—all were in support of the prevailing ideas.

Aside from the libertarian Cato Institute (which published *Patient Power*), the conservative think tanks were just as enthusiastically advocating conventional thinking as the liberal ones. Conservative Republicans were as much on board as liberal Democrats. Historians will record that Hillary Clinton's healthcare reform plan went down to inglorious defeat. What they probably will neglect to say is that a very similar proposal had the support of most Senate Republicans at the time.

The Clinton health reform failed because of White House ineptitude and grass roots resistance. It did not fail because of any major disagreement between the two political parties about health policy.

It was a lonely time. At least for me.

When I took the idea of Health Savings Accounts (HSAs) to Capitol Hill in the early 1990s, only five members of Congress agreed to sign onto a bill creating them. When The Independent Institute published an important book on health policy a few years later, *American Health Care*,[2] they could find only one economist on a university campus anywhere in America who would defend the idea of patients managing their own healthcare dollars.

In retrospect, what we said was not all that radical. Or even all that insightful. What mattered was that we dared to say it. We were like the child who declares that the emperor has no clothes. What we were saying was what thousands of others thought all along, but didn't quite know how to express.

Our book began an intellectual sea change in thinking about health policy. Even today, I meet people who tell me that their entire approach to health policy was shaped and molded by *Patient Power.*

So why do we need a new book? In part because the policy landscape has changed. In the not-so-distant future we may be living with the Affordable Care Act (ACA). In addition, there are four important things I have learned since I wrote *Patient Power.*

First is the importance of liberating doctors. Our focus in *Patient Power* was on freeing the patient. A good part of the book was devoted to the idea that when people are spending their own money they behave very differently than when they are spending other people's money. Give patients control over their own healthcare dollars, we argued, and they will become more careful, prudent consumers of medical care.

All that was true. What I didn't anticipate was that the changes on the supply side of the market would be far more profound than the changes on the demand side. On the consumer side of the market, patients spending their own money will shop, compare prices and decide to buy or not to buy. When you stop to think about it, there's not much more they can do. On the provider side, however, we are unleashing a torrent of entrepreneurial activity that would have been unthinkable only a decade ago.

When patients aren't spending their own money, there is no way doctors can compete for their patronage based on price. When they don't compete on price, they don't compete on quality either. The services they offer will be only those services the third parties pay for and only in settings and ways the third parties have blessed. But give patients control over their own healthcare dollars and the provider community will begin to meet needs in ways the third-party-payer bureaucracies could never have dreamed of. Who do you think is going to be more creative about meeting unmet needs? Executives at a handful of insurance companies? Or 800,000 doctors dealing with real patients day in and day out?

At one point, I was tempted to title this book, *Doctor Power.* Its central message could not be more radically different than the prevailing thinking in the health policy community. The orthodox view is that doctors are the problem. They have too much freedom, we are told. They need to be constrained and told what to do. But the orthodox view is wrong. Doctors are not the problem. They are the solution.

Have you ever heard the phrase, "We are paying for volume, not value"? If not, just attend a few more health conferences and you surely will. The problem with that point of view is that it suggests that we can make things right by changing the way buyers pay for care. Wrong. What we need is a system in which the provider side of the market competes to provide value because it is in their self-interest to attract patients in that way. We will never solve America's healthcare crisis from the buyer side of the market. It can only be solved from the provider side.

Over and over again I have discovered that every center of excellence, every example of exemplary care, every example of high-quality, low-cost medicine originated on the supply side—not the demand side—of the market.

The second thing I missed the last time around was the importance of prices. The single worst public policy decision in all of heath care was the decision to eliminate money prices from the market for medical care. Have you ever wondered why the panhandler on the street corner has a cell phone, but no access to primary care? It's because he can buy a cell phone in a real marketplace, but he can't buy healthcare that way.

As this book goes to press, a new study finds that enrolling children in the Children's Health Insurance Program (CHIP: essentially, Medicaid for children) does not result in their receiving more medical care. But when CHIP pays higher fees to doctors, the children do get more care.[3] Think about that for a minute. We encourage low-income families to enroll their children, usually by making the insurance absolutely free. Many of them drop their private coverage to take advantage of the offer. But we make it illegal for the family to add to CHIP's fees and pay the market rate for their care. They can have free health insurance only if they agree not to purchase the same care everyone else is able to buy.

When we expand a government insurance plan for low-income patients, we are spending billions of dollars in a way that *doesn't* increase their access to care. At the same time, we forbid the enrollees to do the one thing that *would* expand access to care.

Contrast this foolishness with the Food Stamp program. Low-income shoppers can enter any supermarket in America and buy almost anything the market has to offer by adding cash to the "voucher" the government gives them. They can buy everything you and I can buy because they pay the same price you and I pay. But we absolutely forbid them to do the same thing in the medical marketplace.

The third thing I failed to fully appreciate in the earlier book is the second biggest mistake in all of health policy: making it illegal for insurers to charge premiums that reflect real risks. In every other insurance market, insurers try to find people who face important risks and they try to sell them on the idea that it is rational to insure against those risks. In the health field we do the opposite. In most places we make it against the law for a health insurer to charge a fair premium to a person who has above average expected healthcare costs. This means that insurers have an economic self-interest in avoiding people with health problems and in failing to encourage them to seek optimal treatment once they do enroll.

One of the most amazing features of the healthcare sector—both in this country and in other countries—is the persistence of so many unmet needs. Millions of diabetics, asthmatics, people with hypertension, people with high cholesterol, etc., are not getting the drugs they need. Many are not getting medical treatment at all. According to one calculation, if these chronic conditions were being treated optimally, we would double, triple, and even quadruple the number of drugs being dispensed for these and other conditions.[4]

The absence of real prices for health insurance and real prices for medical care combines to completely deter what should be a vibrant market to solve the problems of people with medical problems.

One reason for this policy mistake is erroneous thinking about pre-existing conditions. Ninety percent of all the people with private health insurance in this country are already in a health insurance plan that is legally barred from charging anyone a higher premium because of a pre-existing condition. Once the ACA kicks in, no plan will be able to charge an enrollee a high premium based on health status.

The solution to this problem is not to *outlaw* insurance for pre-existing conditions, but to *legalize* it. In an unfettered market, you would be able to insure against the possibility of developing a pre-existing condition that results in above average premiums, should you need to change health plans. When you enter a new health plan, you and your previous insurer would pay a premium that fully reflects the expected costs you bring to that plan. In such a market, the sick would be just as desirable as the healthy to an insurance company. And there would be an active, entrepreneurial market to find low-cost ways to solve your health problems—in order to lower costs both for you and your insurer.

Notice that both of these policy mistakes share the same basic problem: the suppression of the price system. That is why I chose to title this book, *Priceless*.

It is clearly a double entendre. On the one hand, most of us would probably describe good health as a priceless asset—something money can't buy. On the other hand if something goes wrong and we need help, the system we have erected to correct our problems is also priceless. In a normal market, prices convey information. A high price tells innovators and entrepreneurs the market places a high value on getting a problem solved. It communicates that the reward for finding a solution could be high as well. When the price system is artificially suppressed, that information does not get communicated. Almost all of our problems in health policy stem from this central fact.

There is a fourth factor that I ignored in the earlier work. Normally I do not comment on the motives or the psychological makeup of people I disagree with. I don't want to be guilty of argument ad hominem. Yet through the years I have discovered that the most important differences people have over health policy have little to do with facts, reasoning or logical argument. The most important differences stem from differences in fundamental world views. There are a very large number of people in this field who find the price system distasteful—at least for medical care.

Why is it important to know this? Because most of the health policy community is at least nominally committed to the idea of using pilot programs and demonstration projects to find out what works and what doesn't work. Put differently, most health policy experts are committed to "evidence-based" public policy.

But the truth of the matter is that there is no amount of evidence that is going to convince most of the orthodox health policy community that prices should be allowed to allocate resources in the market for medical care. For well intentioned reasons perhaps, they are emotionally predisposed to favor the suppression of normal market processes.

For better or for worse, I think it is valuable to know this, before the intellectual discussion even begins.

This book could not have been written without my first learning something about health economics, and for that I am most grateful to Gerald Musgrave, who taught me much while we were writing *Patient Power*.

Mark Pauly (Wharton School) helped refine my thinking on how the government should optimally subsidize private health insurance. Our *Health Affairs* article[5] laid out the case for fixed-sum, refundable tax credits and Roth Health Savings Accounts. I think of this as the economists' approach because almost all the health economists I know like the ideas. The tax credit concept we developed has been incorporated in most of the more radical Republican health reform proposals over the past two decades and in some Democratic proposals as well.

Mark, Gerald and University of South Florida professor Philip Porter also helped refine my thinking on managed competition, discussed in Chapter 8.

Almost the whole of Chapter 11 on designing ideal health insurance comes from a paper solicited by Harvard Business School professor Regina Herzlinger, for her book, *Consumer-Driven Healthcare*.[6] Many of the ideas on reforming the malpractice system in Chapter 12 were inspired by the early writings of New York University law professor, Richard Epstein.

Some of the key ideas here also first appeared in *Lives at Risk*,[7] written with Gerald Musgrave and Devon Herrick, and *Handbook on State Health Care Reform*,[8] written with Michael Bond, Devon Herrick, Gerald Musgrave, Pam Villarreal and Joe Barnett. Also important, especially in comparing our own healthcare system to that of other countries, is the National Center for Policy Analysis paper "Health Care Reform: Do Other Countries Have the Answers?",[9] which I wrote with Linda Gorman, Devon Herrick, and Robert Sade.

Readers will note that a number of the graphics and quite a few endnotes in this book refer to studies produced for the National Center for Policy Analysis by Thomas R. Saving and Andrew J. Rettenmaier with the Private Enterprise Research Center at Texas A&M University. Needless to say, I am greatly in their debt. Also important to this book's message is the work I have done over the years with Boston University professor Laurence J. Kotlikoff.

John Goodman's Health Policy Blog has become *the place* where the economic approach to health policy is debated by health policy wonks from across the political spectrum. I have borrowed shamelessly from the posts of fellow bloggers Linda Gorman, Greg Scandlen, John Graham and Devon Herrick, and from like-minded bloggers at other sites, including David Henderson and

Arnold Kling at *Econlog*, Jason Shafrin at *Healthcare Economist* and Avik Roy at *The Apothecary*. But I've also learned from the pushback I get in the comments section from such people as Princeton University health economist Uwe Reinhardt, Don McCanne with the Physicians for a National Health Program, and by Austin Frakt, Aaron Carroll and their colleagues at *The Incidental Economist* blog.

My blog, by the way, would not be possible without the tireless behind-the-scenes work of Amber Jones. In fact, in some ways the blog is more Amber's than it is mine. After all, I just write. She does everything to actually make the blog work. Amber also tirelessly worked on all the many drafts of the manuscript of this book. In fact, without her help this book would not have been published.

I am deeply indebted to my colleague Devon Herrick—especially for many hours spent fact-checking and verifying source material. Also at the NCPA, I am indebted to Courtney O'Sullivan, Joe Barnett and Pam Villarreal.

David Theroux and his colleagues at The Independent Institute have been a pleasure to work with every step of the way. Jaqueline Tasch is a terrific copy-editor, whose careful editing and assiduous attention to detail improved the manuscript considerably.

I hasten to add that any errors of reasoning or judgment are my own.

1

Introduction

FORGET EVERYTHING YOU know about healthcare for a moment. I want to introduce you to a new way of thinking about it.

Our healthcare system is an example of what social scientists call *complex systems.* These systems are so complicated that no one person can ever fully grasp everything that is going on. As individuals, all we ever really see is a small slice of the system. That's usually the part of it we experience.

For example, the typical patient sees a doctor only a handful of times during any given year. A primary care doctor takes care of only about 2,500 patients. These interactions are important, but when we stop to realize that there are 300 million potential patients and 800,000 doctors, it's clear that the perspective of any one doctor or any one patient is extremely limited.

Other markets in our economy are also examples of complex systems, but healthcare is many times more complex than a normal market. The reason: in addition to garden-variety economic forces, the medical marketplace is institutionalized, bureaucratized, and extensively regulated. Doctors are heavily influenced by medical ethics and traditional ways of doing things. Almost everything they do is affected by third-party payer bureaucracies (insurance companies, employers, and government) and by regulations that are inconsistent, voluminous, and complex. They also face the ever-present threat of tort law litigation.

To make matters even more complicated, we have completely suppressed normal market processes in healthcare—in this country and all over the developed world. As a result, in healthcare few people ever see a real price for anything. Employees never see a premium reflecting the real cost of their health insurance. Patients almost never see a real price for their medical care. Even at the family doctor's office, it's hard to discover what anything costs. For something complicated, like a hip replacement, the information is virtually impossible to obtain—at least in advance of the operation.

On the supply side, doctors and hospitals are rarely paid real prices for the services they render. Instead, they are paid on the basis of *reimbursement formulas*. Each payer may have a different formula. Medicare (for the elderly and the disabled) pays one set of fees. Medicaid (for the poor) pays another. BlueCross pays yet a third. All of the other insurers and all of the employer plans may also have separately negotiated fees. As a result, there really is no *market-clearing price* that brings supply and demand together in a way we experience in other sectors. Enormous amounts of money change hands every day in the medical marketplace, but most of the conventional rules of economics do not directly apply.

An interesting characteristic of complex systems is that when you perturb them (by passing a law, for example), there are always unintended consequences. The less you know about the system, the more unpredictable these consequences can be. Economic history provides numerous examples of governments that adopted policies in an attempt to improve things but ended up making the situation worse. Unfortunately, this happens in healthcare all the time.

For example, one of the goals of many public policies adopted in this country and around the world is to remove price as a barrier to care. Ideal health insurance is often said to be health insurance with no deductible or co-payment, making medical care essentially free at the point of delivery. Yet, if patients have no out-of-pocket costs their economic incentive will be to overuse the system, essentially consuming healthcare until the last amount obtained has a value that approaches zero. Also, if patients are not paying money for the services they receive, they're not likely to shop around for the best buy, so doctors, hospitals, and other providers will not compete for patients based on price, They will have no economic incentive to keep costs low—the way producers behave in other markets. To the contrary, the incentive of the providers will be to maximize against the payment formulas in order to enhance their incomes.

Well-intentioned public policies designed to make healthcare affordable for individuals, therefore, have had the surprising effect of causing healthcare spending to become unaffordable for the nation as a whole. Rising healthcare spending is the principal cause of our out-of-control federal deficit. It is bankrupting cities, counties, and state governments. It has created huge unfunded liabilities for some of our largest corporations. It is contributing to the stagnation in worker take-home pay. It can potentially bankrupt the families of individuals who have the misfortune to become ill—even those with health insurance.

Another well-intentioned public policy initiative—adopted by some states—is to try to make health insurance affordable for people with pre-existing conditions by requiring insurers to charge the same premium to all buyers, regardless of health status. Yet, this legislation has the unintended consequence of encouraging people to remain uninsured until they get sick. As healthy people drop out of the market and only people with health problems remain, the premium needed to cover the insurers' cost begins to soar. In the state of New York, this sort of regulation has produced staggeringly high premiums. For a run-of-the-mill individual policy, United Healthcare Oxford charges a premium of $1,855.97 a month, or more than $22,000 a year. For a family, the premium is $5,707.11 per month, or more than $68,000 a year.[1] A policy designed to make insurance affordable, therefore, is pricing thousands of people out of the market.

Federal health programs provide other examples of unintended consequences of public policies foisted on a complex system. In 1965, Congress passed Medicare in an attempt to increase access to healthcare for the elderly and improve their health status. Members of Congress believed they could do so without any material impact on the rest of the healthcare system. Yet MIT professor Amy Finkelstein has discovered that the passage of Medicare had no effect on the health of the elderly—at least as measured by mortality—but the additional spending set off a bout of healthcare inflation for all patients—one that never subsided.[2]

In 2003, Congress passed a Medicare drug benefit, largely out of concern that senior citizens couldn't afford the coverage themselves. Since the new program (Medicare Part D) had no funding source, Congress created a $15.6 trillion unfunded liability for the federal government, looking indefinitely into the future—more than the unfunded liability in Social Security.[3] Yet economist Andrew Rettenmaier discovered that only 7 percent of the benefits actually bought new drugs for seniors. The other 93 percent simply transferred to government (and taxpayers) the bill for drugs the elderly or their insurers were already buying.[4] Only one in every thirteen dollars represented a new drug purchase. Interestingly, the help given to the small number of people who were not otherwise getting medications actually reduced Medicare's spending, as drugs were substituted for more expensive doctor and hospital therapies.[5] But this profit on the truly needy was overwhelmed by the cost of giving the benefit to those who didn't need it—a cost that has created an enormous obligation for current and future taxpayers.

Here are two other unintended consequences of health policies designed to make healthcare free at the point of delivery. In other markets, producers don't compete only on price. They compete on quality as well. In healthcare, however, it appears that when providers don't compete on price, they often don't compete on quality either. That may be one reason why critics find that the quality of care we receive (including the very large number of avoidable errors and other adverse medical events) falls far short of what we would expect in a normal market.

Also, in most markets, we pay for goods and services with both time and money, and producers and sellers understand that we value our time as well as our pocket book. Public policies designed to suppress the role of money as a medium of exchange in the medical marketplace, however, have had the inadvertent consequence of increasing the importance of waiting times and other non-price barriers to care. These efforts to *increase* access to care may well have *decreased* access instead by making people wait longer to get appointments and to see the doctor once they reach her office.

How We Are Trapped

The premise of the book is that most of our problems arise because we are trapped. We are caught up in a dysfunctional system in which perverse economic incentives cause all of us to do things that raise the cost of care, lower its quality, and make access to care more difficult. Perverse incentives are faced by everyone: patients, doctors, nurses, hospital administrators, employees, employers, and so on. As we interact with the system, most of us spot ways to solve problems. We see things we could individually do to avoid waste and make care less expensive, for example. But the system generally penalizes us for doing the right things and rewards us for doing the wrong things. Anything we do as individuals to eliminate waste generally benefits someone other than ourselves.

So what's the answer? Let people out of the trap. Liberate them from the dysfunctionality that is causing us so much trouble.

This message is precisely the opposite of what you are likely to hear from other health policy experts—on the right and the left. The conventional view is that we have too much freedom, not too little. Doctors are said to have too much freedom to provide treatments that are not "best practice" or that are not "evidenced-based." Patients are said to have too much freedom to patronize doctors and facilities with inferior performance records.

Hence, the conventional solution: put even more restrictions on what doctors can do and where patients can go for their care. Ultimately, the conventional answer to the country's health policy problems is to have government tell doctors how to practice medicine and to tell patients what care they can have and where they can get it.

The biggest problem with this approach is that it would leave us even more trapped than we currently are. Incentives would be even more perverse. We would have a plan designed by folks in Washington. But 300 million potential patients, 800,000 doctors, almost 2.5 million registered nurses, and thousands of others working in the system would find it in their self-interest to undermine the plan. My answer is just the opposite. I want all those patients and all those doctors to discover it is in their self-interest to *solve problems*, not *create them*.

Under the conventional approach, every doctor, every nurse, every hospital administrator will get up every morning and ask, "How can I squeeze more money out of the payment formulas today?"

My answer is just the opposite. Under the approach I will recommend, all these people will be encouraged to start each day by asking, "How can I make my service better, less costly, and more accessible to patients today?"

Getting Out of the Trap: Emerging Entrepreneurs

That we need a new way of thinking is almost self-evident. After all, healthcare has been recognized as one of our most important national policy problems for over a quarter of a century. It has spawned thousands of conferences, briefings, speeches, legislative hearings, books, essays, and scholarly articles. It provoked legislation that envisions a complete overhaul of the system in just a few years. Yet even with all of this, we are no closer to a genuine solution to our problems than we were twenty-five years ago.

In complex systems, there are always unmet needs and problems to be solved. The more dysfunctional the system, the more numerous are the unmet needs and the more severe are the problems. In other sectors, needs to be met and problems to be solved are the fertile ground from which entrepreneurs emerge. Where is healthcare's equivalent of a Bill Gates or a Steve Jobs?

The answer: There are literally thousands of entrepreneurs in healthcare. I meet them every day. In fact, I believe I can safely say that there is no serious problem in the business of health that is not already being substantially solved in some way by an entrepreneur somewhere in the system. Unfortunately, these efforts tend to be scattered and limited. Most of the time they run into three major barriers: insurance companies, employers, and government.

These are the three entities that pay most of the healthcare bills. They are the *third-party payers.* (The first two parties are the doctor and the patient.) With respect to healthcare, they tend to be bureaucratic, wedded to tradition, and resistant to change. They are, in a word, the entrepreneur's nemesis.

Take the subject of hospital costs. It is well known that the cost of procedures varies radically from hospital to hospital, as does the quality of care. So why not take advantage of this fact? In this book, I am going to argue that a version of what some call *value-based* health insurance could cut the typical health plan's hospital costs in half. How does it work? The insurer pays the cost of care at a low-cost, high-quality facility (which may require the patient to travel) and only that amount. Patients are free to go to another facility but must pay the full extra cost of their choice.

Now, I wasn't the first person to think of this. In fact, an Austin, Texas-based company, Employer Direct Healthcare, is offering employers a variation on that idea at this very moment. They negotiate rates with select hospitals that are from one-third to one-half lower than what other health insurers are paying. Most insurers are at the opposite end of the smart-buying spectrum, however. BlueCross of Texas, for example, not only does not steer patients to one hospital rather than another, there is not a single hospital in Dallas that is not in its network.

Part of the reason why the insurers are so resistant to cost-reducing innovations is that many of their employer clients are also resistant. The typical client of Employer Direct Healthcare, for example, waives the deductible and co-payment for patients who choose the low-cost, high-quality facilities, but that is the full extent of the financial incentive. A step in the right direction perhaps, but a timid one. An aggressive strategy would be to let the employee pay the full extra cost of their choices.

Of the three third-party payer institutions, government is by far the worst at resisting entrepreneurship—even when the government itself is implementing radical change. As part of the Affordable Care Act (ACA), for example, states are to establish health insurance exchanges, allowing individuals to electronically select their health insurance from among competing plans. The federal government is offering millions of dollars to set up these exchanges. In some states, officials are arguing about how to spend the money, and in other states, they are actually refusing the money on the grounds that it amounts to acceptance of a health reform they do not like.

But why does any state need to spend millions to set up an exchange? Did you know that eHealth already has an electronic exchange, and more than 1 million people have health insurance purchased online through its system? The Obama administration is asking fifty state governments to spend a great deal of money to invent something that a private company has already discovered—and is ready to implement for the government for pennies on the dollar.

The administration is also spending millions of dollars trying to encourage electronic medical records. But did you know that eHealth already offers many of its customers an electronic medical record (including a record of doctor visits, prescriptions taken, etc.), based on insurance payment records?

Although we often associate the term *entrepreneur* with profit seeking, the healthcare field is teeming with innovators who are largely motivated by altruism. Take Dr. Jeffrey Brenner of Camden, New Jersey.[6] In any other field, Brenner would be a millionaire, but because he's in healthcare, he doesn't know how he's going to make ends meet. Like entrepreneurs in every market, Brenner thought outside the box. He discovered an ingenious way of lowering healthcare costs: focus on the "hot spots" of medicine—the high-use, high-spending patients—and solve their problems with unconventional care.

Brenner discovered that of the 100,000 people who used Camden's medical facilities over the course of a year, only 1,000 people—just 1 percent—accounted for 30 percent of the costs. He began with one of them: Frank Hendricks (a pseudonym), a patient with severe congestive heart failure, chronic asthma, uncontrolled diabetes, hypothyroidism, gout, and a history of smoking and alcohol abuse. He weighed 560 pounds. In the previous three years, he had spent as much time inside hospitals as he spent outside them.

Some of what Brenner did to help Hendricks was simple doctor stuff, but a lot of it was social work. For example, Brenner and his colleagues helped Hendricks apply for disability insurance so that he could leave the chaos of welfare motels and have access to a consistent set of physicians. The team also pushed him to find sources of stability and value in his life. They got him to return to Alcoholics Anonymous, and when Brenner found out that Hendricks was a devout Christian, he urged him to return to church. As a result, Hendricks's health improved, and his medical expenses plummeted.

Following that success, Brenner formed the Camden Coalition to apply his methods to more patients. He tells me he can drive down the streets of Camden, point to entire buildings, and say how much the people who live there are costing the taxpayers. By targeting these patients in unconventional ways, Brenner is saving millions of dollars for Medicare and Medicaid. Were others able to do the same thing in other cities, the savings for taxpayers would be huge.

Now for the bad news. How much does Medicare reward Brenner for all the savings he creates for our nation's largest health plan? Zero. How much does Medicaid pay for all the savings it realizes? Not a penny. In fact, Brenner is able to do what he does only because of grants from private foundations.

Getting Out of the Trap: Overcoming Unwise Policies

Like many other providers of low-cost, high-quality care, Brenner and his colleagues leave tons of money on the table when they fail to practice medicine in conventional ways. Of the thousands of tasks that Medicare pays doctors to perform, social work is not among them. Brenner's attempts to get Medicare and Medicaid to pay him in a different way have all drowned in a bureaucratic morass, even as Medicare is spending millions on pilot programs and demonstration projects "to find out what works."

Experiences just like Brenner's are repeated again and again, day in and day out, around the country. No one knows if Brenner's techniques can be replicated (any more than we know if the medical practices of the Mayo Clinic or the

Cleveland Clinic can be replicated). But there's one way to find out: Let Brenner out of the trap. How do we do that? By letting him become rich. Rich? Yes, rich.

The federal government should offer to let Brenner and his colleagues keep twenty-five cents of every dollar they save the government. Then let every other doctor, nurse, social worker, hospital administrator, and so on in the country know that the government is willing to change the way it pays for care. The message should be: If you can save taxpayers money, you can make money—the more money you save us, the more you earn for yourself. Let a thousand millionaires bloom.

Sadly, the trend of federal health policy right now is in the opposite direction. Not only will it not let Brenner out of the trap, it will make the trap more confining. Under the new health reform law, doctors are being encouraged to join Accountable Care Organizations (ACOs), where a federal bureaucracy will virtually dictate the way medicine is practiced.

Brenner, in fact, is trying to get his organization qualified as an ACO. In my opinion, this is a mistake. Under the new rules, bureaucrats will ask: Did Brenner have the prescribed electronic medical record? Did he follow the checklist of inputs ACOs are supposed to follow? Did he manage all of the care—including hospital care? Sadly, the answers are no, no, and no.

It is almost impossible for an entrepreneur to flourish in an environment that fundamentally dislikes entrepreneurship. Fortunately for the innovators, however, patients are paying for more healthcare bills out of their own pockets. And wherever we find health markets dominated by patients paying for care directly, entrepreneurship is thriving.

Getting Out of the Trap: Emerging Markets

In fields as diverse as cosmetic surgery and LASIK surgery, we are discovering that healthcare markets can give patients transparent package prices and that costs can be controlled—despite a huge increase in demand and enormous technological change (of the type we are told increases costs for healthcare generally). For services as diverse as walk-in clinics and mail-order drugs, we are seeing that price competition is possible and that price competition promotes quality competition as well. In the international market for medical tourism, we are discovering that almost every type of elective surgery can be subjected to the discipline of the marketplace; that discipline is increasingly evident within our borders in the emerging market for domestic medical tourism, where patients willing to travel to other cities can find cheaper, higher-quality care.

In each of these cases, new products and new services have cropped up to meet the needs of patients spending their own money. These are products and services that were made possible precisely because the third-party-payer bureaucracies were not standing in the way. If the private sector is left free to continue with such innovations, there is much more to come.

Among the current buzzwords in Washington policy circles are such terms as electronic medical records, medical homes, coordinated care, integrated care, and so on. To hear the policy wonks tell it, the ACA is designed to bring all these new ideas to the practice of medicine—prodded by the guiding hand of government regulators.

But did you know that sensible, workable electronic records systems (including the ability to electronically prescribe drugs) have been in use for over a decade by walk-in clinics, by private telephone and email consultation services, and by concierge doctors (who give their patients more time, more services, and special attention) without any guidance from Washington or from any employer or insurance company? Did you know that sensible, workable medical homes—together with diverse doctors providing integrated, coordinated, low-cost, high-quality care—have been emerging in the private sector for some time, without any federally funded pilot program or any advice, encouragement, or harassment from any third-party payer?

I stress the words *sensible* and *workable* because in the hands of impersonal bureaucracies, shielded from marketplace competition and subject to pressures from every special interest group imaginable, we are likely to get systems that are neither sensible nor workable.

Liberated from the confinement of legal impediments and suffocating bureaucracies, doctors, patients, hospital personnel and profit-seeking entrepreneurs are perfectly capable of solving our most serious health policy problems. All they need is the freedom to be able to do so.

PART I

Why We Are Trapped

2

How Healthcare Is Different

COMPLEX SYSTEMS, by definition, are systems that are too complex for any single individual (or group of individuals) to grasp and understand. What difference does that make? It makes a huge difference.

Most of us wouldn't walk into a chemistry lab and start pouring solutions from one beaker into another—at least if we don't know anything about chemistry. Similarly, we wouldn't walk into a biology lab and start moving substances from one petri dish to another if we're not trained biologists. And if we don't know anything about nuclear power plants, most of us wouldn't walk into one and start pushing buttons.

We wouldn't do any of these things because most of us have common sense. We know intuitively that if we don't know what we are doing in a complex environment, odds are great that anything we do will mess things up.

Not everyone has this common sense-based humility, however. The late Nobel laureate economist, Friedrich Hayek, called the hubris of people who want to tinker with systems they do not understand the "fatal conceit."[1] The term is apt. Just about everything that has gone wrong in health policy can be directly attributed to this very error. In what follows, I want to look more carefully at what goes wrong in health policy and why.

No Reliable Model

For more than 200 years, economists have been studying the complex system we call the economy. How do they do it? They don't try to understand the economy in all its complex detail. Instead, economists use highly simplified models to predict some general effects of parameter changes in ordinary markets. For example, we can say with some certainty that rent controls will cause housing shortages and price supports in agriculture will cause crop surpluses.

Unfortunately, there is no model of the healthcare system that allows us to make anything like these kinds of predictions. In just a few years, ACA will insure an additional 32 million people. In addition, most of the rest of us will have to convert to health plans that have more generous coverage than we now have. We know that when people have more insurance coverage they try to consume more care. But what happens when there is a system-wide increase in demand and no change in supply?

Will the excess demand drive thousands of people to hospital emergency rooms? Will clinics run by nurses start springing up to meet the demand that doctors cannot meet? If service is rationed by increasing the waiting time, will everyone who can afford it turn to concierge doctors, who will be paid extra fees for prompt service? As more doctors become concierge doctors, how will the system manage the even greater rationing problem faced by all those left behind? Will patients start going out of the country—seeking care in the international medical marketplace?

Unfortunately, there is no model that allows us to answer these questions with any confidence.

Why can't we apply ordinary economic models to healthcare markets? One reason is that price doesn't play the same role in healthcare as it does elsewhere in the economy. Although many would like to think that our system is very different from the national health insurance schemes of other countries, the truth is that Americans mainly pay for care the same way people all over the developed world pay for care at the time they receive it—with time, not money.

On the average, every time we spend a dollar at a physician's office, only 10 cents comes out of our own pockets. As a result, for most people, the price of care in terms of the time (getting to and from the doctor's office, waiting in the reception area, waiting in the exam room, etc.) tends to be greater—and probably much greater—than the money price of care.

In general, we have no reliable model to tell us who gets care and who doesn't when the time price of care rises for everyone, as we expect to happen once ACA gets fully implemented.

The Role of Prices

Take a look at Table 2.1, which shows representative prices for a knee replacement for different patients in different settings. The most shocking thing about the table is that prices for essentially the same procedure are all over the map. Here are some obvious questions:

1. How is it that a Canadian can come to the United States and get a knee replacement for less than half of what Americans are paying?
2. Why are Canadians coming to the United States paying only a few thousand dollars more than medical tourists in India, Singapore and Thailand—places where the price is supposed to be a fraction of what we typically pay in this country?
3. Why do fees US employers and insurance companies pay vary by a factor of three to one (between $21,000 and $75,000), when foreign and even some US facilities are offering a same-price-for-all package?
4. Why is the price of a knee replacement for a dog—involving the same technology and the same medical skills that are needed for humans—less than one-sixth the price a typical health insurance company pays for human operations? Why is it less than one-third of what hospitals tell Medicare their cost of doing the procedure is?

It's amazing how often people cannot see the forest for the trees. Think how many volumes have been written trying (and failing) to explain why our healthcare costs are so high. Sometimes the answers to complex questions are more easily found by asking the simplest of questions.

Let's turn to the canine question. When you recover from your knee replacement surgery, let's say you spend two nights in a hospital room. If you are like some patients, you may be enjoying all the comforts of a luxury hotel. Fido recovers in a cage, which presumably costs much less. But even with meals, two nights in a hotel should come in under $1,000. The price difference we are trying to explain is many times that amount.

Then, there is the difference in surgeons' skills. Presumably, the surgeons who operate on humans are more talented and therefore more valuable. But an orthopedic surgeon in Dallas typically gets paid an amount equal to about 10 percent of the $32,500 an insurer pays to the hospital.

Table 2.1. Knee Replacement Costs

Location/Type	**Amount**[1]
Asking Prices	
Hospital Gross Charge[2]	$60,000–$65,000
What Private Insurers Pay	
Range (Dallas)[3]	$21,000–$75,000
Average (Dallas)[3]	$32,500
Medicare (Dallas)[4]	
What Medicare Pays	$16,000–$30,000
Cost Reported to Medicare	$14,627–$15,148
Physician Fees	$1,400–$1,700
Domestic Medical Tourism	
Medibid Rate (US)[2]	$12,000
Canadian Citizen US Cash Price[5]	$16,000–$19,000
International Medical Tourism	
Medibid Rate (overseas)[2]	$7,000–$15,000
Bumrungrad (Thailand) Median Price[6]	$14,916
US dog (Dallas)[4]	$3,700–$5,000

1. Does not include the physician fees, except for the veterinary charge.
2. Source: Medibid.com
3. Source: Group and Pension Administrator, Inc.
4. Source: NCNelink.com
5. Source: North American Surgery Inc.
6. Source: http://www.bumrungrad.comlthailandhospital

I suppose you (as a patient) would get more attention than Fido from nurses and support staff for the one or two days of recovery. Guess how much a nurse gets paid in Dallas? It's about $30 per hour. That is nowhere near the explanation we are searching for.

Let's take the actual cost hospitals tell Medicare they incur for this procedure.[2] It's about $15,000, not including surgeon's fees. But if veterinarians can do it for a third of that amount, it's hard to see why the human hospital cost isn't at least half of what it actually is.

The only explanations I can come up with for why human knees cost so much more are (1) government regulations, (2) malpractice liability, and (3) the inefficiencies created by the third-party payment system. It looks like these three factors are doubling the cost of US healthcare.

Let's take regulations first. In terms of rules, restrictions, and bureaucratic reporting requirements, the healthcare sector is one of the most regulated industries in our economy. Regulatory requirements intrude in a highly visible way on the activities of the hospital medical staff and affect virtually every aspect of medical practice. In *Patient Power*, Gerry Musgrave and I described the burdens faced by Scripps Memorial Hospital, a medium-sized (250-bed) acute care facility in San Diego, CA. Scripps had to answer to thirty-nine governmental bodies and seven nongovernmental bodies.[3] It periodically filed sixty-five different reports, about one report for every four beds. In most cases, the reports were not simple forms that could be completed by a clerk. Often, they were lengthy and complicated, requiring the daily recording of information by highly trained hospital personnel.

Then there is the malpractice system. Estimates place the burden of the system at between 2 percent and 10 percent of the cost of US healthcare. But it's hard to separate out the effects of malpractice from the effects of regulation. Remember, both institutions are trying to do the same thing: reduce the incidence of adverse medical events (no matter how imperfectly). If a hospital fails to follow a regulation and that failure leads to a patient death, the failure would undoubtedly be the basis for a malpractice lawsuit. So the existence of the malpractice system helps encourage compliance with regulations—making them more costly.

Finally, there are the inefficiencies produced by the third-party payment system. I noted in the Introduction that when providers do not compete for patients based on price, they typically do not compete on quality either. In the hospital sector, they tend to compete on amenities instead. The way you compete on amenities is to spend more on amenities. This adds to costs.

Now let's consider medical tourism. If you ask a hospital in your neighborhood to give you a package price on a standard surgical procedure, you will probably be turned down. After the suppression of normal market forces for the better part of a century, hospitals are rarely interested in competing on price for patients they are likely to get as customers anyway.

A foreign patient is a different matter. This is a customer the hospital is not going to get if it doesn't compete. That's why a growing number of US hospitals are willing to give transparent package prices to foreigners, and these prices often are close to the marginal cost of the care they deliver.

North American Surgery (an enterprise that facilitates medical tourism) has negotiated deep discounts with about two dozen surgery centers, hospitals, and clinics across the United States, mainly for Canadians who are unable to get timely care in their own country. The company's cash price for a knee replacement in the United States is $16,000 to $19,000, depending on the facility a patient chooses.[4]

Now here is what is interesting: The same economic principles that apply to the foreign patient who is willing to travel to the United States for surgery also apply to *any patient* who is willing to travel. That includes US citizens. In other words, you don't have to be a Canadian to take advantage of North American Surgery's ability to obtain low-cost package prices. *Everyone can do it.*

US patients willing to travel and able to pay cash may get an even better deal by taking advantage of the online service, MediBid. People register and request bids or estimates for specific procedures on MediBid's website for the services of, say, a physician, surgeon, dermatologist, chiropractor, dentist, or numerous other medical specialists. MediBid-affiliated physicians and other medical providers respond to patient requests and submit competitive bids for the business of patients seeking care. MediBid facilitates the transaction, but the agreement is between doctor and patient, both of whom must come to an agreement on the price and service.

The company facilitated more than fifty knee replacements in 2012. Each request got an average of five bids, with some getting as many as twenty-two. Most prices were between $10,000 and $12,000, and the average was about $12,000.[5]

The implications of all this are staggering. Many US hospitals are able to offer traveling patients package prices that are competitive with the prices charged by top-rated medical tourist facilities around the world. (You don't have to travel to Thailand, after all.) However, I would insert this note of caution: Although a hospital with excess capacity gains by charging the *marginal customer* the marginal cost of care, it may not cover the full costs it needed to stay in business if it charges *every customer* that price. So the prices we are looking at may not be long-run equilibrium prices.

The final question is: Why are US employers and insurers overpaying by so much, and why does the amount they overpay vary so much?

In part, because in the entire medical marketplace, there is no natural evolution to uniform, market-clearing prices, the way markets work in other sectors of the economy. Even MRI scans vary by over 650 percent in a single town. Furthermore, most providers don't even know how to price their services because they don't know what their costs are.[6]

Both the Right and Left Go Wrong

Despite the fact that prices in healthcare do not play the same role as they do in other markets, there is a tendency on both the political right and the political left to ignore this fact.

The right, for example, issues frequent calls to make prices transparent. A number of proposals would even require doctors and hospitals to post their prices. Doctors find these proposals perplexing because they know that there are no *prices* at a typical physician's office. There are only different *payment rates*. What possibly could be gained by posting these rates on the wall? If you are a BlueCross patient, how does knowing what an Aetna patient is paying help you in any way?

On the left, a common view is that health costs are too high because healthcare prices are too high. They believe that the way to control costs is to push prices down. This idea is actually written into the ACA legislation. All kinds of efficiency ideas are included in the new law, but when all else fails—and most knowledgeable people believe that all else will fail—ACA will try to solve the problem of rising Medicare costs by squeezing the providers. Medicare's chief actuary predicts that by the end of the decade, Medicare fees for doctors and hospitals will be lower than Medicaid's.[7] And it may not end there. At least one organization advocates imposing Medicare-type price controls on the entire healthcare system.[8]

The problem with this way of thinking is that prices in healthcare are *symptoms* of problems, not *causes* of problems, in the same way that a high body temperature is a symptom of a fever. Just as it would make no sense to try to treat a fever by lowering the body's temperature, it makes no sense to try to control prices while ignoring why they are what they are. Plus, when we treat symptoms rather than their causes, there are inevitably unanticipated negative consequences. For example, if we tried to impose low fees on every provider for all patients, we would begin to drive the most capable doctors out of the system—into alternative pay-cash-for-care services and perhaps even out of healthcare altogether.

But there is an even more fundamental problem with trying to solve the problem of cost by suppressing prices. The suppression of provider payments is an attempt to shift costs from patients and taxpayers to providers. Even if we get away with it, *shifting costs* is not the same thing as *controlling costs*. Doctors are just as much a part of society as patients. Shifting cost from one group to the other makes one group better off and the other worse off. It does not lower the cost of healthcare for society as a whole, however.

Finally, both the right and the left—but especially the left—too often assume that the ideal price of care for low-income patients is zero. After all, if price is a deterrent to care, doesn't it follow that you maximize access by making healthcare free at the point of consumption? Not necessarily.

Which Matters More: The Time Price or the Money Price of Care?

What I call health policy orthodoxy is committed to two propositions: (1) The really important health issue for poor people is access to care, and (2) to ensure access, waiting for care is always better than paying for care. In other words, if you have to ration scarce medical resources somehow, rationing by waiting is always better than rationing by price.

(Let me say parenthetically that the orthodox view is at least plausible. After all, poor people have the same amount of time you and I have, but a lot less money. Also, because their wages are lower than other people's, the opportunity cost of their time is lower. So if we all have to pay for care with time and not with money, the advantage should go to the poor. This view would be plausible, that is, so long as you ignore tons of data showing that whenever the poor and the non-poor compete for resources in almost any non-price rationing system, the poor always lose out.)

The orthodox view underlies Medicaid's policy of allowing patients to wait for hours for care in hospital emergency rooms and in community health centers, while denying them the opportunity to obtain less costly care at a walk-in clinic with very little wait at all. The easiest, cheapest way to expand access to care for millions of low-income families is to allow them to do something they cannot now do: add money out of pocket to Medicaid's fees and pay market prices for care at walk-in clinics, doc-in-the-boxes, surgical centers, and other commercial outlets. Yet, in conventional health policy circles, this idea is considered heresy.

The orthodox view lies behind the obsession with making everyone pay higher premiums so that contraceptive services and a whole long list of screenings and preventive care can be made available with no co-payment or deductible. Yet, this practice will surely encourage overuse and waste and, in the process, likely raise the time prices of these same services.

The orthodox view lies at the core of the hostility toward Health Savings Accounts (HSAs), Health Reimbursement Arrangements (HRAs), and any other kind of account that allows money to be exchanged for medical services. Yet, it is precisely these kinds of accounts that empower low-income families in the medical marketplace, just as food stamps empower them in any grocery store they choose to patronize.

The orthodox view is the reason so many ACA backers think the new health reform law will expand access to care for millions of people, even though there will be no increase in the supply of doctors. Because they completely ignore the almost certain increase in the time price of care, these enthusiasts have completely missed the possibility that the act may actually decrease access to care for the most vulnerable populations.[9]

The orthodox view is the reason there is so little academic interest in measuring the time price of care and why so much animosity is directed at those who do measure such things. It explains why MIT professor Jonathan Gruber can write a paper on Massachusetts health reform and never once mention that the wait to see a new doctor in Boston is more than two months.[10]

The evidence we will examine in this book suggests that the orthodox view is totally wrong.

The Cost of Non-Price Rationing

The orthodox approach to health policy is obsessively focused on the burdens of price barriers to care, and at the same time inordinately oblivious to the burdens of non-price barriers. Yet non-price barriers to care can be very costly.

In Britain, for example, hundreds of thousands of patients relying on the British National Health Service are waiting months for hospital surgery. Many are waiting in pain. Many are risking their lives by waiting. The cost of such waiting for many of them is undoubtedly greater than the cost (to the government) of their surgery.[11]

Not only is rationing by waiting costly, it is usually socially wasteful. To employ a numerical example, consider a hospital emergency room where people come for free primary care. Let's say the real cost of a doctor visit is $100 per patient, on the average. In a normal market, the market-clearing money price of care would also be $100—and that would be the fee patients pay.

If the services are free, however, a much larger group of patients will try to take advantage of them, including patients who value doctor visits at only $5 or $10. Since demand greatly exceeds supply at a price of zero, the doctor's time is available in this example only to those who are willing to wait the longest. How long will people wait, on the average? Someone who values a doctor visit at $100 will be willing to spend $100 worth of time. (Consider a patient who values his time at his wage rate. If he is paid $20 an hour, he will wait five hours; if he is paid $25 an hour, he will wait four hours, and so on.)

Just as price rationing produces a market-clearing *money price of care*, rationing by waiting time produces a market-clearing *time price of care*. In this example, the market will clear at $100 worth of time for the marginal patient. But remember, other people (probably taxpayers) have to pay the doctor $100 in money. That means that the *care is being paid for twice: once with time and again with money*. Non-price rationing, in this example, effectively doubles the social cost of medical care.

By the way, a surprising number of patients—about one in five, on the average—get discouraged and leave emergency rooms without ever being seen. Just as people at an auction get outbid by others who are willing to pay a higher money price, patients in emergency rooms often get outbid by others who are willing to pay a higher time price for their care.

Six Billion Physician Fees

Even though prices don't have the same meaning in the medical marketplace that they do in other markets, they still have the power to influence provider behavior.

Take Medicare, which has a list of some 7,500 separate tasks it pays physicians to perform. For each task, there is a price that varies according to location and other factors. Of the 800,000 practicing physicians in this country, not all are in Medicare, and no doctor is going to perform every task on Medicare's list.

Yet Medicare is potentially setting about 6 billion physician fees across the country at any one time.

Is there any chance that Medicare can set fees and approve transactions in a way that does not cause serious problems? Not likely.

What happens when Medicare gets it wrong? One result is that doctors face perverse incentives to provide care that is costlier and less appropriate than the care they should be providing. Another result is that the skill set of our nation's doctors becomes misallocated, as medical students and practicing doctors respond to the fact that Medicare is overpaying for some skills and underpaying for others.

Every lawyer, every accountant, every architect, every engineer—indeed, every professional in every other field—is able to do something doctors cannot do. They can repackage and reprice their services. If demand changes or if they discover a way of meeting their clients' needs more efficiently, they are free to offer a different bundle of services for a different price. Doctors, by contrast, are trapped.

Suppose you are accused of a crime and suppose your lawyer is paid the way doctors are paid. That is, suppose some third-party payer bureaucracy pays your lawyer a different fee for each separate task she performs in your defense. Just to make up some numbers, let's suppose your lawyer is paid $50 per hour for jury selection and $500 per hour for making your final case to the jury.

What would happen? At the end of your trial, your lawyer's summation would be stirring, compelling, logical, and persuasive. In fact, it might well get you off scot free if only it were delivered to the right jury. But you don't have the right jury. Because of the fee schedule, your lawyer skimped on jury selection way back at the beginning of your trial.

This is why you don't want to pay a lawyer, or any other professional, by task. You want your lawyer to be able to reallocate her time—in this case, from the summation speech to the voir dire proceeding. If each hour of her time is compensated at the same rate, she will feel free to allocate the last hour spent on your case to its highest valued use rather than to the activity that is paid the highest fee.

Six Billion Tasks

The problem in medicine is not merely that all the prices are wrong. A lot of very important things doctors can do for patients are not even on the list of tasks that Medicare compensates.

In addition, Medicare has strict rules about how tasks can be combined. For example, special-needs patients typically have five or more comorbidities—a fancy way of saying that a lot of things are going wrong at once. These patients typically cost Medicare about $60,000 a year, and they consume a large share of Medicare's entire budget. Ideally, when one of these patients sees a doctor, the doctor will deal with all five problems sequentially. That would economize on the patient's time and ensure that the treatment regime for each malady is integrated and consistent with all the others.

Under Medicare's payment system, however, a specialist can bill Medicare the full fee only for treating one of the five conditions during a single visit. If she treats the other four, she can only bill half price for those services. It's even worse for primary care physicians. They will generally get no payment for treating four additional problems. Since doctors don't like to work for free or see their income cut in half, most have a one-visit-one-condition policy. Patients with five morbidities are asked to schedule additional visits for the remaining four problems with the same doctor or with other doctors. The type of medicine that would be best for the patient and that would probably save the taxpayers money in the long run is the type of medicine that is penalized under Medicare's payment system.

Take Dr. Richard Young, a Fort Worth family physician who is an adviser for the federal government's new medical Innovation Center. As explained by Jim Landers in the *Dallas Morning News*:[12]

> [When Young] sees Medicare or Medicaid patients at Tarrant County's JPS Physicians Group, he can only deal with one ailment at a time. Even if a patient has several chronic diseases—diabetes, congestive heart failure, high blood pressure—the government's payment rules allow him to only charge for one.
>
> "You could spend the extra time and deal with everything, but you are completely giving away your services to do that," he said. Patients are told to schedule another appointment or see a specialist.
>
> Young calls the payment rules "ridiculously complicated."

Consequences of Suppressing Normal Market Forces

Think of a supermarket. There are probably more than a hundred in the city of Dallas alone. I can walk into any of them—in most cases, at any time day or night—and buy thousands of different products. The only wait I experience is at checkout, but express lanes speed that along if I want only an item or two. When I go to purchase something I want, the product is always there. I can't recall an instance when a shelf space offering something I wanted to buy was empty. Further, the products being offered are produced by thousands of different suppliers, and they travel thousands of different routes to get to market. What is true of Dallas is true of every city of any significant size in the country.

Contrast that with the market for medical care, where almost nothing is available at the drop of a hat. Nearly one in four patients has to wait six or more days for a physician appointment. Less than one-third of physician practices have made arrangements allowing patients to see a doctor after hours when the practice is closed. Sixty percent of patients find it difficult to get care after hours or on weekends.[13] Newspaper reports around the country tell horror stories of the consequences of the shortage of cancer drugs and other life-saving pharmaceuticals. Four- and five-hour average waiting times at hospital emergency rooms are not uncommon.

In fact, the few places in healthcare where waiting is not a problem provide services that are peripheral to the orthodox healthcare system. Teladoc promises a physician will return your call within three hours or the telephone consultation is free. Most calls are returned in less than one hour — during which time, you are free to do other things. MinuteClinics in some CVS pharmacies give you an estimated waiting time so you can shop while you wait for your care. Think of these last two examples as services that developed in the part of medical care where normal market processes have not been suppressed.

Everything I purchase in a supermarket is fee-for-service. There is no prepayment of the type that so many favor in healthcare. I pay the market price for what I get. There is *bundling,* to use another popular buzzword. I don't pay extra if I ask an employee for directions. There is no extra charge for the butcher to trim fat off tenderloin. These services are included in the price of the products I buy. But the bundling choices are made by the supermarket, not by the buyers of their products. There is no supermarket equivalent of managed care, integrated care, or coordinated care. Market prices are sending continuous signals to producers of thousands of products all over the world, and these prices accomplish the remarkable feat of making sure that everything we want to buy is on the supermarket shelf at the time we want to buy it.

The vast majority of goods sold in a supermarket are not produced by the supermarket itself, using its own employees. They are produced by independent entities in private practice, to borrow another term from the medical world. Supermarkets meet the needs of millions of people without the necessity of employing all of the people who produce all of the products they offer—unlike the Obama administration's plans to force virtually all doctors to become employees of hospitals.

Supermarkets have electronic inventory and monitoring systems—far more sophisticated than anything you will normally find in medicine. When Sam Walton first started electronic inventory control in his Wal-Mart stores, he did it in order to improve the quality of service and lower prices to attract more customers. Unlike healthcare, electronic inventory systems have emerged quite naturally in the supermarket business, without any government guidelines and without any government subsidies.

Now, you might be inclined to argue that healthcare cannot reasonably be compared to items on a supermarket shelf. Okay. I concede that. One is a product. The other is a service. But consider your Blackberry. Or your iPhone. Or your iPad. In some ways these have similarities with our bodies. Things can go wrong. When they do, we want someone to help fix them.

In my neighborhood, I can walk into almost any phone store (Verizon, Sprint, AT&T, etc.) with no appointment, and most of the time I get service immediately. And the phone store has competitors. Independent phone repair companies are popping up every day. There are even tools on the Internet that help you start your phone repair business.[14] In most places, repair companies are within ten miles of their customers; repairs are done in fifteen minutes or less; and they are usually inexpensive ($40 to $60, say).[15] Shopping malls have phone repair kiosks. Some companies will come to your house to repair your phone.[16]

Consider customer education. Elderly buyers in particular often have difficulty mastering the electronic devices they buy. The market has a solution. Verizon offers its customers free two-hour classes in how to use their iPhones. Yet, I don't know anywhere in Dallas that will give Medicare patients free counseling (or even paid counseling) on how to manage their diabetes. That's unfortunate. This one disease is costing the country $218 billion a year.[17]

Why is the marketplace so much kinder to my iPhone than it is to my body? I would argue that it's because one type of service is emerging in a real market, while the market has been suppressed in the other.

Getting Out of the Trap

Is there a better way? Here's one idea.[18] Instead of having Medicare fix millions of prices for predetermined packages of care, we should allow providers the opportunity to produce better care and cheaper care by repackaging and repricing their services. Everyone on the provider side should be encouraged to make Medicare a better offer. Medicare should accept these offers provided that (1) the total cost to government does not increase, (2) patient quality of care does not decrease, and (3) the provider proposes a reasonable method of assuring that (1) and (2) have been satisfied.

Instead of maximizing against payment formulas, doctors and hospitals would be encouraged to discover more efficient ways of providing care. They would be able to make more money for themselves as long as they save taxpayers money and patients don't suffer.

Can a Free Market in Healthcare Work?

From time to time, I hear policy wonks claim that the market cannot work in healthcare. Usually, they cite a very old article by Stanford University economist Kenneth Arrow, who claimed that the market for medical care is inherently imperfect.[19] True, but most markets are imperfect. The question is: does the market for healthcare work better than a nonmarket for healthcare? I believe the evidence supports an unqualified yes.

Consider some standard complaints that are normally leveled at the current system: that price and quality information is not transparent, that the market is not competitive, that unsustainable rising costs are inevitable, that quality is inadequate, and that providers make inadequate use of technology, including electronic medical records and electronic prescribing. But do these problems exist because of an inherent flaw in healthcare markets? Or do they exist because normal market forces have been systematically suppressed?

As it turns out, healthcare markets seem to work reasonably well wherever third-party payers are not the dominant payers. Wherever patients are paying with their own money, providers always compete on price, and where there is price competition, transparency is never a problem. Moreover, in such markets, we do not find the problem of healthcare inflation that plagues the rest of the system. The real price of cosmetic surgery has actually declined over the past fifteen years. The real price of LASIK surgery has declined by 30 percent over the past decade.[20]

I know of nothing in health economics that would lead a rational person to conclude that markets cannot work in medical care. Indeed, the evidence all points in the other direction: Markets can work much better than our current system, if they are allowed to do so.

Choosing Public Policies for Complex Systems

Most people in health policy do not understand complex systems. They really don't understand social science models either. As a result, when they advocate or enact public policies, they are almost always oblivious to the inevitability of unintended consequences. The idea that a policy based on good intentions could actually make things worse is beyond their comprehension.

Take health policies designed for low-income patients. Through our insistence on pushing low-income families into free public programs and regulating private alternatives out of their reach, the poor often must rely on bureaucratic medical care that is not very responsive to their needs.

This problem is not unique to healthcare. I think it is fair to say that virtually everything we do to try to help low-income families meet essential needs is deeply flawed:[21]

- The cheapest form of housing, for example, is prefabricated housing. Yet zoning regulations outlaw this low-cost form of shelter in almost every large city. Through unwise regulation, we have literally priced many low-income families out of the market for private housing and forced them to turn to public housing instead.
- Through taxi/jitney regulations, we have eliminated private, low-cost transportation alternatives and forced low-income families to turn to public transportation instead (in most places, a bus system that may or may not take people where they most need to go). When they do turn to the private sector (low-income families take more cab rides than the middle class!), they probably pay two or three times the free-market rate.
- In education, government has established a (frequently inadequate) monopoly, paid for in part by taxes borne by the poor. As a result, very few low-income children are able to take advantage of private-sector alternatives.
- Healthcare fits the same pattern. Through our insistence on pushing low-income families into free public programs and regulating private alternatives out of their reach, the poor often must rely on unresponsive, bureaucratic care.

In general, the middle class tends to have access to the benefits of capitalism. The poor must rely on government. The middle class exercises choice. The poor have no alternative to what they are offered. The middle class gets the benefits of competition. The poor are left with public sector monopoly. If middle-class patients are unsatisfied with a doctor or a facility, they can take their dollars and patronize another. The poor tend to be left with whatever doctor or facility is given to them.

No one ever planned for the poor to have services that were inferior, bureaucratic, and unresponsive. These outcomes are the unintended consequences of policies that were often designed to help them.

When dealing with a complex system for which there is no reliable predictive model, the first lesson is to show humility. Restrictions on behavior limit people's ability to meet their own needs and the needs of others. In the absence of better information, we should want people to freely exercise their intelligence, their creativity, and their entrepreneurial abilities to solve problems.

A second lesson is that we should eliminate restrictions on behavior unless there is overwhelming evidence that the limits do more good than harm. This means, for example, allowing low-income families on Medicaid greater access to services whose prices are determined in the marketplace.[22] Also, we should make it easier for nurses, physicians' assistants, and other non-doctor providers to deliver care to low-income patients by relaxing occupational licensing restrictions.[23]

A third lesson is to avoid trying to administer and regulate the system from the top. If we are dealing with a complex system and we don't have a reliable model to predict how it will respond to simple parameter changes, it is more important than ever to avoid trying to solve problems with top-down commands. Instead, we need to begin the process of liberation by working from the bottom up.

Consider a notorious violation of this principle. At one point, leaders in the Soviet Union thought they understood enough about their country's entire economy to manage the whole thing from a central command post. Today, even the Russians admit they were wrong.

A fourth lesson is that complex systems can't be copied. Suppose I said to you: "Let's look around the world, find the economy that seems to work the best, and then replace our own system by copying the one we like better." If you have any sense, you would respond by saying, "Goodman, that is a really dumb idea; don't you know that complex systems by definition can't be copied?"

You would be right. It is a dumb idea. But did you know that is exactly how President Obama talks about healthcare? Time and again he has said, "Let's find out what works and then go do it." This is an approach that is destined to fail before it even begins.

On the supply side, we have the islands of excellence (Mayo, Intermountain Healthcare, Cleveland Clinic, etc.). On the demand side, we have a whole slew of experiments with pay-for-performance and other pilot programs designed to see whether demand-side reforms can provoke supply-side behavioral improvements. And never the twain shall meet.

We cannot find a single institution providing high-quality, low-cost care that was created by any demand-side buyer of care. Not the Centers for Medicare and Medicaid Services (CMS), which runs Medicare and Medicaid. Not BlueCross. Not any employer. Not any payer, anytime, anywhere. As for the pilot programs, their performance has been lackluster and disappointing.[24]

What about other demand-side reforms: forcing/inducing/coaxing providers to adopt electronic medical records, to coordinate care, to integrate care, to manage care, to emphasize preventive care, to adopt evidence-based medicine, and so on? The Congressional Budget Office (CBO) has reviewed the evidence on all these reforms and concluded that the savings will be meager, if they materialize at all.[25]

What Difference Does Healthcare Make?

I now want to shift to a fascinating question, about which there is considerable debate. One person who thinks we are getting a good deal for the money we spend is Harvard University health economist David Cutler.[26] A 45-year-old man alive in 1950 had few effective treatments for today's most common killer, heart disease. At that time, little was spent on treatment or prevention. Today, such a man can expect to spend more than $30,000 (in 2004 dollars) on treatment of heart disease over the course of his remaining life, according to Cutler. The benefit: he can expect to live about 4.5 years longer. At a cost of $6,667 per extra year of life, this is a terrific return on our investment in health. In terms of the benefits of healthcare, we largely get a good deal for what we pay for, he argues. Although medical care consumes a greater portion of our economy than in years past, we get a lot back in return.

The reduction in physical disability is another advance that Cutler attributes to the marvels of modern medical science. Thirty years ago, one-quarter of the elderly population was unable to live independently. Hip and knee replacements and other advances have reduced that number to less than one in five today. That's why the nursing home population has hardly changed in the past couple decades or so, he argues.

Against this view is a growing body of research that is highly skeptical about what we are getting for our healthcare dollars—at least at the margin.

In the previous chapter I noted that although the Medicare program led to an enormous increase in healthcare spending, it apparently had no effect on the life expectancy of the elderly.[27] Some readers may be surprised at that result. If so, I have a few more surprises for you. People with high-deductible health insurance spend about 30 percent less than people with first-dollar coverage; yet, this lower level of spending apparently has no adverse effect on their health.[28] People without health insurance at all spend about half of what insured people spend,[29] but, again, with no obvious impact on their health.[30]

Imagine that you are in an automobile accident. An ambulance rushes to the scene and the emergency medical technicians and then the emergency room doctors save your life. This is the image of heroic medicine that a lot of people project on the entire healthcare system.

But suppose you are choosing to live in one of two cities, and City A spends twice as much on medical care per citizen as City B. City A has more doctors, more medical equipment, more hospital beds; and doctors in that city do more things. Would your life expectancy be longer if you choose to live in City A rather than City B? Probably not.

Researchers have studied this question across the fifty states, across hospital regions, and across Veterans Affairs regions and found that large variations in healthcare spending apparently have little, if any impact on overall population mortality. George Mason University economist Robin Hanson summarizes the literature this way:[31]

> [H]ealth policy experts know that we see at best only weak aggregate relations between health and medicine, in contrast to apparently strong aggregate relations between health and many other factors, such as exercise, diet, sleep, smoking, pollution, climate, and social status.... For example, [one study] found large and significant lifespan effects: a three year loss for smoking, a six year gain for rural living, a ten year loss for being underweight, and about fifteen year losses each for low income and low physical activity (in addition to the usual effects of age and gender).

This conclusion is important to keep in mind as we evaluate the likely impact of health reform. The nation as a whole is probably going to vastly increase the amount we are spending on healthcare. Yet, if we want to improve the nation's health, there may be wiser ways to spend that money.

Who Spends Most of the Healthcare Dollars?

Have you ever read an article in which the writer compares the incomes of the top 1 percent to the bottom 99 percent over the last decade, say? The problem: The author is encouraging you to think that the people in the top 1 percent at the beginning of the decade are the same people who are in the top 1 percent at the end of the decade. But they aren't. People move in and out of this category with surprising frequency. Yet, if they aren't the same people, what's the point of the comparison?

A similar thing happens in healthcare. I frequently see writers say that a small number of people spend most of the healthcare dollars. True. But the small number this year is not the same group of people as the small number last year, or the year before.

As in the case of the income comparisons, readers can be misled into thinking that our healthcare problems boil down to how to take care of a small number of people. Not so. A study by the Agency for Healthcare Research and Quality shows how much fluidity there is among the categories of patients who spend the most healthcare dollars:[32]

- In 2008, 1 percent of the population accounted for about one-fifth of all healthcare spending. Yet the following year, 80 percent of these patients dropped out of the top 1 percent category.
- The top 5 percent of the population accounted for nearly half of all healthcare spending. Yet 62 percent of these patients dropped out of this category the following year.
- Although the top 10 percent spent 64 percent of all healthcare dollars, the following year fewer than half of these patients were still in this category.
- At the other end of the spectrum, the bottom half of the population spent only 3 percent of healthcare dollars. Yet one of every four of these patients moved to the top half the following year.

Here is something else that's interesting:

- The top 10 percent are spending almost two-thirds of all healthcare dollars in any one year.
- Of those who remained in this category for both years, 43 percent were elderly, and another 40 percent were under 18 years of age.

In other words, the persistently sick tend to be young or old. Among the adult, nonelderly population who were in the top 10 percent the first year, almost three of every four were in the bottom 75 percent of spenders the second year.

Why is this important? If a small number of people spent most of the healthcare money and they were the same people year after year, there would not be much point in having a real market for health insurance.

Consider fire insurance. This makes sense only if fires are largely unpredictable and could happen to any homeowner. But suppose that the small percentage of homeowners who experience a fire in any one year are the very same people who experience a fire every year. In such a world, fire insurance would not be very practical. The same thing is true in healthcare.

Most people in health policy view health insurance as just a way to pay medical bills. This book is one of the very few places in all of the health policy literature where you will find a defense of the idea that there is a social need for real health insurance. It is also one of the very few places you will find an argument that we need a real market for health risks to determine the best way to insure against them and to determine what is the best way to partition insurance products between self-insurance and third-party insurance.

The Role of Medical Ethics

One of the most important differences between this book and the conventional literature on health policy is my belief that patients should be encouraged to choose between healthcare and other uses of money. And that's not just for small expenses. I think patients should be encouraged to make choices involving expensive procedures as well. If I'm right, doctors will have to take a new approach to medicine, and in taking this approach, they may have to rethink how they view medical ethics.

The latest edition of the American College of Physicians manual on ethics created quite a stir with the following passage:[33]

> Physicians have a responsibility to practice effective and efficient healthcare and to use healthcare resources responsibly. Parsimonious care that utilizes the most efficient means to effectively diagnose a condition and treat a patient respects the need to use resources wisely and to help ensure that resources are equitably available.

On the right, American Enterprise Institute scholar Scott Gottlieb reacts by writing, "Parsimonious, to me, implies an element of stinginess, and stinginess implies an element of subterfuge."[34] On the left, Aaron Carroll, a professor of pediatrics at Indiana School of Medicine, writes:[35]

> I would fight tooth and nail to get anything—and I mean anything—to save [my own child]. I'd do it even if it cost a fortune and might not work. That's why I don't think you should leave these kinds of decisions up to the individual. Every single person feels the way I do about every single person they love, and no one will ever be able to say no. That's human.
>
> Similarly, I don't think that it's necessarily fair to make it a physician's responsibility. I also want my child's doctor to fight tooth and nail to get anything that might save my child. Many times, physicians have long-standing relationships with patients. Asking them to divorce themselves from the very human feelings that compel them to do anything that might help their patients is not something that I think will necessarily improve the practice of medicine. They also should be human.
>
> So whose job is it? Well, mine for instance. That's what I do as a health services researcher. That's what policy makers should also do....

That's a roundabout way of saying that only the government can ration care the right way.

My view: people in healthcare have become so completely immersed in the idea of third-party payment that they have completely lost sight of the whole idea of agency. Can you imagine a lawyer discussing the prospects of launching a lawsuit without bringing up the matter of cost? What about an architect submitting plans for a building but completely ignoring what it would

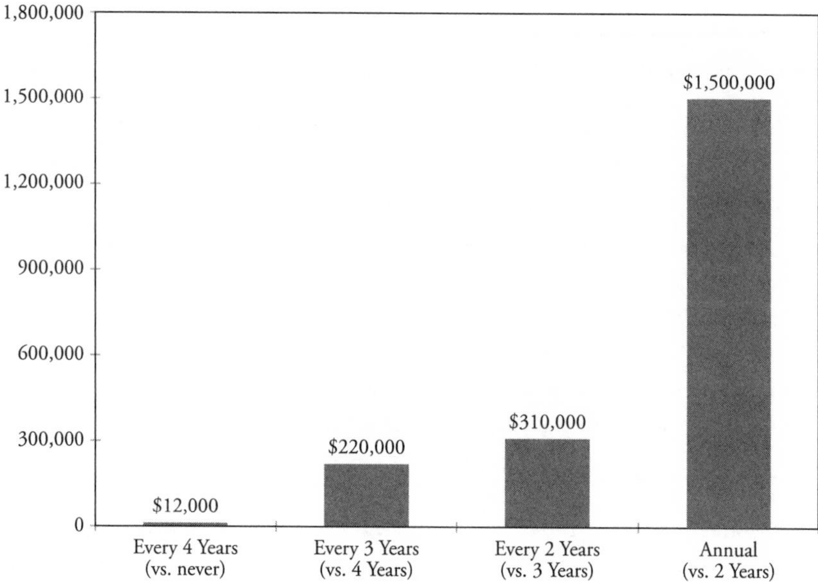

Figure 2.1. Cervical Cancer Tests: Cost per Year of Life Saved (Women Age 20)
Source: Tammy O. Tengs et al., "Five Hundred Lifesaving Interventions and Their Cost-Effectiveness," *Risk Analysis*, June 1995.

cost to build it? Outside of medicine, can you imagine any professional anywhere discussing any project with a client and pretending that money doesn't matter? Of course not.

Then what is so special about medicine? Answer: the field has been completely corrupted by the idea that (a) patients should never be in a position to choose between health benefits and monetary cost, (b) doctors shouldn't have to think about such tradeoffs either, (c) to insulate the patient from having to choose between healthcare and other uses of money, third-party payers should pay all the medical bills, and (d) since no one else is going to think about what anything costs, the third-party payer is the only entity left to decide which services are worthwhile and which ones aren't.

To appreciate how doctors could do the same thing other professionals do in advising patients on how to spend their own money, take a look at Figure 2.1. Armed with this information, what would a responsible doctor tell her patient about Pap smears and how often the patient should get them?

Note that getting a Pap smear every four years (versus never getting one) costs $12,000 per year of life saved, when averaged over the whole population. What the responsible doctor should say is, "In the risk avoidance business, this is a really good buy. Based on choices people like you make in other walks of life, this is a good decision. This type of risk reduction is well worth what it costs."

What about getting the test every three years (versus every four) or every two years (versus every three)? Here the doctor should say, "Now we are moving toward the upper boundary of what most other people are willing to spend to avoid various kinds of risks, when the probabilities are small and the amount of money is also small. So at this point, serious thought needs to be given to whether the test is really worth what it cost."

How about getting the test done every year (versus every two years)? Here the responsible doctor will say, "This is definitely a bad buy (unless there is some specific indication or unless not getting the test is going to keep the patient awake at night). The cost of an annual Pap smear in relation to the amount of risk reduction achieved is way outside the range of choices most people make with respect to other risks."

Notice what is going on here. The responsible doctor, functioning as an agent of a patient who is not familiar with the medical literature and who is not skilled at evaluating risks or trading off risk reduction for other uses of money, advises her patient in these matters. She helps her patient manage both her health and her money—because both are important.

When Dr. Carroll says, "I'd do it even if it cost a fortune and might not work," I am sure he is being sincere. But I am equally sure that is not how he normally makes decisions. It is in fact easy to spend a fortune to avoid small-probability events. The Environmental Protection Agency makes the private sector do it every day. But if an ordinary family tried that, they would end up spending their entire income avoiding trivial risks. And that is not what normal people do.

Here is another example of a money-is-no-object-no-matter-how-improbable-the-prospects-if-life-and-death-are-at-stake choice. This is former White House health adviser, Ezekiel Emanuel, writing in *The New York Times*:[36]

> Proton beam therapy is a kind of radiation used to treat cancers. The particles are made of atomic nuclei rather than the usual X-rays, and

> theoretically can be focused more precisely on cancerous tissue, minimizing the danger to healthy tissue surrounding it. But the machines are tremendously expensive, requiring a particle accelerator encased in a football-field-size building with concrete walls. As a result, Medicare will pay around $50,000 for proton beam therapy for a patient with prostate cancer, roughly twice as much as it would if the patient received another type of radiation.

Emanuel claims there is no evidence the treatment works for prostate cancer—so the therapy is a waste of $25,000. Is he right? I don't know. If you're paying the extra $25,000 out of your own pocket, listen to what the doctors at Mayo have to say (in favor of its use) and then listen to what Emanuel has to say and make up your own mind.

Bottom line: helping patients manage their health dollars as well as their healthcare should be what doctoring is all about.

3

Why People Disagree About Health Policy

HAVE YOU EVER witnessed an argument in which two people just talk past each other? Neither actually seems to grasp or even hear what the other is saying. In fact, they don't even use the same language to describe the issue they are arguing about. Yes, I know. This is a pretty good description of Congress. But it's also a good description of the field of health policy.

When I talk about healthcare, I often use economic terms. For example, I often refer to the *medical marketplace*. I frequently refer to patients as *consumers* and doctors and hospitals as *producers* or *providers* of care, and I talk about the *time price* of care and the *money price* of care. People in health policy rarely use these terms. Randomly pick up almost any book on health policy and see if you can find the term *time price* in the glossary. I bet you can't. Ditto for the word *consumer*.

To me, the economic way of thinking is just common sense. I realize there will be many readers who didn't experience it that way in Econ 101, but stop and think. Wouldn't you be more likely to buy something if the price were lower rather than higher? Of course. Well, that's a commonsensical way of describing the law of demand. Further, all of the economic concepts I will use in this book are commonsensical in just that way. Still, I find that many people don't share my sense of common sense. What follows are some examples.

How Much Should Individual Preferences Matter?

Years ago, Kenneth Arrow, an economist who was joint winner of the Nobel Memorial Prize in Economics in 1972, argued that Pareto optimality[1] (a situation in which everyone is as well off as he can possibly be from his own point of view—given the constraints of the system) is a good thing. Unless you are willing to systematically deny people whatever it is that they want, he said, Pareto optimality would seem to be a value we all should endorse. And almost every economist I know does endorse it.[2]

Yet, in the world of health policy, I can introduce you to a whole slew of folks who are perfectly willing to deny people whatever it is they want. For lack of a better term, I will call them "paternalists."

One of the most controversial decisions made by the Obama administration in implementing its health reform has been the notion that health insurance should cover something almost everyone can easily pay for out of pocket: contraceptives.

Why, you might ask, does this decision have to be made in Washington? Why can't decisions like this be left to individuals and the marketplace? Why not let people who want contraception coverage pay higher premiums and get the coverage they want? Why not let everyone else pay lower premiums? In deciding to intervene, the administration paid a heavy political price. Forcing Catholic universities, hospitals, and charities to provide health insurance that includes free contraceptives (as well as sterilization) produced a reaction that was poignant and hyperbolic.

That the Obama administration was willing to take the heat shows just how strong is the desire of many health reformers to tell everyone else what to do. (As of the time of this writing, the Obama administration has decided to let employers off the hook, but require the health insurance company the employer contracts with to provide free contraceptive services[3]—a distinction economists will find not worth making.)

Interestingly, one of the most controversial decisions made in Hillary Clinton's effort to reform the healthcare system in the 1990s also concerned two other inexpensive procedures: mammograms and Pap smears. In fact, some people believe that her position on these two issues were what finally killed public support for the entire health overhaul.

Fifteen years ago, the experts didn't agree on how frequently women should have these procedures any more than they agree today. I'm sure that when various women asked various doctors they got various answers. And, by the way, there is nothing wrong with that. Whenever there is risk and uncertainty, opinions will differ. That's not the end of the world.

What was the end of HillaryCare, however, was the notion that the White House should decide these questions for every woman in America. When you stop to think about it, that takes a certain amount of chutzpah. It also reflects a degree of meddlesomeness that is really hard for people who are not paternalists to understand. But both the Clinton White House and the Obama White House were staffed by folks who just could not abide the idea of your having a health plan different from the one they think you should have—down to the tiniest detail.

For Hillary and her advisers it came down to this: They decided that sexually active women should have a cervical cancer test every three years, instead of every two. For women in their fifties, they called for a mammogram every other year, instead of every year. And these decisions, unfortunately for Clinton, were different from what most doctors were recommending at the time.[4]

Now the right way to think about all this is very simple. How much does a mammogram cost? About $100, if you pay cash. If you want one, take the money out of your Health Savings Account and go buy it. How often should you do that? Probably as often as it gives you peace of mind. Is not having the test keeping you awake at night? Then spend the $100 and get the test. The same principle applies to contraceptives. If you want them, go buy them.

And what about the tiny, tiny, tiny portion of the population that really can't afford these services? They can go to a community health center or to Planned Parenthood and ask for them for free.

Incidentally, if there were a good social reason to promote contraception, there are three things government can do that are superior to regulating everyone's health insurance: (1) it can add to the millions of dollars it already spends making contraceptives free through county health programs; (2) it could make contraceptives available over-the-counter rather than by prescription; or (3) it could allow pharmacists to do the prescribing (thereby cutting out the expense of a doctor visit), as is done in many countries and was done in the United States before 1938. (I owe these last two points to economist David Henderson.[5])

The Public-Private Double Standard

If a private insurance company denies a breast cancer patient a bone marrow transplant,[6] that's considered a moral outrage—even if the procedure is experimental and is later shown not to work. But if the Arizona Medicaid program denies people organ transplants that do work and do save lives, that is considered an unfortunate budget issue.[7]

If 25,000 British cancer patients die every year because the National Health Service won't buy the drugs that would have prolonged their lives and they cannot afford to pay for those drugs out of their own pockets, that is considered, again, an unfortunate budget problem.[8] But if even one uninsured American dies prematurely because he or she cannot afford those very same drugs, that is ethically unacceptable.

What I am describing is, of course, a double standard. Many people in health policy, for example, viscerally dislike the idea of private Medicare Advantage plans, an alternative chosen by about one in four Medicare enrollees. Instead they would like to see everyone in conventional Medicare—a public plan. You would be amazed at how many otherwise knowledgeable people are completely unaware of the fact that Medicare is not actually run by the federal government. It's run by private contractors, including such private insurers as Cigna and BlueCross.

The view that public insurance is good and private insurance is bad really amounts to saying that when BlueCross is called *Medicare* it is good and altruistic, but when the same company is called *private insurer* it is bad and selfish. It makes no sense, but there are a lot of people who think exactly that way.

Economic Versus Engineering Views of Society

There are two fundamentally different ways of thinking about complex social systems: the *economic* approach and the *engineering* approach.

Social engineers see society as disorganized, unplanned, and inefficient. Wherever they look, they see underperforming people in flawed organizations producing imperfect goods and services. The solution? Let experts study the problem, discover what should be produced and how to produce it, and then follow their advice. Social engineers invariably believe that a plan can work, even though everyone in society has a self-interest in defeating it. Implicitly, they assume that incentives don't matter. Or, if they do matter, they don't matter very much.

Yet to a commonsense observer, incentives seem to matter very much. Complex social systems display unpredictable spontaneous order, with all kinds of unintended consequences of purposeful action. To have the best chance of good social outcomes, people must find that when they pursue their own interests, they are meeting the needs of others. Perverse incentives almost always lead to perverse outcomes.

In the 20th century, country after country and regime after regime tried to impose an *engineering model* on society as a whole. Most of those experiments have thankfully come to a close. By the century's end, the world began to understand that the economic model, not the engineering model, is where our hopes should lie. Yet healthcare is still completely dominated by people who steadfastly resist the economic way of thinking.

As I see it, healthcare is a field that can be described as a sea of mediocrity punctuated by islands of excellence. The islands always spring from the bottom up, never from the top down; they tend to be distributed randomly. They are invariably the result of the enthusiasm, leadership, and entrepreneurial skills of a small number of people. They are almost always penalized by the payment system.[9]

Now if you think like a commonsense economist, you will say, "Why don't we reward, instead of punish, the islands of excellence and maybe we will get more of them?" But if you think like an engineer you will reject that idea as completely unacceptable. Instead, you will try to (1) find out how medicine should be practiced and (2) find out what type of organization is needed for doctors to practice that way, so that (3) you can then go tell everybody what to do.

Here is Harvard Medical School professor Atul Gawande, explaining how medicine should be practiced:[10]

> This can no longer be a profession of craftsmen individually brewing plans for whatever patient comes through the door. We have to be more like engineers building a mechanism whose parts actually fit together, whose workings are ever more finely tuned and tweaked for ever better performance in providing aid and comfort to human beings.

Here is Karen Davis of The Commonwealth Fund, explaining (in the context of health reform) how medical care should be organized:[11]

> The legislation also includes physician payment reforms that encourage physicians, hospitals and other providers to join together to form accountable care organizations [ACOs] to gain efficiencies and improve quality of care. Those that meet quality-of-care targets and reduce costs relative to a spending benchmark can share in the savings they generate for Medicare.

The ACA was heavily influenced by the engineering model. Who, but a social engineer, would think you can control healthcare costs by running pilot programs? They are a prime example of the social engineer's fool's errand.

Can Entrepreneurship Be Copied?

Time and again, President Obama has told us how he intends to solve our healthcare problems: spend money on pilot programs and other experiments, find out what works, and then copy it. He's also repeatedly said the same thing about education. The only difference: In education, we've already been following this approach with no success for twenty-five years.

Still, if the president were right about health and education, why wouldn't the same idea apply to every other field? Why couldn't we study the best way to make a computer or invest in the stock market—and then copy it?

I want to propose a principle that covers all of this: entrepreneurship cannot be replicated. Put differently, there is no such thing as a cookbook entrepreneur.

Let's suppose for a moment that I am wrong. Suppose we could study the behavior of successful entrepreneurs and write down the keys to their success in a book that everyone could read and copy. Consider Bill Gates, Warren Buffett and Sam Walton. If we could discover what they did right, and everyone copied their behavior, then we could all become billionaires. Right? Well, not quite.

Here's the problem: In order for each of us to be a billionaire, we have to each be doing something that produces a billion dollars' worth of goods and services. But if all we're doing is copying action items out of a book, then we are not doing anything special. And if we're not doing anything special, we are definitely not producing a billion dollars of value added.

In mathematics, Gödel's Theorem says that no complex, axiomatic system can be both consistent and complete. What I am proposing is something similar for social science. Although some habits of highly successful people can be identified and copied, not enough of them can be copied for each of us to become highly successful ourselves through copycat behavior alone.

This is Goodman's Nonreplicability Theorem.

In healthcare, it's already been borne out. Scholars associated with the Brookings Institution identified ten of the best hospital regions in the country and then tried to identify common characteristics that could be replicated.[12] There were almost none. Some regions had doctors on staff. Others paid fee-for-service. Some had electronic medical records. Others did not. A separate study of physicians' practices found much the same thing.[13] There were simply not enough objective characteristics that the practices had in common to allow an independent party to set up a successful practice by copycat alone.

By the way, this is not bad news. It is good news. How much fun would life be if we all went around copying what we read in a book?

Health Insurance Versus Healthcare

Do you care whether I have health insurance? If you do care, do you also care if I have other kinds of insurance?

While you're thinking about the initial question, here are a few follow-up questions:

- Do you care whether I have life insurance?
- What about disability insurance?
- Homeowner's insurance?
- Auto casualty insurance?
- Auto liability insurance?
- What about retirement insurance? (A pension or savings plan.)
- Do you care whether I keep my money at an FDIC-insured institution?
- Or whether I bought an extended warranty on my car?
- Or whether I bought travel insurance before taking a scuba-diving trip to Palau? (It pays off if you get sick and can't go.)

There is actually a rational reason (based on economics) why you should care about some of my decisions and not others. Most of us basically don't care whether people insure to protect their own assets (at least we don't care enough to try to make them insure). But we do care about decisions that could create external costs for the rest of us.

Through Social Security, we force people to pay for life insurance benefitting dependent children (who could potentially become wards of the state) but not for a working-age spouse. All but three states force people to have auto liability insurance (covering harm to others) but not casualty insurance (covering their own cars). We basically don't care whether people insure their own homes, but we force them to contribute to retirement and disability schemes to prevent their accidental dependency on all the rest of us.

Here is the principle: Government intervenes in those insurance markets where an individual's choice to insure or not insure imposes potential costs on others. Because of our basic human generosity, we're not going to allow people to starve or live in destitution. So when people don't insure in some areas, society is going to step in and help (where help is needed). Implicitly, we have a social contract that socializes the downside of certain risks. If we leave the upside to individual choice, we have privatized the gains and socialized the losses. When people don't bear the social cost of their risk-taking, they will take more risks than they would otherwise.

Another way to think about the problem is in terms of the opportunity to become a "free rider" on other peoples' generosity. Consider people who have no life insurance (for dependent children), no disability insurance, and no retirement savings program. Because they are not paying premiums or saving for retirement, they can consume all of their income and enjoy a higher standard of living than their cohorts. But if they bet wrong (die while children are still minors, become disabled, reach retirement with no assets), they are counting on everyone else to help them out.

How does all of this apply to health? Considering the extensive interest in insuring the uninsured, you would expect an exhaustive literature. But aside from Robin Hanson's thesis that healthcare is different,[14] there is virtually nowhere you can go to find a rational, well-thought-out, consistent analysis of why you should care whether or not I have health insurance.

If we are concerned that the uninsured will impose an external cost on the rest of us, there is a simple remedy: impose a fine equal to the expected cost of any unpaid medical bills they might incur. Note, however, that uninsured middle-income families are already paying higher taxes because they do not have the tax-subsidized (employer-provided) insurance their neighbors have. Far from being free riders, these families appear to be paying their own way. Of course, the extra taxes the uninsured pay tend to go to Washington, while uncompensated care tends to be delivered locally. This mismatch of revenue and expense is not caused by the uninsured, however. It is the result of government not having its act together.

For high-income families, it's not clear why we should be concerned. People who have, say, $1 million or more in assets—and that's about 1 in every 30 people —can afford to pay their own medical bills without insurance. Also, the argument for intervention becomes weaker the lower a household's income. People who cannot afford health insurance anyway are not willful free riders. They are not making choices that impose new costs on others. So there is no obvious social reason to force them to insure. They will need healthcare from time to time, however.

What is the best way to get healthcare to people with low incomes and few assets? Not Medicaid or state-run Children's Health Insurance Plans (which you can think of as Medicaid for children). Nor is it any other system, inappropriately modeled on the insurance approach to healthcare.

Bottom line: the case for trying to get everyone insured is not an easy one to make. Nonetheless, most people I know in health policy are obsessed with the idea. In fact, they are more concerned with whether people are insured than whether they get healthcare.

Certainly that was the case in Massachusetts. The entire focus of health reform in that state has been on insuring the uninsured. But is anyone getting more care? Not that scholars have been able to verify. Similarly, the entire focus of ACA is on health insurance and getting people insured. But as noted, nothing in the legislation creates more doctors so that more healthcare can be delivered.

Why are so many people in health policy obsessed with health insurance, while remaining almost indifferent about the actual delivery of healthcare? Read on.

Process Versus Results

I've engaged in many, many debates through the years over whether the Canadian healthcare system is better than our own. The reason: I meet a lot of people who advocate *single-payer* health insurance, by which they mean a system in which government pays all the medical bills. There are basically only three genuine single-payer systems in the world: Canada, Cuba, and North Korea.

On such occasions, I point out that (a) the US system is more egalitarian than the Canadian system (and more egalitarian than the health systems of most other developed countries as well), (b) uninsured Americans get as much as or more preventive care than insured Canadians (as many or more mammograms, PSA tests, colonoscopies; see Figure 3.1), (c) low-income whites in the United States are in better health than low-income whites in Canada, (d) although minorities do less well in both countries, we treat our minority populations better than the Canadians do, and (e) even though thousands of people in both countries go to hospital emergency rooms for care they can't get anywhere else, people in our emergency rooms get treated more quickly and with better results than people in Canadian emergency rooms.

Now I know what you are wondering. Have I ever convinced anyone to change his mind with such arguments? What I discovered after many frustrating conversations was that people who like the way healthcare is organized in Canada do not like it because of any particular result it achieves. They like it because they like the process.

In Canada, what care you receive, where you receive it, and how you receive it is not determined by individual choice and the marketplace. It is determined collectively. For some people, that's an end in itself.

[For more on the comparison between US and Canadian healthcare, interested readers may consult the sources for Figure 3.1, especially the works by former Congressional Budget Office Director June O'Neill and her husband, Dave O'Neill.]

Source for chart, "Patients Spending More than 20 Minutes with Their Doctor": Karen Donelan et al., "The Cost of Health System Change: Public Discontent in Five Nations," *Health Affairs* 18 (1999): 206–216. doi: 10.1377/hlthaff.18.3.206; Source for charts on mammogram, cervical cancer screening and prostate test: June E. O'Neill and Dave M. O'Neill, "Who are the Uninsured? An Analysis of America's Uninsured Population, Their Characteristics and Their Health," Employment Policies Institute, June 2009, http://epionline.org/studies/oneill_06-2009.pdf; Source for charts on colonoscopies: June E. O'Neill and Dave M. O'Neill, "Health Status, Healthcare and Inequality: Canada vs. the US," NBER Working Paper No. 13429, September 2007, http://www.nber.org/papers/w13429.

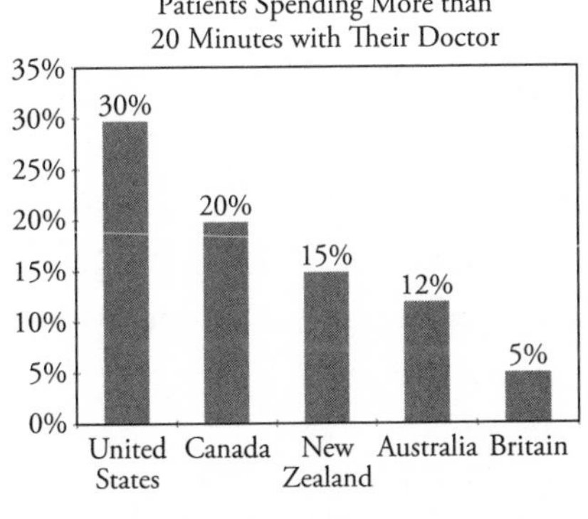
Patients Spending More than
20 Minutes with Their Doctor
35%
30%
25%
20%
15%
10%
5%
0%
30%
20%
15%
12%
5%
United States
Canada
New Zealand
Australia
Britain

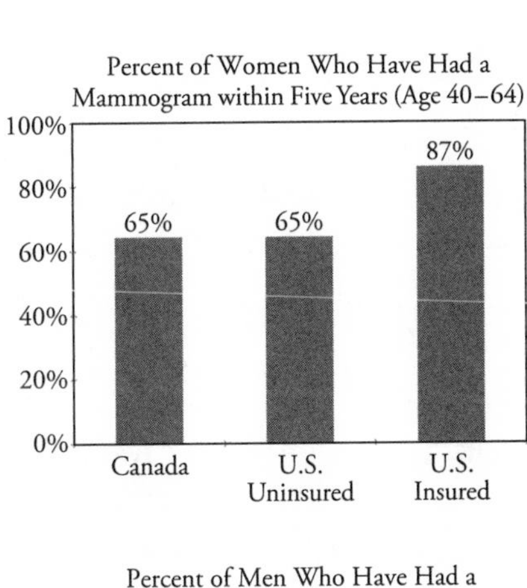
Percent of Women Who Have Had a
Mammogram within Five Years (Age 40–64)
100%
80%
60%
40%
20%
0%
65%
65%
87%
Canada
U.S. Uninsured
U.S. Insured

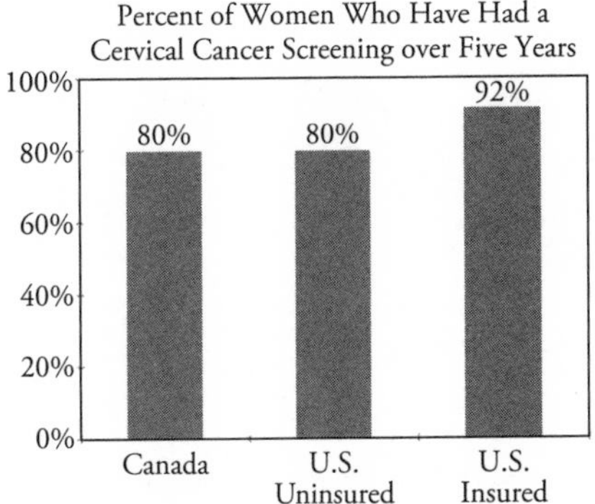
Percent of Women Who Have Had a
Cervical Cancer Screening over Five Years
100%
80%
60%
40%
20%
0%
80%
80%
92%
Canada
U.S. Uninsured
U.S. Insured

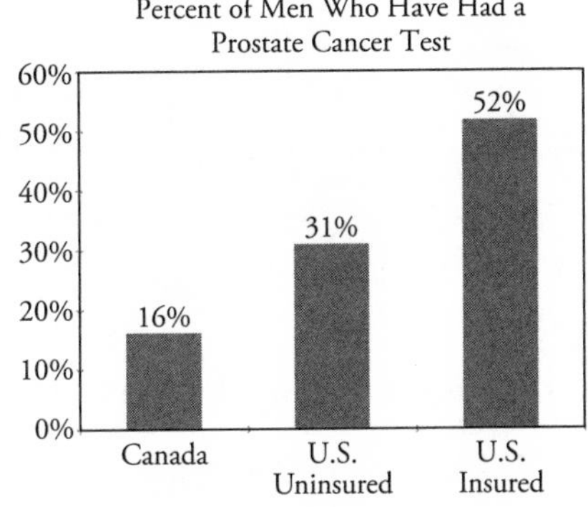
Percent of Men Who Have Had a
Prostate Cancer Test
60%
50%
40%
30%
20%
10%
0%
16%
31%
52%
Canada
U.S. Uninsured
U.S. Insured

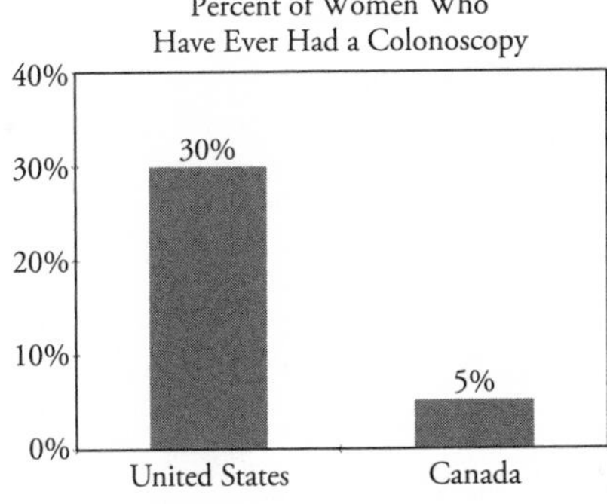
Percent of Women Who
Have Ever Had a Colonoscopy
40%
30%
20%
10%
0%
30%
5%
United States
Canada

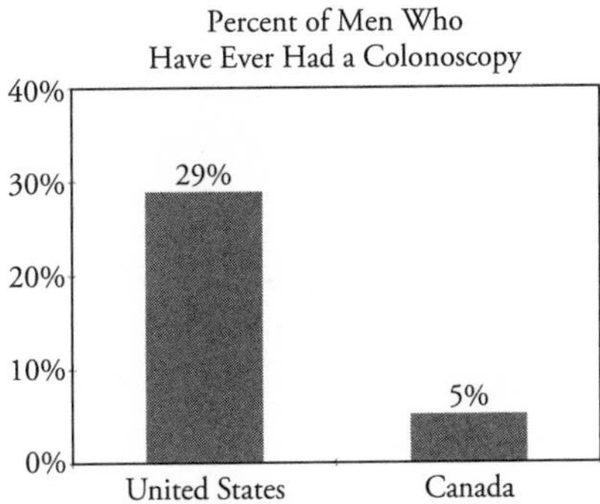
Percent of Men Who
Have Ever Had a Colonoscopy
40%
30%
20%
10%
0%
29%
5%
United States
Canada

Figure 3.1

Institutionalized Altruism

One of the most important tenets of public choice economics is the observation that we do not become different people when we leave the private sector and enter the public square. We do not become less selfish, for example, when we leave the supermarket and enter the voting booth. Nor do we become more selfish when we leave the voting booth and return to the supermarket. We are the same people—just as altruistic or just as selfish—in both realms. Nonetheless, some would have us see the marketplace as institutionalized selfishness and political systems as institutionalized altruism. Put differently, they romanticize politics and demonize the marketplace—failing in both cases to see reality as it really is.

This is the underlying reason why so many people in health policy believe that for-profit hospitals or for-profit insurance companies should not exist. In fact, profit is the opportunity cost of capital and that cost has to be borne, even by entities called nonprofits.[15]

Romanticizing Health Reform

Consider Donald Berwick, President Obama's recess appointee to run Medicare and Medicaid, on his way out of office in the fall of 2011. For starters, he claimed that the Affordable Care Act "is making healthcare a basic human right."[16] Then he went on to say that because of the new law, "we are a nation headed for justice, for fairness and justice in access to care."[17]

In fact, there is nothing in the legislation that makes "healthcare a right." Nor is there anything in the new law that makes the role of government more just or fair. To the contrary, a lot of knowledgeable people (not just conservative critics) predict that access to care is going to be more difficult for our most vulnerable populations. That appears to have been the experience in Massachusetts, which President Obama cites as the model for the new federal reforms. True enough, Massachusetts cut the number of uninsured in that state in half through then-Governor Mitt Romney's health reform. But while expanding the demand for care, the state did nothing to increase supply. More people than ever are trying to get care, but because there has been no increase in medical services, it is more difficult than ever to actually see a doctor.

Far from being fair, the new federal health law will give some people health insurance subsidies that are as much as $20,000 more than the subsidies available to other people at the same level of income.

Right after the passage of the Affordable Care Act, Obama administration health advisers Robert Kocher, Ezekiel Emanuel, and Nancy-Ann DeParle announced that the new health reform law "guarantees access to healthcare for all Americans."[18]

In fact, nothing in the act guarantees access to care for *any* American, let alone *all* Americans. Far from it. Again, take Massachusetts as the precedent. The waiting time to see a new family practice doctor in Boston is longer than in any other major US city.[19] In a sense, a new patient seeking care in Boston has less access to care than new patients everywhere else.

Reformers in other countries also tend to romanticize their accomplishments. With the enactment of the British National Health Service after World War II, the reformers claimed that they had made healthcare a right. The same claim was made in Canada after that country established its single-payer Medicare scheme. Yet in reality, neither country has made healthcare a right. They didn't even come close. Neither British nor Canadian citizens have a right to any particular health service. They may get the care they need, or they may not. Sadly, too often they do not.

There is almost a religious quality to the way some people think and talk about healthcare.

Imagine a preacher, a priest, or a rabbi who gets up in front of the congregation and gets a lot of things wrong. Say he misstates facts, distorts reality, or says other things you know are not true. Do you jump up from the pew and yell, "That's a lie"? Of course not. But if those same misstatements were made by someone during the work week you might well respond with considerable harshness. What's the difference? I think there are two different thought processes that many people engage in. Let's call them "Sunday morning" thinking and "Monday morning" thinking. We tolerate things on Sunday that we would never tolerate on Monday. And there is probably nothing wrong with that, unless people get their days mixed up. In my professional career I have been to hundreds of health policy conferences, discussions, get-togethers, and so on, where it seemed as though people were completely failing to connect with each other. At one point it dawned on me that we were having two different conversations. All too often I was engaged in Monday morning thinking, while everyone else was engaged in Sunday morning thinking.

If people don't come to their convictions by means of reason, then reason isn't going to convince them to change their minds. This principle applies to healthcare, just as it does to other fields.

PART II

The Consequences of Being Trapped

4

What Being Trapped Means to You

SELF-INTEREST IS A very powerful motivator. As Adam Smith explained over 200 years ago, it is not through altruism or charity that we get most of our needs met.[1] Our needs get met because producers and sellers find it in their financial self-interest to do so. But suppose you find yourself in an institutional environment where normal market forces have been systematically suppressed and where perverse incentives are the norm. Suppose other people find it in their self-interest not to meet your needs—or even to do things that turn out to be harmful to you.

That is the direction in which the healthcare sector has been headed for several decades.

How Much Do You Trust Your Doctor?

The primary reason we seek any professional advice is because of what economists call asymmetry of information. They know more than we do. The lawyer knows more about law. The accountant, more about accounting. The engineer, more about engineering. And so forth. Not only do we come to the relationship with a knowledge deficit, it's usually very difficult for us to detect whether the advice we are getting is the best advice or even whether it is accurate.[2]

That's why agency is so important. When we are represented in court, we want a lawyer who puts our interest first, not the interest of a prosecutor or of an opponent in a civil suit. When we have a tax problem, we want our accountant to be our representative, not the representative of the IRS. The same principle holds for medicine.

The ideal doctor is one who is our agent—not just in dealing with disease, but in dealing with the complicated, complex institution we call the healthcare system. The problem is that health insurance undermines the very agency relationship that would best serve our needs. Because the typical insurance contract reduces the out-of-pocket cost of care to patients, they have a perverse incentive to overconsume healthcare. Because the same contract pays doctors according to the number of visits, tests, and procedures they order, they have a perverse incentive to overtreat.

In order to control costs, therefore, insurers typically engage in all manner of techniques to control and limit the choices patients and doctors have. That includes controls over the drugs we can take, the tests we can have, and even the doctors and facilities we have access to. Third-party payers have enormous power to limit our choices because they have the power to pay or deny payment of medical bills. Even if their decisions are challenged and subsequently reversed, third-party payers can impose significant time and money costs on any doctor or patient who doesn't follow their rules.

Physicians who practice medicine in this environment learned long ago that they are not free to be the unfettered agents of their patients. For example, if you are insured by BlueCross, your doctors will tend to view BlueCross as their customer, rather than you. They will look to BlueCross rules and procedures to determine what drugs to prescribe, what tests to order, and when and if surgery is to take place. On the other hand, if you are an Aetna patient, they will tend to view Aetna as their customer and they will tend to look at Aetna's rules and procedures in making treatment decisions.

The danger is that instead of serving as *your* agent, doctors will become agents of third parties—insurance companies, employers, Medicare, Medicaid, and so on. To the degree that this occurs, the third party's needs become more important than the patient's needs. And remember, the primary need of the third party is to avoid spending too much money on you.

How far could this disturbing trend go? Further than you might think. Medicare recently announced that it will start paying more to hospitals that follow a dozen procedures, including administering antibiotics prior to surgery and anticlotting medication to heart attack patients.[3] It will pay less to hospitals that don't comply. The same thing is about to happen to doctors. Those who comply on up to 194 different metrics—including adopting electronic medical records—will get higher compensation.[4] Those who resist will get less. These are examples of a much larger trend: Washington telling the medical community how to practice medicine. This is happening even though a recent study[5] finds little relationship between the inputs Medicare wants to pay for and such outputs as patient survival, and even though the latest pilot programs show that paying doctors[6] for performance doesn't improve quality.

Remember the words *evidence-based care.* They are likely to be very much a part of your future. To its advocates, evidence-based care follows medical treatment guidelines and protocols developed by experts, based on the scientific literature—as reported in medical journals and scholarly reports. If all doctors follow the same protocols, they argue, patients with similar conditions will be treated the same way. Wide variations in the practice of medicine would be replaced by uniform, standardized treatments.

Don't you want your doctors to base their advice on scientific evidence? Don't you want them to follow guidelines that have been written by reputable scholars who have surveyed all the relevant literature? So what's not to like? A lot, it turns out. Think about the calendar you keep on your laptop or your cell phone. It's probably an invaluable aide to help you organize your life. Now suppose that instead of being your servant, the calendar becomes your master. What if there were a rule that says you can't do anything during the week unless it is on the calendar by Sunday. Call this "calendar-based scheduling." Instead of being an aide, the calendar would quickly become an oppressive barrier to your freedom of action.

The same principle applies in medicine. Protocols and guidelines can be helpful or harmful, depending on how they are used. And there are six reasons why such guidelines—in the wrong hands—can reduce the quality of care you receive.

First, in most areas of medicine, there are no treatment guidelines, and where there are, they are often unreliable, conflicting, and incomplete. Even for something as seemingly straightforward as deciding when women should get mammograms, the advice is conflicting.[7] If insurers have to choose among conflicting and inconsistent guidelines, which ones do you think they will choose? The ones that cost them less money, of course.

Second, even well-established guidelines are inevitably written for the average patient. But suppose you are not average. Are doctors free to step outside the protocols and give you care based on their training, knowledge and experience? Or will they be pressured to stick to the cookbook, regardless of how the patient fares? Health plans always say that doctors are free to step outside the guidelines if they have good reason for doing so. But if they have to fill out multiple forms and jump through many hoops to make this possible, they will be tempted to conform to the guidelines even if that's not the best choice for you.

Third, guidelines are often written by people who are not disinterested. One study found that 56 percent of the doctors who helped write guidelines for treatment of heart ailments had potential conflicts of interest.[8] These conflicts are more common than is generally realized. Writing in *The New York Times*, University of Texas law professor Ronen Avraham notes:[9]

> Guidelines produced by insurance companies sometimes put their interests first. Malpractice insurers, for example, may recommend yearly mammograms, even if they are not necessary, because they bear the costs of lawsuits for late diagnoses of breast cancer—and not the costs or health risks of the extra mammograms. Moreover, the nonprofit groups behind many other guidelines have traditionally depended on pharmaceutical and medical device companies to finance their work. Last year, the Council of Medical Specialty Societies issued a new code of conduct seeking to stop these industries from sponsoring the development of guidelines, but there are still too many loopholes, and thousands of guidelines produced before the reform[s] are still in circulation.

In one particularly egregious case, Eli Lilly and Co. funded medical guidelines for the treatment of a deadly infection in an effort to boost sales of a drug with questionable benefits.[10]

Fourth, evidence-based guidelines are based on studies, and these studies often exclude entire segments of the population. For example, a large number of studies on patients with heart failure excluded elderly patients, even though most of the people who have this problem are elderly.[11] If you are an elderly patient, do you want your doctor to follow procedures that were based on studies of patients thirty or forty years younger than you are? According to Don Taylor, a health policy analyst at Duke University, it is not at all unusual to exclude patients with certain characteristics and conditions from clinical trials, while the patients who are excluded are still subjected to the guidelines after the trial is over.[12]

Fifth, the "gold standard" of medical research is the randomized controlled trial. But Steven Goldberg has catalogued all kinds of reasons why even these experiments are often poor guides for practitioners dealing with real patients:[13]

> In the field, where researchers are dealing with specific communities of people with virtually unlimited and sometimes indeterminate or hidden characteristics, creating truly random experiments is maddeningly difficult, time-consuming and expensive.

Finally, the whole idea behind guidelines and protocols is that it is appropriate to treat patients with similar conditions the same way. But individuals are individuals. They don't always respond to treatments the same way. For substance abuse, for example, there apparently is no such thing as a protocol that works for diverse groups of patients.[14]

Evidence-based guidelines could be a boon to medical practice, helping doctors do their jobs. One place where standardization seems to be working remarkably well, for example, is at Geisinger Health Systems in central Pennsylvania. Doctors there follow forty specific steps before performing elective heart bypass surgery, and the operation is cancelled if even one step is overlooked. The system is so efficient that it offers patients a ninety-day warranty—any mistakes that require readmission are taken care of gratis![15]

When these tools developed by outside entities substitute for the doctors' judgments, however, patients are likely to be the losers.

How Much Do You Trust Your Employer?

Here is how most people approach the labor market: they search for a job they like, with health insurance tacked on as a fringe benefit. But here is how some other people approach the labor market: They search for the health insurance they need and agree to the other terms of the job in order to get it.

I first became aware of this second type of person in conversations with a major retailer, who discovered that a person who was way overqualified was working in the company mailroom. The reason: The employee's daughter required $500,000 a year of medical care—all paid for by the company's generous health plan. (See a similar problem at Starbucks.[16]) It's hard not to sympathize with a father who goes to great lengths to take care of his daughter. But regulations that try to force companies to pay for social problems like this one are having unintended consequences for everyone else.

Under federal law, employers can't deny employment or health insurance to people on the grounds that they are likely to need a lot of medical care. Nor can they charge a higher premium to employees based on their health status. These regulations are changing the relationship between employers and their employees. With the current regulations in place, for example, a rational employer has strong incentives to find legal ways to attract employees who are healthy and avoid those who are sick, other things being equal. And that's just what they appear to be doing.

A PricewaterhouseCooper study finds that 73 percent of employers offer wellness programs. Of those with more than 5,000 workers, 88 percent do. But why offer wellness benefits? Such programs cannot possibly pay for themselves—unless they are targeted at the minority of employees with a serious need to change their lifestyles. Preventive medicine may be a wise investment for the individual, but it rarely reduces overall healthcare costs for an employer.[17]

A more likely motive is to create a culture of healthy living. Such a culture is likely to attract new employees who are . . . well . . . healthy. (People who smoke or are overweight and out of shape do not fit in well with people who workout in the gym every day.)

Apparently no company wants to admit this not so subtle goal. The politically correct position is to claim that the company is trying to encourage *everyone* to be healthier. But what difference does the motive really make if the end result is the same?

Moreover, discriminating in favor of the healthy and discriminating against the sick are just two sides of the same coin. As *The Economist* noted:[18]

> A growing number of Healthways' clients want to use sticks as well as carrots. . . . At Safeway, a grocery chain, the premium that employees pay for their health insurance falls if they keep their weight and cholesterol under control. In other words, the unhealthy are penalized. GE first offered incentives to employees who stopped smoking; now those who still smoke must pay $650 more for their health insurance. Companies may be nudging now, but in future they may shove.

Another technique employers are using is to make their overall structure of benefits increasingly less attractive to people with expensive health problems. A typical employer plan these days, for example, will provide first-dollar coverage for checkups and preventive care (expenses most employees could have easily paid out of pocket) but leave employees vulnerable for a large share of catastrophic costs. As Julie Appleby pointed out in *USA Today*:[19]

> To try to control spending, some employers are requiring patients to pay a percentage of the cost of specialty drugs—from 25 percent to 33 percent or more—rather than a flat dollar co-payment. Surveys show that 13 percent to 17 percent of employers have added a "specialty" category to their drug benefits, and more are likely to adopt them, given that more than 600 specialty drugs are in development.

These costs can total tens of thousands of dollars in out-of-pocket spending for cancer patients. And they do more than just shift costs to employees. They encourage prospective employees with a health problem to look for work elsewhere.

Increasingly, the health plans employers offer defy all of the traditional principles of rational insurance, which require people to pay out of their own pockets for the expenses they can afford but protect them against catastrophic costs they cannot afford.

Here is the sad bottom line: perverse incentives created by federal regulations are destroying the relationship between employees and their employers as well as any possibility of obtaining the kind of health insurance most people want and need.

How Much Do You Trust Your Insurer?

Dennis Haysbert is the actor I remember best for playing the president of the United States in several of the Jack Bauer *24* seasons. You probably know him better as a spokesman for Allstate. In one commercial, he is standing in front of a town that looks like it has been devastated by a tornado. He begins by saying, "It only took two minutes for this town to be destroyed," and he ends by saying "Are you in good hands?" Allstate also has a "mayhem" series, featuring all kinds of things that can go wrong.

Allstate isn't alone. Nationwide has a clever commercial in which catastrophe is caused by a Dennis-the-Menace-type kid. In a State Farm ad, a baseball comes through a living room window. Nationwide's "life comes at you fast" series features all kinds of misadventures. And of course, the Aflac commercials are all about unexpected misery.

A print advertisement I like is sponsored by Chubb. It shows a man fishing in a small boat, with his back turned to a serious hazard. He is about to go over a waterfall that looks like it's the size of Niagara Falls. Here's the caption: "Who insures you doesn't matter. Until it does."

Now here is my question to you: Have you ever seen a commercial for health insurance that focused on why you actually need health insurance? That is, have you ever seen a health insurance commercial that told you that you need a really good insurer in case you get cancer, heart disease, AIDS, or some other potentially fatal disease that is expensive to treat?

My bet is that you haven't. In fact, I bet you don't see many health insurance commercials at all. One place where a lot of people do see health insurance television and print ads, though, is Washington, DC, in the late fall. This is the period of "open season" when federal employees have the opportunity to choose a new health plan. Once a year, members of the Federal Employees Health Benefits Program (FEHBP) can choose among a dozen or more competing health plans. At this time, participating insurers compete to lure new customers, using print and television ads.

Unlike the casualty insurer commercials, however, the health insurance ads are never focused on what can go wrong. They are all focused on what can go right. Instead of picturing victims of cancer or heart disease, they show photos of young families with healthy children. The implicit message: if you look like the family in this photo, we want you.

The contrast could not be more stark. Casualty insurers are trying to sell you insurance based on your need for their product. Their implicit message is: we know you don't think about insurance until something goes wrong, and that's when you are going to need us. Health insurers, on the other hand, never even talk about why you might actually need their product—unless by "need" you mean services that healthy people want (wellness checkups, preventive care, exercise facilities, etc.).

So what's going on?

The short answer is: The casualty insurance market is a real market in which real insurance is bought and sold. The health insurance market, by contrast, is an artificial market in which the product being exchanged is not real insurance at all. To a large extent, it is prepayment for the consumption of healthcare.

In the casualty market, each buyer pays a premium that reflects the expected cost (and risk) that the buyer brings to the insurance pool he is entering. Insurers compete to sell the *insurance features* of their product because that is what buyers are buying. Federal employees, by contrast, never pay a premium that reflects their expected cost. What they are buying is the opportunity to consume care with other people's money. As a result, health insurers compete to sell the *consumption features* of their product, and they are interested in selling only to people who don't plan to consume very much.

Why is the FEHBP so important? Because it is the managed competition model for how insurance will be bought and sold in health insurance exchanges under ACA.

In the federal system, insurers must charge every enrollee the same premium—regardless of health status. This gives them strong incentives to attract the healthy and avoid the sick. Furthermore, the perverse incentives do not end after enrollment. Health plans have strong incentives to overprovide to the healthy (to keep the ones they have and attract more) and underprovide to the sick (to discourage the arrival of new ones and the departure of the ones they already have).[20]

As noted, the easiest way to overprovide to the healthy is to offer services that healthy people consume: preventive care, wellness programs, free checkups, and so on. The way to underprovide to the sick is to strictly follow evidenced-based protocols and to be slow to approve expensive new drugs and other therapies. Beyond that, a health plan can underprovide to the sick and discourage their enrollment by not including the best cardiologists and the best heart treatment centers in the plan's network, by not having the best oncologists and the best cancer treatment centers in the network, and so on.

What has been the experience of the federal employees program? Some evidence indicates a backing away from expensive procedures, with the government's approval. But perverse incentives are held in check somewhat by the Office of Personnel Management (OPM), which operates like a large human relations department. Similarly, where managed competition has been implemented for state employees, for university employees, and for employees of large corporations, the employer usually acts to try to prevent the worst abuses.

What would happen, though, if the OPM went away and the FEHBP were opened up to everyone in Washington, DC, in addition to the federal employees? What I would expect is a big mess—with insurers having perverse incentives to undertreat the sick and no one there to stop them from acting on those incentives. Of course, there are countervailing forces: professional ethics, malpractice law, and regulatory agencies among them. But ask yourself this question: Would you want to eat at a restaurant that you know in advance does not want your business? You should think the same way about health plans.

With the advent of ACA, these perverse incentives will be set in place nationwide. Tens of thousands of employees will leave their employer plans and enter a no man's land where the healthy will be desirable and the sick will be vulnerable. Those with serious health problems will find they no longer have an employer who acts as a protector and defender. Their problems will be made worse by the inexorable federal pressure on the health plans to keep premiums from rising, so as to contain the expense of the taxpayer-funded premium subsidies.

But, you may ask, won't federal regulators step in to protect the seriously ill from undertreatment and other abuse? Unfortunately, the government's incentives to do that will be very weak.

How Much Do You Trust the Government?

Just as noneconomists think wages can be set at any level, some people think that any public policy is possible. If wages are judged to be too low, the noneconomist thinks that's because the business owner is hardhearted. If a public policy is judged insufficiently generous, the person unfamiliar with public choice thinks that public officials are hardhearted. In both cases, the error is the same: the belief that decision makers have enormous discretion when, in fact, they have very little.

The Politics of Spending Decisions

In a typical health insurance pool, about 5 percent of enrollees will spend 50 percent of the money. About 10 percent will spend nearly two-thirds.[21] The numbers differ a bit from group to group, but in any given year, a small number of people spend most of our healthcare dollars.

Now suppose you are a Minister of Health. Can you afford to spend half of all healthcare dollars on 5 percent of the voters? Even if they survive to the next election, they may be too sick to get to the polls and vote for your party.

From a political point of view, the answer is clearly "no." The inevitable political pressure is to skimp on care for the sick to spend on benefits for the healthy. Put differently, the politics of medicine pushes decision makers to underprovide to the sick so they can overprovide to the healthy.

That is why it is easier to see a primary care physician in Britain than it is in the United States but harder to see a specialist and much harder to access expensive technology. In the 1970s, the British invented the CAT scanner and for a while supplied half the world's usage (probably with government subsidies). But the National Health Service bought very few CAT scanners for use by British patients. The British (along with the United States) also invented renal dialysis, but today Britain has one of the lowest dialysis rates in all of Europe.[22]

Similar observations apply to Canada, where services for the relatively healthy are ubiquitous and expensive technology is scarce. PET scanners, for example, can detect metabolic cancer about a year earlier than an MRI scanner. At last count, the United States had more than 1,000 PET scanners, while the Canadian Medicare system (with one-fifth our population) had only twenty-four.[23]

The Politics of US Medicare

In the US Medicare program, policymakers achieve through patient cost sharing what other countries achieve through the rationing of services: They punish the sick to reward the healthy. For example, although basic Medicare pays for many minor services that most seniors could easily afford to purchase out of pocket, it leaves the elderly exposed to thousands of dollars of catastrophic costs. This is exactly the opposite of how insurance is supposed to work.

Medicare's hospital deductible is $1,156. Seniors experiencing an extended stay lasting more than two months, however, are required to pay $289 per day in cost sharing. This increases to $578 per day after three months, and Medicare pays nothing in hospital costs for patients who stay more than five months.[24]

When the federal government began regulating Medigap insurance (which fills the gaps in Medicare), Congress forced insurers to follow the same pattern. Medigap must pay small bills, but seniors can still experience thousands of dollars in out-of-pocket costs.[25]

The pattern is repeated in the new Medicare prescription drug program (Part D). A "donut hole" exposes the relatively sick to significant out-of-pocket expenses for no other reason than the political desire to provide first-dollar coverage to the relatively healthy. In 2012, the maximum deductible for a Medicare Part D plan is $320. Once the deductible has been met (not all plans have a deductible), Medicare Part D pays 75 percent of the next $2,610 in drug spending until total drug expenditure is $2,930. The donut hole reflects drug spending that falls between $2,930 and $4,700. Until 2012 it was the responsibility of the enrollee to pay *all costs* inside the donut hole. The Patient Protection and Affordable Care Act created a new benefit in 2012 that pays for 50 percent of the costs. After $4,700 in total drug spending, Medicare Part D enrollees pay only a modest co-pay of $2.60 and $6.50 for each prescription. The donut hole is slated to close by 2020, however.[26]

The Medicaid Exception

It is not uncommon for Medicaid programs to underpay doctors and overpay hospitals. Or they underpay hospitals less than they underpay doctors. In either case, this limits the availability of doctor-provided primary care and drives low-income patients to hospital-based services. How can we explain this apparent exception to the pattern described above?

If low-income people don't vote, or if they always vote for the same party, politicians won't compete for their votes. That means the only significant political pressure comes from providers; and hospitals seem to be much better at pursuing their interests in politics than doctors.

5

Why Do We Spend So Much on Healthcare?

AT LAST COUNT, the United States was spending more than $8,000 a year on healthcare for every man, woman, and child in the country. That's more than $24,000 for a family of three, and it represents almost one-fifth of all consumption spending. Is it necessary to spend this much? If not, why are we doing it? What happens if we continue? How can we stop?

The Path We Are On

For the past 40 years, healthcare spending has been rising at twice the rate of growth of our income. You don't have to be an accountant, a mathematician, or an economist to realize that this is unsustainable. If the cost of something you are consuming is growing twice as fast as your income, eventually it will crowd out everything else in your budget. In fact, if we continue on the path we are currently on, healthcare will crowd out all other forms of consumption by about midcentury. When today's young people reach retirement age, they will have nothing to eat, nothing to wear, and no place to live. But they will have an enormous amount of healthcare. Clearly, that's not where anyone wants to end up.

Long before healthcare spending crowds out every other form of consumption, it will threaten to bankrupt the federal government and most state and local governments as well. This is not a uniquely American problem by the way. Other countries are experiencing similar growth. In fact, the rate of growth of real per capita healthcare spending in the United States for the past four decades

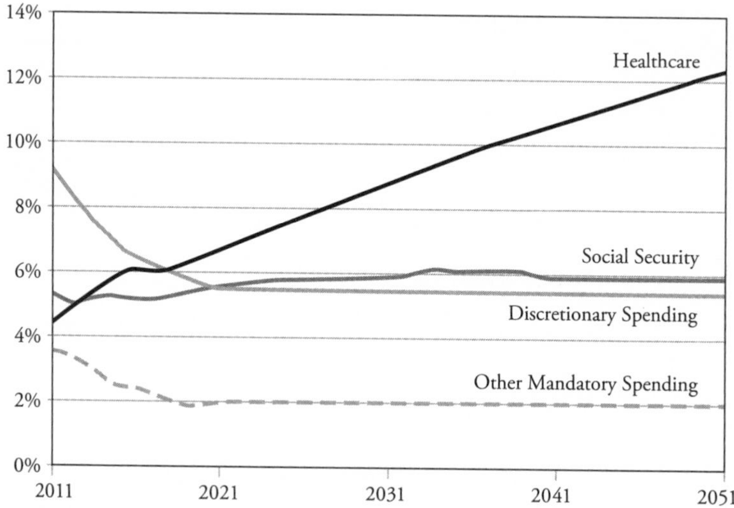

Figure 5.1. Federal Government Spending (as a percent of GDP)
Sources: Calculations by G. William Hoagland (CIGNA) and Congressional Budget Office.

has been right in the middle of the European average. The whole developed world is traveling up a spending path that everyone regards as unsustainable.[1]

One consequence of that is out-of-control federal deficit spending for as far as the eye can see. For much of the last decade, the debate over the need to control entitlement spending has largely focused on Social Security. But if Social Security were our only problem, we could probably muddle through with minor changes. In terms of unfunded liability, however, Medicare is six times the problem of Social Security. And Medicaid is almost as big as Medicare.

Take a look at Figure 5.1. It shows that healthcare will consume more than half of the federal government's budget by mid-century.[2] Moreover, this chart, based on Congressional Budget Office data, assumes that health reform (ACA) will significantly restrain the growth of Medicare. If that turns out to be an incorrect assumption, the picture will look even more dire.

In terms of the numbers, the 2009 Social Security Trustees (pre-ACA) report estimated the unfunded liability in Social Security and Medicare at $107 trillion, looking indefinitely into the future.[3] That's the amount of money we've committed to spend over and above the premiums and dedicated taxes these programs are expected to receive, and it's about six and a half times the size of the entire US economy. Of that amount, Medicare's unfunded liability is about $89 trillion. If we throw in Medicaid, disability insurance, and other entitlement programs (treating them all as implicit promises to current and future generations), the total unfunded liability is in excess of $200 trillion.[4] Again, the bulk of it is healthcare.

Why We Are on an Unsustainable Path

To people who subscribe to the health policy orthodoxy, the riddle of modern healthcare is: Why are health costs rising so fast? To me the riddle is: why isn't health spending rising even faster?

Every time you and I spend a dollar at a physician's office, only 10 cents is coming out of our own pockets, on the average.[5] The remainder is paid by a third party—an employer, an insurance company, or government. That means our incentive is to consume healthcare until it's worth only 10 cents on the dollar to us. That's enormously wasteful. It means we are consuming healthcare that is worth 10 cents when with the same money we could have consumed something worth a dollar. Why do we do that? Because we are trapped. We are in a third-party payer system with use-it-or-lose-it benefits. Most of the time our health plan doesn't give us the option to buy less healthcare and more of something else.

With the advent of ACA, our incentives will become even worse. A long list of preventive services will be made available without any co-payment or deductible. Yet if the cost of these services to us is zero at the time we consume them, our incentive will be to consume them until the last bit is almost worthless.

Some Type A personality readers may be skeptical of the idea that people will overuse the healthcare system. Are we talking about a few hypochondriacs? Or, are we talking about ordinary people? The latter. In Florida, for example, the waiting rooms of many specialist doctors are gathering places for senior citizens who take the occasion to socialize and enjoy each other's company.

First-dollar health insurance coverage means healthcare is free or almost free at the time we obtain it. When something is free, our incentive is to consume it so long as it furnishes any value at all. Yet the reality is that these services are not costless. In fact, the way our system functions, they are very expensive. So although we consume care as though it were free, we all end up paying a very steep price through higher premiums and higher taxes.

As a practical matter, once we pay insurance premiums, that money is combined with everyone else's premiums in a pool. Once the money is in the pool, it is no longer "ours." In fact, when we draw from the pool, we are spending everybody's money. Moreover, the only way to get benefits from the health insurance pool is to spend money on medical care.

If you and I are in the same insurance pool, consider how many ways there are for me to spend your money:

- If my wife and I decide to have another child and we have fertility issues, there's always in vitro. Cost: $20,000.
- If we decide not to have a child, there is always a vasectomy or tubal ligation. Cost: $1,000 to $7,000.
- If I decide my thinning hair needs to be a bit bushier, there's Propecia at an annual cost of $842.
- If my testosterone level isn't in sync with my idealized vision of my own virility, there is Androgel ($831/year).
- If my unhealthy diet leads to diabetes, many of those costs will become "ours" as well (average annual extra cost = $7,000).

Notice I haven't even mentioned yet the normal diagnostic screenings (PSA test, colonoscopy, etc.). They cost money as well. Then, let's say that over time, I abuse my body with alcohol, tobacco, drugs, fatty foods, lack of exercise, and so on. I know that others will pay my medical costs—mainly from first dollar—once I get old enough to qualify for Medicare.

We Don't Have Too Many Unmet Healthcare Needs; We Have Too Few

The single greatest mistake in all of health policy is the belief that people should always get healthcare as long as it provides some positive benefit. Ask yourself this question: Does that principle hold for any other good or service? When you enter a supermarket, do you buy every item that could possibly quench you thirst or quell your hunger? Or do you leave some desirable items on the supermarket shelf? When you walk in a clothing store, do you buy every piece of apparel that could possibly meet your wardrobe needs? When you buy a house, do you buy one large enough to meet every possible need you may have for comfortable shelter? Or do you purchase a house that is more affordable?

Well, if you are unwilling to apply the principle to food, clothing, or shelter, why would you insist on it in healthcare? I believe we could spend our entire national income on healthcare, not by frittering money away, but by spending it on goods and services that even in small ways could improve the odds of better health. Here are some examples of how we could do that:

- The Cooper Clinic in Dallas offers an extensive checkup (with a full body scan) for about $4,000. Its clients include high-profile individuals. Yet if everyone in America took advantage of this opportunity, we would increase our nation's annual healthcare bill by nearly one-half.[6]
- Americans purchase nonprescription drugs about 12 billion times a year, according to a calculation by Simon Rottenberg some time ago, and almost all of these are acts of self-medication. Yet if everyone sought professional advice before making such purchases (as they probably would if there were no time or money cost), we would need twenty-five times the number of primary care physicians we currently have.[7]
- Some 1,100 tests can be done on our genes to determine if we have a predisposition toward one disease or another.[8] In 2010, the charge for a full gene mapping was around $50,000.[9] Yet if every American incurred that expense the total would exceed the country's entire GDP. (The price is currently falling, but at almost any price, the potential for spending is enormous.[10])

Notice that in hypothetically spending all of this money, we have not yet cured a single disease or treated an actual illness. We are simply collecting information. If in the process of searching, we actually found something that warranted treatment, we could spend even more.

Cost-Control Policies That Don't Work

If you were to compare the approach to controlling healthcare spending advocated in this book with the conventional writings of orthodox health policy analysts, you would find very few words in common. The orthodox approach would discuss the need for managed care, integrated care, coordinated care, home-based care, evidenced-based care, electronic-medical-records-based care, and many other kinds of care. These are all part of the toolkit that the Obama administration envisions using via pilot programs, special subsidies, rules, regulations, and other means.

What About ACA?

I don't plan to say very much about these ideas in this book because (1) they are simply the latest fads, (2) many have already been tried before with little or no success, (3) the results of all the federal pilot programs are turning out to be lackluster or negative,[11] (4) the Congressional Budget Office has announced (for the third time) that all of these ideas are not going to save money,[12] (5) the administration's preferred organizational form of healthcare delivery—the Accountable Care Organization—has been rejected by the nation's leading health plans, including those that the administration points to as examples of high-quality, low-cost service,[13] and (6) I have too much respect for your time and your intelligence.

In theory, you can make a reasonable argument for each of these ideas. Who can deny that piecemeal medicine, with dozens of doctors making independent decisions about various aspects of a patient's care, is likely to be wasteful? Wouldn't it be better if the doctors all got together and coordinated their decisions? Doesn't integrated care make more sense than nonintegrated care? Wouldn't integrated care be easier if there were a medical home that kept all the patient records in one place? Wouldn't it all be more efficient if all the doctors could go to a computer screen and see what every other doctor has done to the patient and is planning to do?

I don't have a problem with any of this. In fact, in this book, I point to examples where some of this actually works. My problem is that *wherever I find any of these techniques working, they originated on the supply side of the market, not the demand side.*

Whenever these ideas are foisted on physicians by a government pilot program or by some other third-party payer bureaucracy, they not only don't work, they often backfire. Electronic medical records and other electronic information systems seem to work, and work well, when they are adopted by doctors to solve their specific problems. (After all, isn't that how information systems get adopted in the rest of the economy?) They do not work well when they are designed and imposed by the buyers of care.

As this book goes to press, there is very little in the academic literature that gives much hope that any demand-side reforms envisioned by ACA are going to lower cost or improve quality. What about grading hospitals based on the quality of care? One recent study finds that Medicare's reporting has had almost no impact on mortality.[14] Another survey finds that quality report cards not only don't work, they may do more harm than good.[15] What about paying for results? The latest study of pay-for-performance finds that doesn't work either.[16] Accountable Care Organizations? The latest results show no reason to be hopeful.[17] Electronic medical records? The latest survey of all the academic literature shows they don't improve quality or reduce costs.[18] Indeed, a new study in *Health Affairs* found that when doctors can easily order diagnostic tests online, they tend to order more tests — increasing costs.[19]

The fundamental problem in healthcare is that people in the system face perverse incentives. If we want to change the perverse outcomes, we must change the incentives that lead to them. The orthodox health policy community is dead set against discussing fundamental incentives. So there is really nothing left for them to do but discuss the latest fads—and all the ideas listed above are fads that have replaced the last generation of fads and will be replaced in a few years by another generation of fads.

Recently, former White House health adviser Ezekiel Emanuel explained on national television that the ACA legislation "contained every single cost control idea proposed by every serious health policy expert." Sad, but true—from his point of view. And here is another unfortunate truth: After every one of these ideas has been implemented, we will still be left with a system in which no one—no patient, no doctor, no employer, no insurer, and no government official—will be choosing between healthcare and other uses of money. And if no one is making those choices, healthcare spending will keep on rising in the future with all the relentless persistence it has shown in the past.

What About the Pilot Projects?

As noted, the entire ACA approach to controlling costs and improving quality in Medicare (and ultimately, for the healthcare system as a whole) is based on running pilot projects. Will this approach work? A recent report by the Congressional Budget Office gives us little reason to be hopeful.[20] Over the past two decades, Medicare's administrators have conducted two types of demonstration projects.

Disease management and care coordination demonstrations consisted of thirty-four programs that used nurses as care managers to educate patients about their chronic illnesses, encouraged them to follow self-care regimens, monitored their health, and tracked whether they received recommended tests and treatments. The primary goal was to save money by reducing hospitalization. With respect to these efforts, the CBO finds:

- On average, the thirty-four programs had little or no effect on hospital admissions.
- In nearly every program, spending was either unchanged or increased relative to the spending that would have occurred in the absence of the program.

Value-based payment demonstrations consisted of four programs in which Medicare made bundled payments to hospitals and physicians to cover all services connected with heart bypass surgeries. With respect to these, the CBO finds that "only one of the four . . . yielded significant savings for the Medicare program" and in that one, Medicare spending only "declined by about 10 percent."[21]

So why is none of this working? Probably because it all involves people on the demand side of the market trying to take the place of entrepreneurs who would ordinarily be on the supply side in any other market. Successful innovations are produced by entrepreneurs, *challenging* conventional thinking—not by bureaucrats *trying to implement* conventional thinking. There are lots of examples of successful entrepreneurship in healthcare. There are very few examples of successful bureaucracy. Can you think of any other market where the buyers of a product are trying to tell the sellers how to efficiently produce it?

Megan McArdle, a senior editor for *The Atlantic*, has produced an impressive analysis of all of the reasons why pilot programs in general (not just in healthcare) tend to fail.[22] In a word, she says, things that work and work well in a pilot project cannot be replicated in the larger real world. Why? Because "promising pilot projects often don't scale."[23]

> They don't scale even when you put super smart people with expert credentials in charge of them. They don't scale even when you make sure to provide ample budget resources. Rolling something out across an existing system is substantially different from even a well-run test, and often, it simply doesn't translate.

Here are five obstacles to be overcome:

- Sometimes the success of the earlier project is simply a result of random chance, or what researchers call the Hawthorne Effect, named after a study in which workers became more productive no matter what the stimulus—a change from the ordinary, or the mere act of being studied.
- Sometimes the success is due to what you might call a "hidden parameter," something that researchers don't realize is affecting their test.
- Sometimes the success is due to high-quality, fully committed staff, whose work won't be duplicated by folks who are just looking for a job and don't see the pilot project goal as their life's mission.
- Sometimes the program becomes unmanageable as it gets larger.
- Sometimes the results are due to survivor bias—the subjects who stay in the project are very different from the random population.

On this last point, McArdle explains:

> This is an especially big problem with studying healthcare and the poor. Healthcare, because compliance rates are quite low (by one estimate I heard, something like three-fourths of the blood pressure medication prescribed is not being taken nine months in) and the poor, because their lives are chaotic and they tend to move around a lot, so they may have to drop out, or may not be easy to find and re-enroll if they stop coming. In the end, you've got a study of unusually compliant and stable people (who may be different in all sorts of ways) and oops! that's not what the general population looks like.

On the whole, there is a big difference between the real world and the world of the pilot program, says McArdle:

> [R]eal world applications are . . . not an awesome pilot project with everyone pulling together and a lot of political push behind them; they're being rolled out into a system that already has a very well established mindset, and a comprehensive body of rules.

Before leaving this section, it is worth noting that there have been three pilot projects that actually worked very well:

- In 1996, federal legislation allowed a certain number of people to have high-deductible health insurance, coupled with a tax-free Medical Savings Account. The program was so successful that 2003 legislation allowed the entire nonelderly population to have access to what are now called Health Savings Accounts.
- Another pilot program in the 1990s established Cash and Counseling demonstrations, which allowed homebound, disabled Medicaid enrollees to manage their own budgets. The success of this program led to its expansion across the country.
- A third successful pilot program allowed outpatient surgery under Medicare.

How do these projects differ from the many failures? Medical Savings Accounts (MSAs) had already been tested in the marketplace by Golden Rule Insurance Company before the pilot program ever began. Outpatient surgery was similarly the outgrowth of private entrepreneurial experimentation. In fact, it never was subjected to a government-sponsored pilot program. The first freestanding (not hospital-based) surgery center was opened in Phoenix in 1970 by Drs. Wallace Reed and John Ford. They had to sell the idea to the legislature, medical boards, and insurance companies.[24] Medicare didn't start paying for these services until more than a decade later. The Cash and Counseling Program was a private/public collaboration, with the Robert Wood Johnson Foundation being the principle instigator (and partial funder).

Perhaps even more important, all three of these success stories are really examples of liberation. MSAs allow patients the freedom to manage their own healthcare dollars, and no two patients are likely to be managing their money in the same way. Cash and counseling allows the homebound disabled to manage their own budgets. Outpatient surgery allows the supply side of the market to find cheaper ways of providing minor surgery. In other words, these successful pilot programs were not designed to discover behavior that could be copied. They were designed to discover how to let people make their own decisions.

Is Price-Fixing the Answer?

Despite the rhetoric from Washington, the Obama administration isn't counting on any of the new cost control fads to actually work. At least for Medicare, it has a fallback position: price controls. Should the pilot programs and other reforms fail to slow the growth of Medicare spending, embedded in the new law is the authority given to an independent commission to reduce the fees paid to doctors, hospitals, and other providers. In fact, the Office of the Medicare Actuary is so convinced that the fads won't work that it doesn't even bother to estimate the effects of these efforts. Instead, the actuaries assume that the only way that Medicare's cost growth can be kept in line with the requirements of the health reform legislation is by limiting payments to providers. Yet, lowering fees to providers can have devastating effects on the accessibility of care for patients.

Price controls usually backfire. The reason: their only goal is to shift costs from buyers to providers rather than introduce any real efficiencies into the system. The following case study is a recent example of that.

Price-Fixing Case Study: Drug Shortages

Jenny Morrill is a Kinston, New York, mother and former arts administrator who has been battling ovarian cancer since 2007. When she went for her chemotherapy treatment in June 2011, the nurse greeted her with good news and bad news. The good news: she was responding well to the drug Doxil. The bad news: the hospital had no more Doxil to give her. Morrill was not alone. By November 2011, the plant that produced the drug completely shut down, leaving 7,000 US patients without access to its life-saving properties.[25]

Doxil is not the only drug that patients cannot get. American hospitals and physicians are facing an unprecedented shortage of commonly used drugs, and the

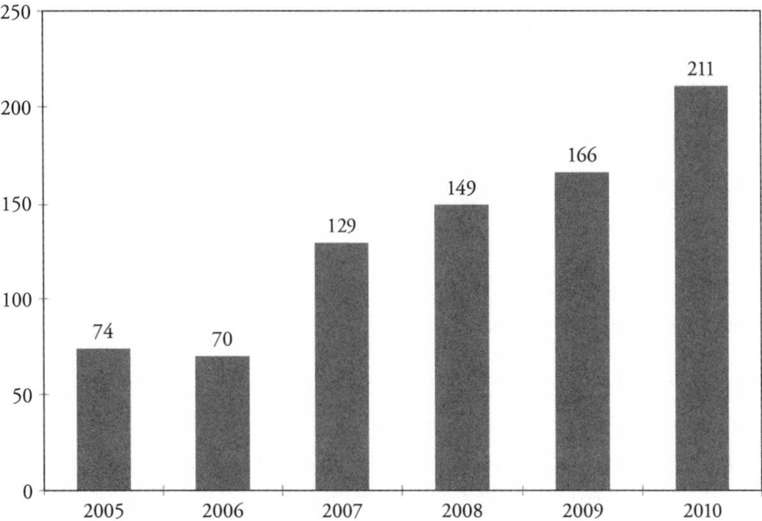

Figure 5.2. Newly Reported Drug Shortages
Source: Drug Information Service, University of Utah, 2010.

problem has been escalating for several years. (See Figure 5.2.) Some patients have died as a result. Others are trying to get by on inferior substitute therapies.

In one survey, nine in ten anesthesiologists reported experiencing a shortage of at least one anesthesia drug.[26] Another survey found that more than 40 percent of the thirty-four generic oncology drugs on the market were in short supply.[27] There are no reliable substitutes for most of these drugs. Most are generic injectable medications that have been on the market a long time and are commonly used in hospitals, emergency rooms, and cancer treatment centers.

The American Hospital Association recently reported that virtually all the community hospitals it surveyed had experienced a drug shortage in the previous six months. Two-thirds of hospitals had experienced a shortage of cancer drugs; 88 percent were short on pain medications; and 95 percent were lacking anesthesia drugs needed for surgery.

Hospitals have responded in a variety of ways, including delaying treatment, giving patients less effective drugs, and providing a different course of treatment than the one recommended. Indeed, about 82 percent of hospitals surveyed reported at least occasionally delaying a treatment because of a drug in short supply. (See Figure 5.3.)

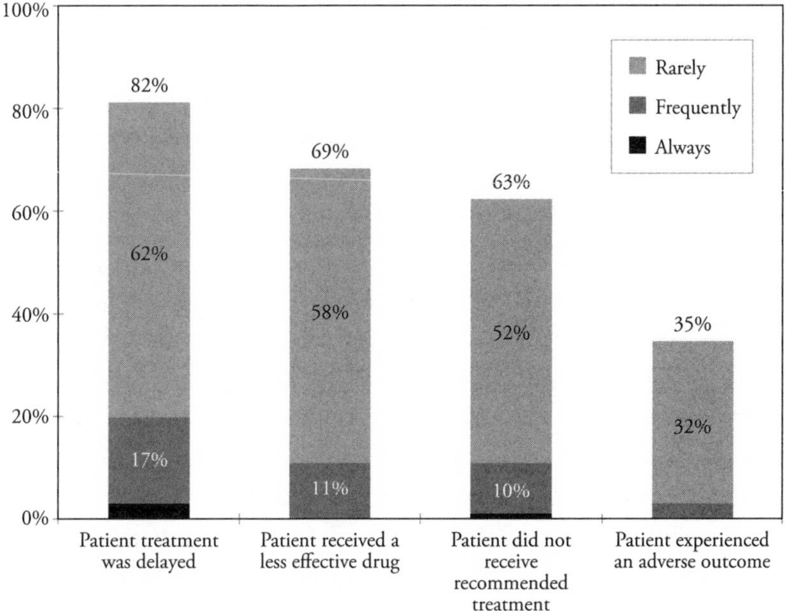

Figure 5.3. Percent of Hospitals Reporting the Impact on Patient Care as a Result of a Drug Shortage

Source: American Hospital Association analysis of survey data from 820 non-federal, short-term care acute hospitals collected in June 2011.

Although there are many reasons for the shortages, according to Ezekiel Emanuel (who in addition to being a former White House adviser is also an oncologist), only about 10 percent of shortages are due to a lack of raw materials needed to manufacture the drugs.[28] A more important source of the problem is government policy.

Problem: Output Controls. About half of the shortages of injectable drugs are due to production problems, and part of the reason for that is Food and Drug Administration (FDA) regulatory policy.[29] The FDA has stepped up its efforts to ensure that drug manufacturing processes and facilities meet its quality standards by instituting a zero tolerance policy. By way of enforcement, the agency levies fines and forces manufacturers to retool both domestic and foreign facilities. Regulations not only slow the production at particular facilities, they make it difficult for competitors to take up the slack. If a shortage develops because the FDA shuts down a competitor's plant, for example, a manufacturer must seek FDA approval to increase output and alter its production timetable. This slows down adjustments in production.

The Drug Enforcement Agency (DEA) also has a regulatory role because minute quantities of controlled substances are often used to make other drugs.[30] Its regulations are also inflexible. For example, if a shortage develops, a manufacturer that has reached its preauthorized production cap cannot respond by increasing output without DEA approval.

Problem: Medicare Part B Price Controls. Some drugs that are administered by physicians—such as chemotherapy drugs or anesthesia during surgery—are paid for through Medicare Part B. Government price controls prevent the prices of these drugs from adjusting in response to shortages, increases in manufacturing costs, or increases in demand. Normally, the market price of a product rises when it is in short supply, attracting competing manufacturers. However, the Medicare Modernization Act (MMA) of 2003 effectively limited the amount by which the price of the drug could rise in response to market conditions over a given period.

This pricing policy gives physicians an incentive to use newer patented drugs, even when older generic drugs are just as effective—or even more effective.[31]

Problem: Inability to "Brand" Generic Drugs. Regulations also limit the ability of drug makers to tout quality or communicate quality improvements to potential customers. This makes it difficult for drug makers to differentiate their products from competitors' products and gain from improving quality. As a result of these and other regulations, firms cannot recoup investments they make in improving the quality of the manufacturing process.[32]

Problem: 340B Price Controls. The little known federal 340B drug rebate program also contributes to shortages. This program forces drug manufacturers to give discounts to outpatient clinics and hospitals that treat a high number of indigent or Medicaid patients, to Public Health Service hospitals and clinics, and to certain Federally Qualified Health Centers. Currently, the law requires manufacturers to give these facilities a 23.1 percent rebate off the average price for brand-name drugs and 13 percent for generic drugs on qualifying outpatient use.[33]

The Affordable Care Act will expand the number of hospitals and clinics that qualify for rebates. The number of participating facilities has already grown from about 8,000 in 2002 to more than 14,000 in 2010. It is estimated that nearly 20,000 are eligible under ACA.[34] According to a US Government Accountability

Office report, nearly one-third of US hospitals qualify for 340B drug discounts.[35] Proposals to expand these discounts to inpatient facilities would further exacerbate the shortages—as would proposals to require rebates for Medicare enrollees who are also dual-eligible for Medicaid.

Furthermore, manufacturers that increase brand-name drug prices faster than the Consumer Price Index are required to rebate the excess amount. This means they have little incentive to purchase new equipment to maintain or improve their manufacturing processes. As a result, some drugs become less and less profitable over time.

Is Government Provision the Answer?

A small but vocal group on the left believes that single-payer national health insurance is the answer to the problem of escalating healthcare costs. Some would like to copy Canada's healthcare system. Others would like to enroll everyone in Medicare. The Physicians for a National Health Program, for example, claims that Medicare has lower administrative costs than private insurance and is able to use its monopsony (single-buyer) power to suppress provider fees.[36] The group favors "Medicare for all" and endorses a bill to do just that by Representative John Conyers.[37]

Columnist Paul Krugman, writing in *The New York Times,* also argues this way.[38] Krugman, along with others, touts the slower growth rate in the Canadian healthcare system (also called Medicare).[39] In separate editorials, both Krugman[40] and former Secretary of Labor Robert Reich[41] have joined the call for Medicare for everyone. What's wrong with this idea?

Is Medicare Really Public Insurance?

Let's begin with a fundamental point that almost everyone tends to ignore. Medicare is not actually managed by the federal government. In most places, Medicare is managed by private contractors, including such entities as Cigna and BlueCross. Further, there is nothing particularly special about the way Medicare pays providers. Private insurers tend to use the same billing codes, and their payment rates are often pegged as a percentage of Medicare rates.

Does Medicare Have Lower Administrative Costs?

What about the claim that Medicare's administrative costs are only 2 percent, compared to 10 percent to 15 percent for private insurers? The problem with this comparison is that it includes the cost of marketing and selling insurance as well as the cost of collecting premiums on the private side but ignores the cost of collecting taxes on the public side. It also ignores the substantial administrative cost that Medicare shifts to the providers of care.

Studies by Milliman[42] and others[43] show that when all costs are included, Medicare costs more, not less, to administer. Further, raw numbers show that, using Medicare's own accounting, its administrative expenses per enrollee are higher than private insurance.[44] They are lower only when expressed as a percentage—but that may be because the average medical expense for a senior is so much higher than the expense for nonseniors. Also, an unpublished, ongoing study by Milliman finds that seniors on Medicare use twice the health resources as seniors who are still on private insurance, everything equal.[45]

Ironically, many observers think Medicare spends too little on administration, which is one reason why one out of every ten dollars of Medicare spending is lost to fraud.[46] Private insurers devote more resources to fraud prevention and find it profitable to do so.

Are Medicare Costs Growing More Slowly?

What about the claim that Medicare's cost per enrollee is growing more slowly? The Congressional Budget Office (Figure 5.4) has calculated spending in excess of GDP growth for the public and private enrollee populations. As the figure shows, Medicare has been growing faster than the private sector. For that matter, Medicaid has also been growing faster.

As the CBO acknowledges, its comparison is far from perfect. The "other" category includes the uninsured as well as out-of-pocket spending by Medicare enrollees. Still, there is no reason to believe that overall spending would have been lower if the entire country had been in Medicare for the past 35 years.

Looking forward, the CBO believes that Medicare will grow more slowly than the private sector. It will grow a lot more slowly if the provisions of the Affordable Care Act are implemented without any changes. Under the act,

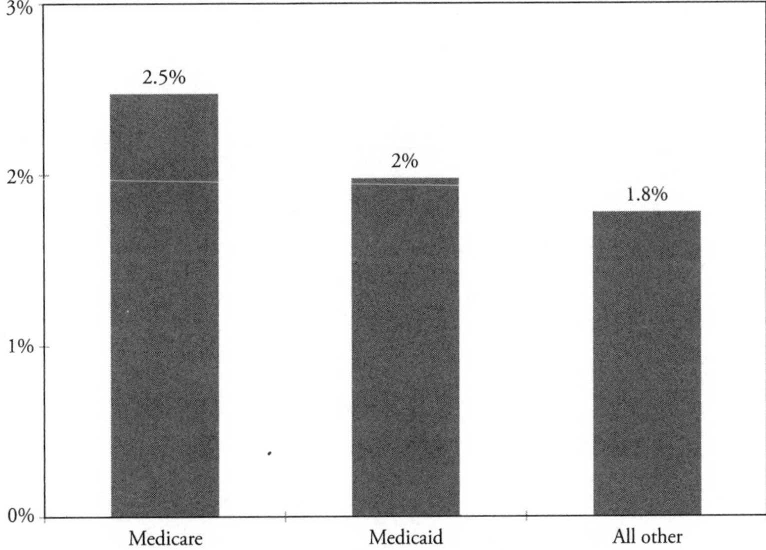

Figure 5.4. Excess Cost Growth in Healthcare Spending (1975 to 2008)
Source: Congressional Budget Office. "The Long-Term Budget Outlook," June 2010 (Revised August 2010).

Medicare will suppress provider fees so much that real per capita Medicare spending will grow no faster than real per capita GDP. Yet, the rest of the healthcare system will be growing at twice that rate. As the Office of the Actuary has explained, this means greatly reduced access to care for the elderly and the disabled.[47] A two-tiered system will likely emerge before this decade is out. Because of the political ramifications of all this, most Washington insiders believe the Medicare spending cuts will never materialize.

What About the Argument That Government Can Use Its Power as a Single Buyer to Suppress Providers' Fees?

There are five problems with it.[48]

First, we don't buy healthcare in a national market. We buy locally. And in local markets, private entities are often as big, or bigger, than Medicare (the auto companies in Detroit, for example, or the mine workers and their employers in West Virginia). There is nothing the US government can do that a lot of private companies and unions cannot also do. Similarly, if Canada is seen as the ideal, nothing is stopping the auto companies and the UAW from creating a global budget and rationing care for autoworkers just as the Canadians do it. That they choose not to do so is telling.

Second, there are negative consequences from unduly suppressing provider fees. Doctors can leave the city, the state, or even the country. Able people can also avoid the profession altogether. If we paid doctors only the minimum wage, for example, medicine would attract only those people who can earn no more than the minimum wage doing something else. The suppression of provider payments ultimately harms patients as highly qualified providers exit the market. The effects of price controls in healthcare will be similar to their effects in other markets.

Third, the suppression of provider payments shifts costs from patients and taxpayers to providers. Shifting costs, however, is not the same thing as controlling costs. Providers are just as much a part of society as patients. Shifting costs from one group to the other makes the latter group better off and the former worse off. It does not lower the cost of healthcare for society as a whole, however.

Fourth, the argument overlooks the fact that public insurance in a democracy is ultimately subject to pressures at the ballot box. Providers get to vote, too. They also can make campaign contributions and lobby. Patients can also exert political pressure. Political competition in a democracy constrains public policy in much the same way that economic competition constrains the behavior of private firms in the marketplace.

Finally, if it really were desirable to have everyone pay low prices, we do not need to enroll everyone in Medicare to achieve that outcome. We could instead impose Medicare-type price controls on the entire healthcare system. In fact, one organization advocates that very thing.[49] Doing so would run into all the problems listed above, however.

Do Other Countries Have the Answer?

The conventional wisdom in health policy is that the United States spends far more than any other country and enjoys mediocre health outcomes. This judgment is repeated so often and so forcefully that you will almost never see it questioned. And yet it may not be true.

Indeed, the reverse may be true. We may be spending less and getting more.

The case for the critics was bolstered recently by a new Organization for Economic Co-operation and Development (OECD) report that concluded:[50]

> The United States spends two-and-a-half times more than the OECD average health expenditure per person . . . It even spends twice as much as France, for example, a country which is generally accepted as having very good health services. At 17.4 percent of GDP in 2009, US health spending is half as much again as any other country, and nearly twice the average.

Similar claims were made in a *New York Times* editorial by Ezekiel Emanuel, who added that we are not getting better healthcare as a result.[51] The same charge was aired at the *Health Affairs* blog by Obama Social Security Advisory Board appointee Henry Aaron and health economist Paul Ginsburg.[52] It is standard fare at columnist Ezra Klein's blog at *The Washington Post*,[53] at *The Incidental Economist* blog,[54] and at The Commonwealth Fund.[55] It is also unquestioned dogma for *New York Times* columnist Paul Krugman.[56]

What are all these people missing? On the spending side, they are overlooking one of the most basic concepts in all of economics.

When you and I buy something, the cost to us is the price we pay for it. But that is not necessarily true for society as a whole. The social cost of something may be a whole lot more or a whole lot less than what people actually spend on it, and that is especially true in healthcare.

As previously noted, in the United States and throughout the developed world, the market for medical care has been so systematically suppressed that no one ever sees a real price for anything. In the United States, for example, a typical doctor is paid by all the different third-party payers. These fees do not count as real market prices, however. Instead, they are artificial payments that often reflect the bargaining power of the various payer bureaucracies. When government accountants sum up all the spending on healthcare, therefore, they are adding artificial price-times-quantity for all the separate transactions to arrive at a grand spending total.

Here is the kicker: since each separate purchase involves an artificial price, no one knows what the aggregate number really means. To make matters worse, other countries are more aggressive than we are at shifting costs and hiding costs.

They use their buying power to suppress the incomes of doctors, nurses, and other medical personnel much more than the United States does, for example. In addition, formal accounting ignores the cost of rationing in other countries. In Greece, patients spend nearly as much on bribes and other informal payments as they do on formal costs such as insurance co-pays.[57] Yet, these bribes do not show up in the official statistics. Bottom line: in comparing international spending totals, we are usually comparing apples and oranges.

Let's take doctor incomes and government healthcare programs. One way to pay doctors is to pay market prices—whatever fees are necessary to induce them to voluntarily provide medical services. Another way is to draft them and pay them little more than a minimum wage—as the government has done in the past in times of war. Obviously, the second method involves a lot lower spending figure. But to economists, the social cost is the same in both cases.

The reason? To economists, the social cost of having one more man or woman become a doctor is the next best use of that person's talents. Instead of becoming a doctor, the pre-med student might have become an engineer, say, or an architect. So what society as a whole must give up in order to have one more doctor is the loss of the engineering or architectural goods and services the young man or woman would otherwise have produced. This cost, called *opportunity cost,* is independent of how much doctors actually get paid.

The principle also applies to other medical personnel and to buildings and equipment. The opportunity cost of a hospital, for example, is the value of a commercial office building or some other use to which those same resources could be put.

The concept of opportunity cost allows us to see that if we don't trust spending totals in the international accounts, there is another way to assess the cost of healthcare. We can count up the real resources being used. Other things equal, a country that has more doctors per capita, more hospital beds, and so on is devoting more of its real income to healthcare than one that uses fewer resources—regardless of its reported spending.

On this score, the United States looks really good.[58] As Table 5.1 (from the latest OECD report[59]) shows, the United States has fewer doctors, fewer physician visits, fewer hospital beds, fewer hospital stays, and less time in the hospital than the OECD average. We're not just a little bit lower. We are among the low-

Table 5.1. Where the United States Health System Does Less than Other Countries

	United States	Rank compared with OECD countries	OECD average
Practising physicians	2.4 per 1,000 population	26th	3.1 per 1,000 population
Doctor consultations	3.9 per capita	29th	6.5 per capita
Hospital beds	3.1 per 1,000 population	29th	4.9 per 1,000 population
Hospital discharges	130.9 per 1,000 population	26th	158.1 per 1,000 population
Average length of stay in hospitals	4.9 days	29th	7.2 days

Source: OECD Health Data 2011.

est in the developed world. In fact, about the only area where we spend more is on technology (MRI and CT scans, for example), as shown in Table 5.2.

Almost a decade ago, Mark Pauly, a professor of healthcare management at the University of Pennsylvania's Wharton School, estimated the cost of healthcare across different countries based on the use of labor (doctors, nurses, etc.) alone.[60] The finding: the United States spends a lot less than such northern European countries as Iceland, Sweden, and Norway and even less than Germany and France.

What about outcomes? Do we get more and better care for the resources we devote? Here the evidence is mixed. As Table 5.2 shows, we replace more knees per capita than any other country. On the other hand, if you think that there are too many tonsillectomies and Caesarean births, our ranking there (2nd and 8th, respectively) may be less admirable. Table 5.3 shows five-year cancer survival rates. The United States basically leads the world.

Studies show almost no relationship between aggregate spending on health and population mortality. Lifestyle, environment, and genes have far more influence on life expectancy than anything doctors and hospitals are doing.

Table 5.2. The United States versus Other Countries

	United States	**Rank compared with OECD countries**	**OECD average**
MRI units	25.9 per million population	2nd	12.2 per million population
MRI exams	91.2 per 1,000 population	2nd	46.6 per 1,000 population
CT scanners	34.3 per million population	5th	22.8 per million population
CT exams	227.9 per 1000 population	2nd	131.8 per 1,000 population
Tonsillectomy	254.4 per 100,000 population	2nd	133.8 per 100,000 population
Coronary angioplasty	377.2 per 100,000 population	3rd	187.6 per 100,000 population
Knee replacements	212.5 per 100,000 population	1st	118.4 per 100,000 population
Caesarean sections	32.3 per 100 live births	8th	25.8 per 100 live births

Source: OECD Health Data 2011.

Nonetheless, life expectancy statistics are a favorite of the critics, since Americans don't score very high. Interestingly, one study found that if you remove outcomes that doctors have almost no impact on—death from fatal injuries (car accidents, violent crime, etc.)—US life expectancy jumps from No. 19 in the world to No. 1, as shown in Table 5.4.[61]

The general consensus of the literature, however, is that there is virtually no relationship between total healthcare spending and life expectancy across countries.[62]

This isn't to say we don't have problems. There is a lot of evidence of waste and inefficiency in US healthcare. Still, it's not clear that we have any reason to feel inferior to the rest of the world. Read on.

Table 5.3. 5-Year Relative Survival Rates for Various Cancers, from the CONCORD Study (2008)

Country	Breast Women	Colorectal Men	Colorectal Women	Prostate	Average
United States	83.9%	59.1%	60.2%	91.9%	73.8%
Canada	82.5%	55.3%	58.9%	85.1%	70.5%
Australia	80.7%	56.7%	58.2%	77.4%	68.3%
Austria	74.9%	52.7%	55.1%	86.1%	67.2%
Germany	75.5%	50.1%	55.0%	76.4%	64.3%
Sweden	82.0%	52.8%	56.2%	66.0%	64.3%
Netherlands	77.6%	53.6%	55.1%	69.5%	64.0%
Iceland	79.0%	49.5%	54.0%	69.7%	63.1 %
Japan	81.6%	61.1%	57.3%	50.4%	62.6%
Finland	80.2%	52.5%	54.0%	62.9%	62.4%
Italy	79.5%	79.5%	52.7%	65.4%	62.1 %
Norway	76.3%	51.1%	55.3%	63.0%	61.4%
Spain	77.7%	52.5%	54.7%	60.5%	61.4%
Ireland	69.6%	46.0%	50.0%	62.8%	57.1 %
Portugal	72.2%	46.5%	44.7%	47.7%	52.8%
UK	69.7%	42.3%	4.7%	51.1%	52.0%
Denmark	73.6%	44.2%	47.7%	38.4%	51.0%
Switzerland	76.0%	N/A	N/A	N/A	N/A

Source: Michael P. Coleman et al., "Cancer survival in five continents: a worldwide population-based study (CONCORD)," *Lancet*, July 17, 2008. doi:10.1016/S1470-2045(08)70179-7.

What the Right and the Left Don't Understand About Healthcare in Other Countries

There is no topic in healthcare that is more misunderstood than what other countries are doing. At both ends of the political spectrum, the mistake is the same: the belief that other healthcare systems are radically different from our own. They aren't.

Table 5.4. National Life Expectancy: 1980 to 1999 (with and without fatal injuries)

Rank	OECD Nations	Actual Mean Life Expectancy (including fatal injuries)	OECD Nations	Standardized Mean Life Expectancy (without fatal injuries)
1.	Japan	78.7	United States	76.9
2.	Iceland	78.0	Switzerland	76.6
3.	Sweden	77.7	Norway	76.3
4.	Switzerland	77.6	Canada	76.2
5.	Canada	77.3	Iceland	76.1
6.	Spain	77.3	Sweden	76.1
7.	Greece	77.1	Germany	76.1
8.	Netherlands	77.0	Denmark	76.1
9.	Norway	77.0	Japan	76.0
10.	Australia	76.8	Australia	76.0
11.	Italy	76.6	France	76.0
12.	France	76.6	Belgium	76.0
13.	Belgium	75.7	Austria	76.0
14.	United Kingdom	75.6	Netherlands	75.9
15.	Germany	75.4	Italy	75.8
16.	Finland	75.4	United Kingdom	75.7
17.	New Zealand	75.4	Finland	75.7
18.	Austria	75.3	New Zealand	75.4
19.	United States	75.3	Czech Republic	75.1
20.	Denmark	75.1	Ireland	75.0
21.	Ireland	74.8	Spain	74.9
22.	Portugal	73.9	Slovak Republic	74.4
23.	Czech Republic	72.2	Greece	74.4
24.	Slovak Republic	71.6	Portugal	74.3
25.	Poland	71.5	Hungary	74.3
26.	Korea	71.1	Korea	73.3
27.	Mexico	70.9	Poland	73.2
28.	Hungary	69.7	Mexico	72.8
29.	Turkey	64.4	Turkey	72.0

Source: Organization of Economic Co-operation and Development.

Take the United States and Canada. I would say that the healthcare systems of these two countries are 80 percent the same. In both countries, third-party payers pay the vast majority of medical expenses. In both countries, the third parties pay by task. In Canada, when patients see a physician, it's free. In the United States, it's almost free. In both countries, normal market forces have been completely suppressed. Healthcare in both places, therefore, is bureaucratic, cumbersome, wasteful, inefficient, and unresponsive to consumer needs.

One reason so many people get misled is that in Canada, government is the third-party payer, whereas in the United States, about half of all spending is private. The mistake is assuming that there is a substantial difference between public and private insurance in the United States. There isn't. As we have seen, Medicare in the United States is managed almost everywhere by private contractors, and much of Medicaid is privately managed as well. Furthermore, one out of every four Medicare enrollees and a substantial majority of Medicaid enrollees are enrolled in private health plans, even though government is paying the bill. Most of the time, private insurers pay providers the same way that the government pays. They use the same billing codes and pay for essentially the same services the same way.

Moreover, private insurance in the United States is so heavily regulated that there is no important difference between the public and the private sector. Our public insurance looks just like the socialized insurance we find in Canada. But so does our private insurance. Indeed, what we call private insurance in this country is little more than private-sector socialism.

One more thing to keep in mind: in the United States, we do not have one health system. We have many. In addition to Medicare and Medicaid, there is the VA health system, CHAMPUS (for military families), the Indian Health Service (which is apparently even worse than Medicaid),[63] all the employer plans (running the gamut from "mini-med" plans[64] to cradle-to-the-grave coverage), a whole host of special labor union plans, and, of course, garden-variety health insurance. There is far more difference *within* US healthcare than there is difference *between* the US and other countries.

The pluralism of US healthcare is important to keep in mind in thinking about health reform. Suppose you are dissatisfied with the way the healthcare system is working in your city or your locality, and you are curious about whether somewhere in the world people have found a better way of doing things. Odds are that you are going to find better answers *somewhere within* the United States than *outside* of it.

People on the left and right who are prone to stress the differences between US healthcare and the healthcare of other countries invariably ignore the 80 percent commonality and focus on the remaining 20 percent. On the left, the focus is usually on the ways we appear to be worse; on the right, the focus is usually on the ways we appear to be better. But even here the differences are narrowing, and I expect that trend will continue.

Doctors who object to managed-care interference with the practice of medicine in this country will not be pleased to learn that everything that is happening here is finding its ways to other countries as well. Indeed, US insurance companies are contracting with governments in other countries to export what they do here to other places.[65] People who are concerned about rationing by waiting time in other countries had better brace themselves. Waiting times are growing in the United States as well. Figure 5.5, for example, shows the percent of patients whose wait for elective surgery is four months or more. As for global budgets, a lot of state Medicaid programs already have them, and they may go system-wide in Massachusetts in the near future.[66]

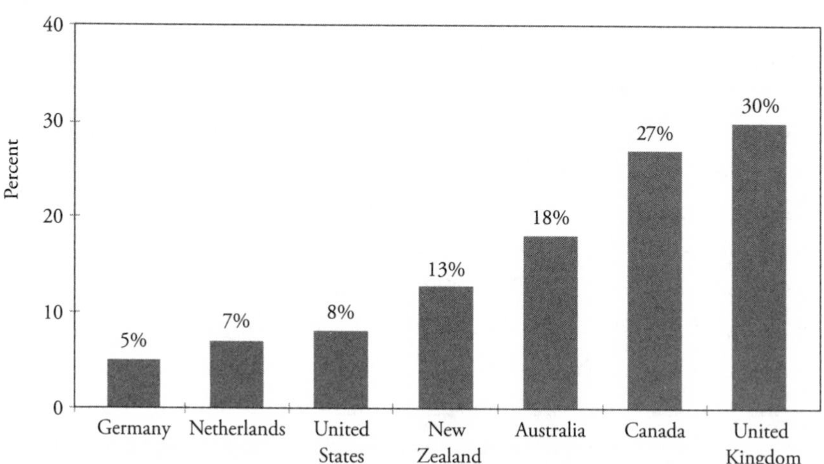

Figure 5.5. Percentage of Patients waiting for Elective Surgery (four months or more)

Source: Karen Davis, Cathy Schoen, and Kristof Stremikis, "Mirror, Mirror on the Wall: How the Performance of the US Health Care System Compares Internationally," The Commonwealth Fund, June 2010.

Another way in which people get misled is in assuming that differences in health outcomes are mainly due to how the medical bills are paid. Yet, differences in health outcomes are far more related to lifestyle, culture, and personal behavior. The United States is an incredibly heterogeneous country—especially in contrast to the homogeneous populations of most Europeans countries. Transplant the US population to France and replace the indigenous population there, and I suspect that in a short period of time, the French healthcare system would come to resemble the system we have in America today. Conversely, transplant the French population to this country to replace all the Americans, and in short order, I suspect that our healthcare system would come to resemble what you see in France today.

Differences in outcomes are very often due to differences in the people involved. Too often, these differences are wrongly ascribed to differences in the payment systems.

A Radically Different Approach: I Cut Healthcare Spending in Half

Before leaving this chapter, I want to make sure that readers understand that we know a lot more than you may think we know about how to reduce healthcare spending. Most health policy analysts and most health policy discussions are focused on all the gimmicks and techniques that won't work. But there are techniques that will work. If we employ them, it appears that we could reduce US healthcare spending per capita to about the same level as the average developed country, in nominal terms.

But wait a minute. In making this claim, aren't I guilty of the same "fatal conceit" that I warned against? How do I know what will work? Actually, I don't know. What I do know is that certain kinds of incentives motivate others to find out what works for them. I have no idea what the healthcare system would look like once we started doing these things. I do know that the following incentive systems show great promise:

- Let patients pay for all routine primary care and all diagnostic screening tests from a Health Savings Account that they own and control.

- Create special HSA accounts for the chronically ill and encourage providers of integrated, coordinated care to compete in an unrestricted market for their patronage.
- Let all elective inpatient care be subject to a type of value-based insurance involving domestic medical tourism—with the third party paying only what the care would cost at low-cost, high-quality facilities and with the patients paying all the additional costs if they choose to seek care from other facilities.

We'll explore ways to implement these ideas in the coming chapters.

6

Why Is There a Problem with Quality?

THERE ARE A lot of indications that the quality of care patients receive is not nearly as good as it should be. In fact, in a RAND study, emergency room patients were judged to have received optimal care only half the time.[1] Critics found problems with the study,[2] but most observers would agree that the quality of care patients receive could be much better.

How Safe Is Your Hospital?

Hospitals are dangerous places to be. By one estimate, as many as 187,000 patients die every year for some reason other than the medical condition that caused them to seek care.[3] Another study estimates that the healthcare system causes 6.1 million injuries a year, including hospital-acquired infections that afflict one in every twenty hospital patients.[4] In a *Health Affairs* study, my colleagues Pamela Villarreal and Biff Jones and I estimated the economic cost of the loss of life and limb from adverse medical events at between $393 billion and $958 billion in 2006 dollars. This is equal to between $4,000 and $10,000 a year for every household in America.[5] By this reckoning, every time the healthcare system spends a dollar healing us, it causes up to 45 cents worth of harm.

Of course, the system also does a lot of good. In fact, the good is many, many times greater than the harm. Still, the cost of adverse medical events is so huge we would be foolish not to try to find ways to make it smaller.

In our study, we accepted previous estimates that the odds are as high as one in 200 that a patient will die for some reason other than the medical condition that caused him to seek care in the first place. A newer study places those odds at 1 in 100.[6] The lowest risk I have seen places the odds at 1 in 500.[7] By comparison, some federal regulatory agencies view any chance of death lower than 1 in 1 million as unacceptable.[8]

My colleague Linda Gorman has carefully reviewed the various studies of "preventable" adverse events (medical errors) and believes the error rate is overstated. She also points to international evidence that the US hospital error rate is lower than the comparable rate in Canada, Britain, and New Zealand.[9] Even so, the evidence suggests that US hospitals are not nearly as safe as they could be or should be.

That brings us to some crucial questions. Why don't hospitals with better safety records compete for patients based on those records? Why doesn't competition force all hospitals to improve their safety standards? More generally, why doesn't quality competition in healthcare work like quality competition in other markets?

Why Don't More Hospitals Complete on Quality?

Go to the website of the Detroit Medical Center and you will learn that its facilities are ranked among the "nation's best hospitals" by *US News & World Report* and that they have won other awards. The Detroit Medical Center has some of the "best" heart doctors, it is "tops" in cancer care, and it ranks among the "nation's safest hospitals."[10] Three of its hospitals, for example, meet standards established by The Leapfrog Group, an organization established by large employers and funded by the Business Roundtable to advise on healthcare quality. Two have received Leapfrog's "top hospital" award.[11]

The Detroit Medical Center's website informs you that the DMC "is dedicated to staying ahead of the crowd when it comes to the quality of our care.... If you want a hospital with walking trails or a day spa, go someplace else," the site advises. "Just don't expect the latest in patient safety technology. Because 100-percent medication scanning is only at DMC."

Why aren't more US hospitals competing for patients in the same way the Detroit Medical Center does? Why isn't Detroit Medical Center competing more aggressively? Some hospitals in India, Thailand, and Singapore, for example, disclose their infection, mortality, and readmission rates and compare them to such US entities as the Cleveland Clinic and the Mayo Clinic.[12] Clearly, the Detroit Medical Center is also competing on the time price of care. It guarantees an appointment within seventy-two hours for MRI scans and promises to report to your doctor within twenty-four hours after the procedure. So why doesn't it also compete on the money price of care by posting fees patients can expect to pay?

How We Pay for the Three Dimensions of Care

Think of healthcare as having three dimensions: a quantity dimension (e.g., the units of service third-party payers typically pay for, such as office visits, diagnostic tests, etc.), a quality dimension (e.g., such factors as lower infection, mortality, and readmission rates, etc.), and an amenities dimension. By increasing the quality of care and the amenities surrounding that care, providers can make their basic services more attractive to patients, provided they have an incentive to do so.

As in the market for other goods and services, people pay for care with both time and money. What makes healthcare unusual is that for most patients, the time price of care is a greater burden than the (out-of-pocket) money price of care—since third-party payers pay all or almost all of the provider's fee. For primary care, emergency room care, ancillary services, and an increasing number of traditional hospital services, time is the principal currency patients use to purchase healthcare in the United States, just as it is in other developed countries.

Market Equilibrium

In a third-party payment system, the provider's fee, including the money price paid by the patient, tends to be set by an entity outside the doctor-patient relationship. For a given unit of service and a given total fee, that leaves a time price, quality, and amenities. Of these three variables, however, only two are typically visible or inferable. The quality variable is normally hidden. As patients respond to what is visible and move back and forth among providers, there will be a tendency toward uniform wait times and uniform amenities. (Think of these as the market clearing time price and the market clearing level of amenities.) Or, if there is a trade-off between waiting and amenities, the rate of substitution will tend to be uniform.

There are no natural equilibrating forces bringing about uniform quality of care, however. As long as quality differences remain invisible, they can persist without affecting the patients' demand for care. This is consistent with the findings that the quality of care varies considerably from provider to provider and facility to facility, as well as the discovery that variations in the quality of care delivered are unrelated to the kind of insurance people have or even whether they are insured at all.[13] (Note, however, that most measures of quality are measures of inputs, not outputs; at least one study finds there is little relationship between these inputs and such outputs as reduced mortality;[14] and some have questioned whether even hospital mortality rates are reliable indicators of quality.[15])

Effects on Quality of Care

Lack of quality competition is in part the result of certain characteristics of healthcare quality. What we call core quality is not a variable at all. It is the result of other decisions made by the providers. Since the vagaries of medical practice are many and since the decision calculus of doctors will often differ, this allows for considerable quality differences. Beyond this core level, quality improvement is a decision variable, and improvements are costly. However, since it is difficult and costly for patients to secure quality data on their own, information about quality typically comes only from the providers.

Such communications are unlikely, however, unless by means of quality improvements, providers are able to shift demand (and, therefore, revenue), sufficient to pay for those improvements. In general, this is not the case.

But why don't providers with superior quality take advantage of that fact and advertise it to patients? In other words, why doesn't quality competition arise in healthcare the way it does in normal markets? Consider two cases.

How Health Insurance Undermines Quality Competition: Doctors

Imagine a health market where supply is restricted and where demand exceeds supply at a zero (or nominal) money price—both for the market as a whole and for individual providers. Under these conditions, which roughly describe most primary care practice, the provider's time will tend to be rationed by waiting. Improvement in the quality of care (if perceived or communicated) will potentially increase demand—maybe even attracting new patients. However, the increased demand will be initially reflected in increased waiting (higher time price), which in turn will cause some of the initial group of patients to see the doctor less often. On the other hand, a decrease in quality of care (again if perceived or communicated) will diminish demand and lead to shorter waits (a lower time price), thus inducing some of the remaining patients to see the doctor more often.

Since the doctor's time is already fully allocated, and since the fee is fixed, in neither circumstance will the physician's revenue be much affected. The same principle applies to amenities. In the face of rationing by waiting, amenity improvements will not in general increase the provider's income, and amenity degradation will not in general decrease it.

So in comparing two practices—one that predominantly relies on price rationing to clear the market and one that relies on rationing by waiting, we would expect both amenities and quality of care to be higher in the former than in the latter.

"I practiced for 30 years without knowing how long patients waited to see me," says Robert Mecklenburg, a doctor who is now at Virginia Mason Medical Center in Seattle.[16] Can you imagine the owner of a retail outlet in any other market admitting that he has no idea how long his customers wait before being served? In a normal market, a storeowner with that attitude would not survive for ten minutes.

How Health Insurance Undermines Quality Competition: Hospitals

Unlike the market for physician care, in most places, the hospital market is characterized by relative freedom of entry. How the hospital competes is likely to be influenced by the type of third-party payment it receives. With mainly Medicaid patients, where reimbursement rates barely cover the cost of care, the hospital's incentive is to keep its rooms fully booked and avoid excess capacity. Under these circumstances, there will be little incentive to improve the quality of care or the amenities surrounding that care.

On the other hand, hospitals whose patients mostly have private insurance may find that third-party reimbursement rates more than cover the cost of care. These facilities can afford to have excess inventory (empty beds)—so that supply exceeds demand. Unable to compete for patients by lowering money prices and with time prices bumping up against a minimum constraint, providers have an incentive to compete by providing higher quality and more amenities. How will they respond?

Some of the literature on hospital economics suggests that quality improvement is quite expensive and that dollar-for-dollar, amenity improvements will increase hospital revenues by more than quality improvements.[17] This is coupled with surveys that find patients more sensitive to amenity changes than to quality changes.[18] (Of course, this latter finding may reflect only the fact that hospitals aren't really trying to communicate quality information.)

These observations suggest that in vying for additional patients, hospitals have an incentive to invest more in amenity changes than in quality changes; and this appears to be what hospitals do. To appreciate what your health insurance premiums are buying these days, consider the following:[19]

> Concierge service. Jacuzzi tubs. Bacon-wrapped scallops or New York strip steak prepared by professionally trained chefs and brought to your room.
>
> These amenities can be found at most new hospitals in Colorado and across the country. Gone are the days of sterile, white hallways, fluorescent lights and cloth curtains separating patients in the same room. The newest hospitals offer bountiful natural light, warm-colored walls and floors, soothing art and private patient rooms with large windows and relaxation videos.
>
> Sky Ridge Medical Center in Lone Tree features fireplaces on every floor. Children's Hospital Colorado in Aurora offers video games in patient rooms. The cafeteria at the new $435 million St. Anthony Hospital in Lakewood includes a soda machine that can make 100 different types of drinks.

Of course, there are also other ways hospitals compete for patients. Take Provena St. Joseph Medical Center in Joliet, Illinois. Recently, the hospital sent postcards promoting lung cancer screening for current or former smokers over age 55. As *Kaiser Health News* explains:[20]

> Provena didn't send the mailing to everyone who lived near the hospital, just those who had a stronger likelihood of having smoked based on their age, income, insurance status and other demographic criteria.
>
> The nonprofit center is one of a growing number of hospitals using their patients' health and financial records to help pitch their most lucrative services, such as cancer, heart, and orthopedic care. As part of these direct mail campaigns, they are also buying detailed information about local residents compiled by consumer marketing firms—everything from age, income, and marital status to shopping habits and whether they have children or pets at home.

Needless to say, the hospital is looking for prospective customers covered by BlueCross or a large employer plan. Medicaid and the uninsured need not apply. Patients, by the way, are often surprised to learn that hospitals can get such detailed information about their health condition and insurance coverage.

The Market for Amenities

Writing in *The New York Times*, Nina Bernstein observes that some hospital rooms are like the Four Seasons:[21]

> The bed linens were by Frette, Italian purveyors of high-thread-count sheets to popes and princes. The bathroom gleamed with polished marble. Huge windows displayed panoramic East River views. And in the hush of her $2,400 suite, a man in a black vest and tie proffered an elaborate menu and told her, "I'll be your butler."
>
> It was Greenberg 14 South, the elite wing on the new penthouse floor of New York-Presbyterian/Weill Cornell Hospital. Pampering and décor to rival a grand hotel, if not a Downton Abbey, have long been the hallmark of such "amenities units," often hidden behind closed doors at New York's premier hospitals. But the phenomenon is escalating here and around the country, healthcare design specialists say, part of an international competition for wealthy patients willing to pay extra, even as the federal government cuts back.

Sure this is unusual, but it may be more common than you think:

> Many American hospitals offer a V.I.P. amenities floor with a dedicated chef and lavish services, from Johns Hopkins Hospital in Baltimore to Cedars-Sinai Medical Center in Los Angeles, which promises "the ultimate in pampering" in its $3,784 maternity suites. The rise of medical tourism to glittering hospitals in places like Singapore and Thailand has turned coddling and elegance into marketing necessities, designers say.

Yet interestingly, hospitals are not anxious to advertise these services to the general public. New York-Presbyterian, for example, would not answer questions about its V.I.P. services and declined a reporter's request for a tour. Moreover, all this is occurring in space-starved New York, where many regular hospital rooms are still double-occupancy, although singles are now the national standard for infection control and quicker recovery.

Like competitors in any market, for hospitals competing in the amenities market, the customer is always right:

> "We pride ourselves on getting anything the patient wants. If they have a craving for lobster tails and we don't have them on the menu, we'll go out and get them," [said] William Duffy, Mount Sinai Medical Center's director of hospitality.

And the appearance of quality, if not the actuality, is maintained:

> "I'm perfectly at home here—totally private, totally catered," [Nancy Hemenway, a senior financial services executive] added. "I have a primary-care physician who also acts as ringmaster for all my other doctors. And I see no people in training—only the best of the best."

Is Price Competition the Key to Higher Quality?

In our third-party-payer health insurance system, the price for care is typically set by entities external to the doctor-patient relationship. As a result, providers rarely compete for patients based on money prices. But if lack of price competition is normally associated with lack of quality competition, could the reverse be true? Do providers who compete for patients on price also compete on quality? There is a lot of evidence that they do.

Quality Competition in Health Markets Without Third-Party Payers

In those healthcare markets where third-party payment is nonexistent or relatively unimportant, providers almost always compete for patients based on price.

Where there is price competition, transparency is almost never a problem. Not only are prices posted (e.g., at walk-in clinics, surgicenters, etc.), they are often package prices, covering all aspects of care (e.g., cosmetic surgery, LASIK surgery, etc.), and therefore easy for patients to understand.

Wherever there is price competition, there also tends to be quality competition. In the market for LASIK surgery, for example, patients can choose traditional LASIK or more advanced custom Wavefront LASIK. Prices vary with type of procedure and where it is performed, ranging from less than $1,000 to more than $3,000 per eye.[22]

Even when providers do not explicitly advertise their quality standards, price competition tends to force product standardization. This reduced variance is often synonymous with quality improvement. Rx.com, for example, initiated the mail-order pharmacy business, competing on price with local pharmacies by creating a national market for drugs. Industry sources maintain that mail-order pharmacies have fewer dispensing errors than conventional pharmacies.[23] Walk-in clinics, staffed by nurses following computerized protocols score better on quality metrics than traditional office-based doctor care and have a much lower variance.[24]

In general, medical services for cash-paying patients have popped up in numerous market niches where third-party payment has left needs unmet. It is surprising how often providers of these services offer the very quality enhancements that critics complain are missing in traditional medical care. Electronic medical records and electronic prescribing, for example, are standard fare for walk-in clinics, concierge doctors, telephone, and email consultation services, and medical tourist facilities in other countries.[25] Twenty-four/seven primary care is also a feature of concierge medicine and the various telephone and email consultation services.

Waiting Times and Amenities

Competition in the provision of amenities is also common in the niche markets. Cancer Treatment Centers of America takes third-party payment, but its patients usually have to travel some distance to get to its facilities—at both inconvenience and expense. To attract them, the Centers go to great lengths to ensure the comfort of its patients and facilitate the needs of accompanying family members—offering services similar to what medical tourist facilities offer in other countries (they also post their cancer survival rates).[26]

In general, providers who compete on price are competing to lower the money price of care. Where this occurs, they tend to compete to lower the time price as well (hence the term "MinuteClinic"). Teladoc promotes its services by publishing the response times (a doctor's return call) for its clients. Most concierge doctors promise same-day or next-day appointments. Some diagnostic testing services make the test results available to patients online within 24 to 48 hours.[27]

In general, these markets do not appear to be fundamentally different from non-healthcare markets. Competition tends to produce more uniformity of fees and waiting times than would otherwise be the case. Similarly, quality competition also tends to produce either uniform quality or a uniform trade-off between money prices and quality.

Reverse Medical Tourism

In the international tourism market, when people travel for their care, quality is almost always a factor. Cost often is also a factor—either because the patient is paying the entire bill out of pocket or because the patient and a third-party insurer have an arrangement that allows both to profit from the travel. More generally, we have seen that price and quality competition tend to complement each other.

Is it possible to replicate this experience in the domestic hospital marketplace? Even without a major policy change, developments are under way. By one estimate 430,000 nonresidents a year enter the United States for medical care.[28] As noted, some Canadian firms are able to obtain package prices for Canadians seeking medical care at US hospitals.

Moreover, you do not have to be a foreigner to benefit from domestic medical tourism. Colorado-based BridgeHealth International offers US employer plans a specialty network with flat fees for surgeries paid in advance that are 15 percent to 50 percent less than a typical network. North American Surgery, Inc., has negotiated deep discounts with 22 surgery centers, hospitals, and clinics across the United States as an alternative to foreign travel for low-cost surgeries. As noted, the cash price for a hip replacement in the network is $16,000 to $19,000, making it competitive with facilities in India and Singapore.[29]

One reason why so little is known about the domestic medical tourism market is that hospitals prefer that most of their patients not know about it. The reason: they are often offering the traveling patient package prices not available to local patients. That occurs because the hospital is only competing on price for the patients who travel.

If traveling patients begin to make up a large percent of a hospital's caseload, however, medical tourism has the potential to change the hospital's entire business plan.

That brings us back to Detroit Medical Center. An explanation for the center's emphasis on quality competition may be its interest in competing for traveling patients—both internationally and within the United States. The Detroit Medical Center draws about 300 international patients a year.[30] For robotic prostate cancer surgery, it has attracted 600 patients from 50 states and 22 countries. Although its website does not post prices, if you are an international patient, you are promised cost estimates and package pricing.

The Detroit Medical Center also advertises the availability of rooms and suites for family members on campus, their willingness to book rooms for the family at area hotels, free parking, and other amenities.

Furthermore, it may be no accident that such facilities as the Cleveland Clinic and the Mayo Clinic also attract large numbers of patients who travel. High-quality care and medical tourism seem to go hand in hand.

Recap

A major reason why healthcare quality varies is because of the third-party payment system. Four critical aspects of healthcare delivery are interrelated: the underlying cost of care, wait times, amenities, and quality. Those four aspects are rivals for managers' attention and organizational resources. In competitive markets, they will tend to be brought into an equilibrium reflecting their value to the consumer. In healthcare markets, the lack of price competition at the patient level leads to greater quality variation than would occur otherwise. This finding is consistent with the observed characteristics of markets with little out-of-pocket payment and has important policy implications.

In general, any move to promote price competition will probably promote quality competition indirectly.

7

Why Is There a Problem with Access to Care?

HERE IS THE conventional wisdom in health policy: access to healthcare is determined by price, and this is unfair to low-income families. Because they lack the resources to pay for health insurance, thousands of people do not get the healthcare they need. To solve the problem, we need to provide the poor with health insurance that requires very little out-of-pocket spending—one of the goals of ACA.

Here is the alternative vision elaborated in this book:

- The major barrier to care for low-income families is the same in the United States as it is throughout the developed world: the time price of care and other non-price rationing mechanisms are far more important than the money price of care.
- The burdens of non-price rationing rise as income falls, with the lowest-income families facing the longest waiting times and the largest bureaucratic obstacles to care.[1]
- ACA, by lowering the out-of-pocket money price of care for almost everybody while doing nothing to change supply, will intensify non-price rationing and may actually make access to care more difficult for those with the least financial resources.

Interestingly, the current recession provides a natural experiment that tests these two opposing visions.

A Natural Experiment

According to a recent report from the Center for Studying Health System Change, middle-class families are responding to bad economic times by cutting back on their consumption of healthcare. They are postponing elective surgery, forgoing care of marginal value, and making more cost-conscious choices when they do get care. This reduction in demand is freeing up resources, which are apparently being redirected to meet the needs of people who face price and non-price barriers to care. From 2007 to 2010:[2]

- The percentage of the population experiencing an unmet healthcare need actually fell from 7.8 percent to 6.5 percent.
- The percentage of people who say they have delayed care fell from 12.1 percent to 10.7 percent over the same period.

During the recession, the money price barrier to care actually rose among the uninsured, although the increase was not statistically significant. Yet, over the same period, the number of people experiencing access problems because of waiting and other non-price barriers was almost cut in half (falling from 40.3 percent to 24.1 percent). Specifically, the number of people who "could not get an appointment soon enough" fell from 34.6 percent to 24.4 percent; the number who "could not get there when the doctor's office was open" fell from 28.4 percent to 22.7 percent; those who said "it takes too long to get to the doctor's office" fell from 17.5 percent to 11.5 percent; and those who "could not get through on the telephone" fell from 16.1 percent to 10.7 percent.

Here is something even more interesting. Suppose that in an attempt to increase access to care, we add one more doctor, one more nurse, or one more clinic. Who is likely to benefit? The study implies that the higher your income, the greater the likelihood you will gain. During the recession, for example, the percentage of people experiencing an unmet need with income at 400 percent of the poverty level ($43,000 for an individual or $89,000 for a family of four) or above was more than cut in half. Yet, among those with incomes below 200 percent of poverty ($22,000 and $45,000 respectively), the percentage of those with unmet needs actually rose.

Think (metaphorically) of a waiting line for care. The lowest-income families are at the end of that line. The longer the line, the longer they will have to wait. If you do something to shorten the line, you will be mainly benefitting higher income people who are at the front.

Why is that? I believe that many of the skills that allow people to do well in the market are the same skills that allow them to do well in non-market settings.[3] High-income, highly educated people, for example, will find a way to get to the head of the waiting line, whether the thing being rationed is quality education, healthcare, or any other good or service. Low-income, poorly educated individuals will generally be at the rear of those lines.

And that raises an interesting question: Are low-income patients deterred more by money prices or by non-price barriers to care? Another recent study suggests that it may be the latter.

Although most states try to limit Medicaid expenses by restricting patients to a one-month supply of drugs, North Carolina for a period of time allowed patients to have a three-month supply. Then the state reduced the allowable one-stop supply from one hundred days of medication to thirty-four days and at the same time raised the co-payment on some drugs from $1 to $3. Think of the first change as raising the time price of care (the number of required pharmacy visits tripled) and the second as raising the money price of care (which also tripled).

Researchers discovered that tripling the time price of care led to a much greater reduction in the needed drugs obtained by chronically ill patients than a tripling of the money price, all other things remaining equal.[4] This study pertained to certain drugs and certain medical conditions. But suppose the findings are more general. Suppose that for most poor people and most healthcare, time is a bigger deterrent than money. What then?

If the study findings apply to a broad array of health services, it appears that the orthodox approach to getting health services to poor people is as wrong as it can be. It implies that everything we have been doing in health policy to make healthcare accessible for low-income patients for the past 60 years is completely misguided.

How Much Does Health Insurance Affect Health?

There have been a number of claims that lack of insurance is life threatening. The most recent and well known is an Institute of Medicine (IOM) study claiming that 18,000 people die every year because they do not have health insurance.[5] Using a similar methodology, a study for the Physicians for a National Health Program expanded that number to 44,789.[6] Families USA, a nonprofit advocacy group, went as far as to predict the number of deaths by state.[7] "More than eight people die each day in California because they don't have health insurance," the organization asserts.[8] Careful analysis by such scholars as the former Congressional Budget Office director June O'Neill[9] and health economist Linda Gorman[10] find these studies are defective.

Helen Levy and David Meltzer, scholars with an interest in healthcare, found that most studies that attempt to find a causal link between health insurance and health status were poorly designed. They conclude that, although health insurance can make a difference to selected subpopulations of people, for most people, the effect is very modest.[11] In a more thorough study, former Clinton adviser Richard Kronick found that insurance had virtually no effect on mortality rates.[12]

Moreover, in the decision about where to invest finite resources to improve health outcomes, universal coverage may not be the low-hanging fruit. Michael Cannon, the director of health policy studies at the Cato Institute, points out that if improving health status is the primary goal, there is no evidence that universal coverage would accomplish this any better than, say, boosting education or expanding community health centers. If saving lives is the primary goal, the IOM's own estimates suggest that reducing preventable medical errors would save far more lives than boosting health coverage.[13]

Is Health Insurance a Requirement for Access to Healthcare?

The conventional wisdom among health experts across the ideological spectrum is that people need health insurance to get good healthcare. Indeed, to some politicians the terms "no healthcare" and "no health insurance" are interchangeable. Almost as widely accepted is the view that some health plans are a ticket to better healthcare than others. But a RAND Corporation study shatters those assumptions:[14]

- Among people who seek care (actually see a doctor), RAND researchers found virtually no difference in the quality of care received by the insured and uninsured.
- They also found very little difference in the care provided by different types of insurance—Medicaid, managed care, fee-for-service, and so forth.

Unfortunately, the care everyone received was less than ideal. The study concluded that patients received recommended care only about half the time.

The implication is that reforming the supply side of the medical marketplace is far more important than getting everyone on the demand side insured.

For people who have a hard time imagining a world in which health insurance does not matter, consider the case of Parkland Memorial Hospital in Dallas, Texas. Both uninsured and Medicaid patients enter the same emergency room door and see the same doctors. The hospital rooms are the same, the beds are the same, and the care is the same. As a result, patients have no reason to fill out the lengthy forms and answer the intrusive questions that Medicaid enrollment so often requires.

Furthermore, the doctors and nurses who treat these patients are paid the same, regardless of patients' enrollment in an insurance plan. Therefore, they tend to be indifferent about who is insured by whom, or if they're even insured at all. In fact, the only people concerned about who is or is not enrolled in what plan are hospital administrators, who worry about how they will cover the hospital's costs.

At Children's Medical Center, next door to Parkland, a similar exercise takes place. Children who are uninsured and children covered by Medicaid or the Children's Health Insurance Program all enter the same emergency room door; they all see the same doctors and receive the same care. Interestingly, at both institutions, paid staffers make a heroic effort to enroll people in public programs—even as patients and their families wait in the emergency room for medical care. Yet, they apparently fail to enroll eligible patients more than half the time. After patients are admitted, staffers valiantly go from room to room to continue this bureaucratic exercise. But even among those in hospital beds, the failure-to-enroll rate is significant—apparently because it has no impact on the care they receive.

Do Medicaid and CHIP Improve Access to Care?

It is an article of faith in the conventional health policy community that the goal should be to enroll low-income families in health plans with no price barriers to care. Even if there are non-price barriers to care, the conventional wisdom is that rationing by waiting time is always better than rationing by price. That is why Medicaid and CHIP were created. So how well is this approach to healthcare working? One recent study found that enrolling children in CHIP did not result in more medical care. The one thing that apparently does increase access to care is paying physicians higher fees.[15] Yet, ironically Medicaid and CHIP enrollees are not allowed to pay out-of-pocket to supplement the government fee schedule and pay the same prices other patients pay. There are also other problems.

Eligible But Not Enrolled

An estimated one of every three uninsured people in this country is eligible for a government program (mainly Medicaid or CHIP) but is not enrolled.[16] Either they haven't bothered to sign up, or they did bother and found the task too daunting. Going all the way back to the Democratic presidential primary, ACA was always first and foremost about insuring the uninsured. Yet, at the end of the day, the new health law is going to insure only about 32 million people out of more than 50 million uninsured. Half that goal will be achieved by new enrollment in Medicaid. But if you believe the Census Bureau surveys, we could enroll just as many people in Medicaid by merely signing up those who are already eligible.

Why don't eligible people take the trouble to enroll. All they have to do is fill out a form or, in the case of many hospital emergency rooms, let someone else fill out the form for them. That they demur implies that patients view enrollment in a public health insurance plan as unlikely to result in better care or less out-of-pocket cost.

All of this suggests that what matters most—especially to low-income families—is access to care, not health insurance. On paper, Medicaid coverage appears more generous than the benefits the vast majority of Americans receive through private health insurance. In theory, Medicaid enrollees can see any doctor or enter any facility and pay nothing. In practice, things are different.

Another possible explanation for the failure to enroll is that millions of people are discouraged by all the bureaucratic obstacles to enrollment. Writing in *Health Affairs*, health policy stalwart Alain Enthoven and healthcare executive Leonard Schaeffer discuss what people encounter when they try to sign up for free health insurance from Medi-Cal (California Medicaid) in the San Diego office:[17]

> Of the 50 calls made over a three-month period, only 15 calls were answered and addressed. The remaining 35 calls were met by a recording that stated, "Due to an unexpected volume of callers, all of our representatives are currently helping other people. Please try your call again later," followed by a busy signal and the inability to leave a voice message. For the 15 answered calls, the average hold time was 22 minutes with the longest hold time being 32 minutes.

This study was conducted by the Foundation for Health Coverage Education (FHCE), a nonprofit organization dedicated to helping the uninsured enroll in available health coverage programs. The head of FHCE's national call center reports that his staff has taken hundreds of calls from people who have tried in the past to enroll in Medicaid but who found the process so complicated and difficult that they simply quit trying.

What about doctors and hospitals? Can't they help poor people sign up for public programs and isn't it in their self-interest to do so? Turns out that medical providers have just as much difficulty with the Medicaid bureaucracy as the patients do:[18]

> [I]t routinely takes more than 90 days for the state to enroll uninsured patients into public programs. This is because it is the patient's responsibility to apply directly to the state program to receive the needed documentation for hospital reimbursement. Once treatment is provided and the medical incident is over, it is difficult to ensure that the patient continues with the enrollment process.

Can you imagine Aetna taking 90 days to sell someone an insurance policy? What about WellPoint? Or BlueCross?

Another problem is the Medicaid payment rates. They are so low that California hospitals frequently don't even bother to try to enroll patients who come to the emergency room, unless they're admitted to the hospital:[19]

> [P]ublic program reimbursement is often so low that hospitals are more likely to only seek reimbursement for patients who are eligible for public coverage that fall into the "treat and admit" category rather than those patients who enter the emergency room with minor emergencies or

illnesses. Furthermore, hospitals estimate that they receive as low as 9 percent of fully-billed charges for Medi-Cal patients. Therefore, the providers have little financial incentive to encourage patient enrollment in public programs.

Insured Without Access to Care

Nearly one-third of doctors do not accept any Medicaid patients and, among those who do, many limit the number they will treat. Access to care at ambulatory (outpatient) clinics is also limited for Medicaid patients, as is access to specialist care. According to a *New York Times* investigation on access to care in New York City:[20]

- A child on Medicaid with an irregular heartbeat was not able to see a cardiac specialist for nearly four months.
- The parents of a boy needing corrective ear surgery were told the wait could be as long as five years.
- At specialty clinics run by teaching hospitals, Medicaid patients often have to wait one to three hours for a five- to ten-minute appointment with a less-experienced medical resident or intern.

The problem is not limited to New York City. The *Denver Post* reported that the University of Colorado Hospital refused Medicaid patients and that Medicaid enrollees face six- to eight-month waits for appointments at specialty clinics.[21] In Washington state, a 45-year-old Seattle woman admitted to a hospital with a triple fracture of her ankle waited nine days for a doctor to agree to take her case because none of the orthopedic surgeons on staff would accept Medicaid.[22]

A central element in most state healthcare reform plans is an effort to enroll people who are eligible in public insurance programs, even while they are at public health clinics and in hospital emergency rooms. But why? Does anyone seriously believe that filling out forms in hospital emergency rooms is going to lead to more care or better care? In fact, it may lead to worse care.

It almost certainly leads to worse care if the availability of free care from the state leads families to drop their private insurance coverage. And it could lead to serious discontinuities of coverage as people's eligibility seesaws back and forth with changes in their income.

Eligible, Ineligible, and Then Eligible Again

One of the biggest problems with any insurance plan that makes eligibility conditional on income is that eligibility potentially changes every time income changes:[23]

- Two-thirds of all the children in the United States were eligible (based on family income) for Medicaid or CHIP at some point between 1996 and 2000.
- One in five children were eligible for both programs at some point, and 73 percent of children eligible for CHIP over the whole period were eligible at some time for Medicaid.

What this means is that public coverage is available sporadically as family income rises and falls, leading to significant discontinuities in coverage. In fact, one study concludes that the main reason why 6 million children are eligible but not enrolled in Medicaid and CHIP is due to changes in eligibility.[24] Also, children with discontinuous coverage are thirteen times as likely to experience delayed care as children who are continuously insured, according to another study.[25]

This problem, by the way, will become much worse under ACA. That's because eligibility for two separate, highly subsidized programs will depend critically on family income: Medicaid and subsidized insurance in the soon-to-be-created health insurance exchanges. According to one study of the problem, within six months, more than 35 percent of all adults with family incomes below 200 percent of the federal poverty level will experience a shift in eligibility from Medicaid to an insurance exchange, or the reverse. Within a year, 50 percent, or 28 million, will.[26]

In contrast to spending money on programs for which people's eligibility constantly changes, a better strategy is income support. Under this approach, the government offers a subsidy to be applied to private insurance. As family income rises and falls from year to year, the subsidy falls and rises in an offsetting way. (Or, in the case of a fixed-sum tax credit, the subsidy remains constant as income changes.) As a result, there is no reason for the underlying health insurance to change.

Case Study: Healthcare Without Insurance in Dallas

Let us return to Parkland Memorial Hospital in Dallas. This hospital delivers 16,000 babies a year—more than any other hospital in the nation. Almost all the mothers are uninsured. The vast majority are Hispanic (82 percent) and illegal (70 percent). By almost any definition, these mothers are "at risk."[27] But among those who take advantage of Parkland's prenatal program (more than 90 percent), the infant mortality rate is only half the national average.[28]

How does Parkland do it? By being very good at what it does. Despite being a publicly funded health delivery system, Parkland operates what Regina Herzlinger of Harvard University has described in other contexts as a "focused factory." They are so good at delivering babies, they produce an annually updated, internationally praised textbook on how to deliver babies, and their methods are being copied in Britain and other countries.[29]

However, Parkland's methods will not satisfy everybody. Prenatal care is delivered in clinics staffed by nurses, not doctors, and midwives rather than obstetricians handle the deliveries. Like public hospitals in Toronto and London, Parkland is perpetually overcrowded. In fact, it is not unusual to find patients on beds in hallways.

If all of Parkland's 16,000 expectant mothers were enrolled in Medicaid or had private insurance, however, the experience might be worse. Prenatal care delivered by nurses and deliveries performed by midwives—rather than doctors—might not be allowed under many states' Medicaid rules. Under typical state insurance regulations, patients with private coverage are encouraged to see obstetricians, where the cost is higher and the overall quality of the pregnancy/delivery episode might not be as good because of fragmented care.

Bottom line: if the goal is high-quality, low-cost care for at-risk expectant mothers, clearly the Parkland system should be continued and its replication encouraged in other cities instead of trying to replace it with a health insurance scheme.

In fact, the Parkland model could easily be expanded to other services. MinuteClinics and other walk-in clinics, for example, are staffed by nurses following computerized protocols. They charge half as much as a typical general practitioner, and a Minnesota study concluded that the quality in these clinics matches the quality of conventional care for routine problems. There is also probably far less variation in practice patterns.[30]

It is easy to imagine providing subsidized care at walk-in clinics located in shopping malls, drugstores, and other places convenient for low-income patients. People would be encouraged to get low-cost, high-quality care for a wide range of services (such as flu shots, strep throat, and allergies). Note that walk-in clinics are an alternative to health insurance. Indeed, walk-in clinics exist only because so many patients pay for routine care out of their own pockets. There would be no walk-in clinics if BlueCross were paying all the bills.

Although Parkland is quite good at some things, it is not as good at others. As is the case with many other inner-city public hospitals, patients who do not face life-or-death emergencies can wait hours for care in Parkland's emergency room. A migraine headache patient might wait all day. In fact, almost any non-emergency service involves inordinate waiting. Getting a refill on a phoned-in prescription, for example, can typically take three days. By contrast, Dallas-area Walgreens stores refill prescriptions in less than an hour, and some Walgreens outlets will do it in the middle of the night.

The Impact of Universal Coverage

Now let's turn to healthcare in Massachusetts, where reform under former Governor Mitt Romney provided the model for ACA. How well is reform working in Massachusetts? According to the latest survey by the Massachusetts Medical Society:[31]

- New patients must wait more than a month before they are able to see a family doctor; and the wait to see an internist averages forty-eight days.
- More than half of all family doctors and more than half of all internists are not accepting new patients at all.

Of special interest is what has happened to the people who were newly insured as a result of health reform. As Figure 7.1 shows:

- Whereas 87 percent of family doctors accept Medicare patients, only 56 percent accept patients enrolled in Commonwealth Care (subsidized insurance sold in the exchange).

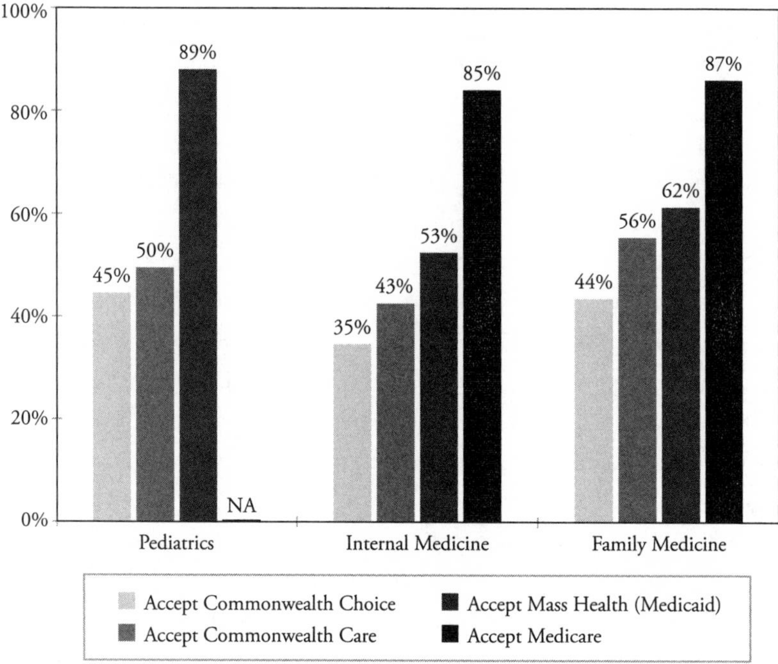

Figure 7.1. Percent of Massachusetts Doctors Who Accept Patients
Source: "2011 Patient Access to Health Care Study: A Survey of Massachusett's Physicians' Offices" (Survey conducted by Anderson Robbins Research for the Massachusetts Medical Society), 2011.

- Only 44 percent accept patients in Commonwealth Choice (unsubsidized insurance sold in the exchange).
- Although 85 percent of internists accept Medicare patients, the fraction that accepts Commonwealth Care or Commonwealth Choice are 43 percent and 35 percent, respectively.

In Massachusetts, this is called "access to care."

Under ACA, about 32 million people will be newly insured, and if economic studies are correct, they will try to double their consumption of medical care.[32] The act inexplicably forces middle- and upper-middle income families to have more coverage than they might have preferred—a long list of preventive services with no deductible or co-payment. Once they have it, certainly some of them will use it. Yet nothing in the act increases supply to meet the anticipated demand.

Instead, we can expect a rather large increase in non-price rationing—as waiting lines grow at the family doctor's office, the emergency room, and everywhere else. In such an environment, people in a health plan that pays the lowest fees will be pushed to the end of the waiting lines. These include the elderly and the disabled on Medicare, low-income families on Medicaid, and (if Massachusetts is a guide) people with subsidized insurance in the newly created health insurance exchanges.[33]

Ironically, ACA may end up hurting the very people many ACA supporters thought they were going to help.

National Health Insurance and Access to Care

One of the most persistent myths in health policy—both in this country and around the world—is the idea that making healthcare free at the point of delivery will (a) create genuine equality of access to care and (b) be especially beneficial to low-income and disadvantaged groups. Study after study has refuted this notion.

Take the British National Health Service (NHS). Since its establishment, a little over 60 years ago, Britain's ministers of health have consistently assured Britons that they were leaving no stone unturned in a relentless quest to root out and eliminate inequalities in healthcare. But more than thirty years into the program (in the 1980s), an official task force (the Black Report) found little evidence that access to healthcare was any more equal than when the NHS was started.[34] Almost twenty years after that, a second task force (the Acheson Report) found evidence that access had become less equal in the years between the two studies.[35]

Across a range of indices, NHS performance figures have consistently shown widening gaps between the best-performing and worst-performing hospitals and health authorities, as well as vastly different survival rates for different types of illness, depending on where patients live. The problem of unequal access is so well known in Britain that the press refers to the NHS as a "postcode lottery" in which a person's chances for timely, high-quality treatment depend on the neighborhood or "postcode" in which he or she lives.[36] "Generally speaking, the poorer you are and the more socially deprived your area, the worse your care and access is likely to be," says *The Guardian,* a staunch defender of socialized medicine.[37] Scholarly studies of the issue have come to similar conclusions. For example, a study by the Joseph Rowntree Research Trust published in 2000 found discrepancies between geographical locations for all causes of death:[38]

- Nonelderly Britons living in areas with the worst-performing hospitals were 42 percent more likely to die on any given day than the average for Britain as a whole.
- The nonelderly population living in regions with the best-performing hospitals were 24 percent less likely to die than the average for Britain as a whole.
- Overall, the study found that if healthcare inequality were merely decreased to 1983 levels, some 7,500 premature deaths among people younger than sixty-five could be avoided each year.

Other research reinforces these conclusions:

- One study found that if the proportion of cancer-related illnesses and deaths were the same in Britain's lowest socioeconomic groups as in the most affluent, there would be 16,600 fewer deaths from cancer each year.[39]
- The British Heart Foundation (BHF) found that the premature death rate for working-class men is 58 percent higher than non-working-class men.[40]
- The BHF estimates that more than 5,000 working-class men under the age of sixty-five die of coronary heart disease each year in Britain because of variations in healthcare access for different socioeconomic groups.[41]

The British results are not unique. In most countries with waiting lists for care, the poor wait longer than the wealthy and powerful. For example, a survey of Ontario physicians found that more than 80 percent of physicians, including 90 percent of cardiac surgeons, 81 percent of internists, and 60 percent of family physicians, had been personally involved in managing a patient who had received preferential access on the basis of factors other than medical need. When asked about those patients most likely to receive preferential treatment, physicians reported that 93 percent had personal ties to the treating physician, 85 percent were high-profile public figures, and 83 percent were politicians.[42]

Other studies have reached similar conclusions. One study found that the wealthy and powerful in Canada have significantly greater access to medical specialists than the less well-connected poor.[43] A University of Toronto study found that high-profile patients enjoy more frequent services, shorter waiting times, and greater choice in specialists.[44]

These results are well known in health policy circles, but the conventional view is that they are aberrations that demonstrate a lack of diligence in pursuing an important social goal. In fact, they are the expected result of substituting non-price rationing for the marketplace. In the United States, access to cell phones (for which everyone pays the market price) is far more equal than access to healthcare (for which no one pays a market price).

What Britons and Canadians have is not insurance in any real sense of the word. What they have is an imperfect system of free care. In fact, the US system is actually more egalitarian than the systems of many other developed countries, with the *uninsured* in the United States, for example, getting more preventive care than the *insured* in Canada.[45]

Absent government intervention, people tend to purchase insurance for rare, high-dollar events that could be financially devastating. By contrast, they tend to self-insure (and pay out of their own pocket) for small-dollar, routine costs that are easily managed. Casualty insurance for an automobile covers expensive accidents, not oil changes.

In Britain and Canada, this principle is turned on its head. Citizens of these countries have ready access to free, routine primary care and tend to see general practitioners more often than do US citizens. But the British and Canadians have less access to specialists and sophisticated diagnostic tests (such as CAT scans, MRI scans, and PET scans).[46] They have even less access to expensive medical interventions, such as kidney dialysis or transplants.[47] Moreover, when the British go into the private market to buy services they cannot get from their National Health Service, and when Canadians come to the United States for services they cannot get from their Medicare system, they are in no sense insured for those costs. Instead, they must pay out of pocket.

In response, about 11 percent of the British population buys real insurance on top of the system of free care to provide financial protection against the out-of-pocket costs of expensive care they are forced to purchase on their own.[48] Canada outlaws private insurance for treatments covered by the government plan, so people must essentially self-insure for these costs.[49]

Finding a Better Way to Create Healthcare Access

Consider a low-income population, including perhaps illegal immigrants, who will need help from others to pay for almost any kind of healthcare beyond the most basic and inexpensive. In this scenario, the idea behind the British system may not be all bad. In fact, virtually every country south of the US border (with the exception of Argentina and possibly Chile) provides free healthcare to the population at large. However, everyone in these countries who achieves even a modest standard of living goes to the private sector for healthcare, buying private health insurance in many cases.

The trouble with all of these systems is that government-provided monopoly care tends to be inefficient and wasteful, marked by highly variable quality and access. Those adjectives also seem to be an apt description of federally funded community health centers, favored by both the Bush and the Obama administrations. Not only does the government tell these centers what they can do and how they can do it down to the minutest detail, health economist Linda Gorman discovered that in Colorado, these centers actually cost more than what doctors charge middle-class patients in the private sector.[50]

Since free or highly subsidized care is already largely available in the United States, what is needed is not an alternative to free care but a way to subject the free care system to market forces. Reflecting again on the experience of Parkland's baby-delivery focused factory, the suppliers of care need to be given appropriate incentives so that they realize economic gains from producing higher quality, low-cost care and realize economic losses if they produce the opposite.

A special type of insurance plan might be of value. This plan would not really be insurance at all. Instead, it would put money that is likely to be spent anyway into the hands of patients—perhaps through a vehicle similar to a Health Savings Account—and make providers compete for those dollars.

8

Why Can't You Buy Real Health Insurance?

AS WE HAVE seen, in the casualty insurance market the product that is being bought and sold is real insurance: protection against catastrophic loss. In contrast, what is being bought and sold in healthcare is not really insurance at all. In fact, to a large extent health insurance is pre-payment for the consumption of healthcare. What difference does this make?

How Health Insurance Is Different

Coverage and Risk

Casualty insurance almost always insures against a risky event. By definition, a risky event is an event that is not under control of the person who is insured. Homeowners' insurance, for example, pays for damage caused by wind, hail, fire, and so on. But it does not pay for the normal wear and tear that is the product of normal household living. Automobile insurance pays for collisions. It does not pay for oil changes, tire rotation, or other routine maintenance.

Further, to ensure that the damage covered is the result of a risky event not under the control of the insured, casualty insurance typically has a deductible. A $1,000 deductible, for example, makes the car owner responsible for the cost of the typical minor fender benders. By adjusting the amount of the deductible, drivers can decide how much risk they're willing to accept for relatively small dollar damages. The reason: the cost of insurance for small-dollar damages is quite high in relation to the cost of insurance for rare, high-dollar damages. In general, the higher the deductible the less you have to pay per dollar of coverage.

Health insurance stands in stark contrast to these practices. The typical employer plan, for example, covers general checkups and such routine screenings as mammograms, Pap smears, and prostate cancer tests. These are expenses that may be recommended but are not the result of some unpredictable event. In addition, health insurance typically pays for such events from the first dollar. A number of employer plans, for example, cover routine primary and preventive care with no deductible or co-payment. Under ACA, this practice will be required by law.

Even more surprising, many of the employer plans that pay for routine care from the first dollar leave employees exposed to tens of thousands of dollars of out-of-pocket expenses in the case of catastrophic illness. In other words, these plans pay for routine expenses that most families could easily pay themselves, while leaving them exposed to large bills that they cannot afford.

Obligation to Pay

In other insurance markets, the insurer is obligated to pay for damages, once the risky event has occurred and the damages have been realized. For example, life insurers are obligated to pay a death benefit to the survivors, once the death has occurred. No insurer insists that a widow continue to pay premiums long after her husband is deceased. Similarly, the homeowner's insurer is responsible for paying for damage from a fire, once the fire has occurred. No insurer insists that owners continue to pay premiums long after the house has burned down—unless they want to insure another house.

Health insurance is different. Health insurance typically pays for medical expenses only so long as the patient continues to pay premiums. Suppose you get cancer and begin chemotherapy and other treatments. As long as you and your employer continue to pay health insurance premiums, the insurer will pay the cost of the care (minus your co-payments). But suppose you quit your job, say, because you are too sick to work. Then you will eventually lose your employer's coverage, and at that point, the insurer will cease paying for the cost of your care.

This unique feature of health insurance is the primary reason why people have a problem with pre-existing conditions in the health insurance marketplace. Most chronic health problems (diabetes, asthma, cancer, heart disease, etc.) do not arise while people are uninsured. They arise when people and their employers are paying premiums. In a mobile labor market, however, people leave their jobs. When they seek new insurance, they discover that the new insurer either won't insure them or insists on excluding coverage for the pre-existing condition.

In popular discussions of this problem, the tendency is to blame the new insurer, but this condemnation is surely misplaced. Remember, the person with the pre-existing condition has been paying premiums (perhaps for many years) to the original insurer. Does it make sense to allow the original insurer to collect all the premiums but force the new insurer to pay all the bills?

Payments for Loss

A third unique feature of health insurance relates to how and why insurance payments are made. If your car is totaled in an accident, the insurance company doesn't insist that you pay to have it repaired in a specific way. It simply writes you a check for the value of your loss. If your home is destroyed by a tornado, the insurer does not insist that you build it back as it was—brick by brick. Instead, it writes you a check for the value of your loss.

Modern health insurance, by contrast, does not write checks to patients based on the value of their losses. Instead, health insurers write checks to doctors, hospitals, and other providers, based on services they provide. Instead of reimbursing us for losses, health insurance pays for healthcare consumption, and the amount it pays depends on how much we consume.

By way of analogy, if life insurance were structured like health insurance, my wife would not receive a check when I die. Instead, the life insurer would pay only for expenses related to my death: the cost of my funeral, autopsy, cremation, and so on.

The Key Relationship

This leads us to the fourth difference between health insurance and other forms of insurance. In a very real sense, health insurance is not fundamentally about a relationship between the insurer and the insured. It's about a relationship between the insurer and the healthcare providers.

Home insurers are not in the roofing business. Automobile insurers are not in the car repair business. But modern health insurance is very much in the business of healthcare. In fact, it originally began not as a way to compensate patients for their losses, but as a way to make sure providers got paid for the services they rendered. In such a world, the providers came to view the third-party payers, rather than patients, as their clients. In the worst case, patients became merely an excuse for submitting bills to third-party payers. Then, as healthcare costs began to escalate to unreasonable levels, health insurers got into the business of supervising doctor behavior and then into the business of managing care.

The Evolution of Health Insurance

To appreciate what happened to health insurance you have to know something about how government regulations have affected the entire healthcare marketplace. In the United States, the seeds of the current regulatory environment were sown in the middle of the nineteenth century, at the very first meeting of the American Medical Association (AMA). The doctors who attended that convention were deeply disturbed by the fact that anybody could hang out a shingle and call himself a "doctor," regardless of training or skills. So they sought medical practice statutes (occupational licensing laws) at the state level and were largely successful in achieving them in most of the states by the early part of the twentieth century.

From medical practice statutes, the profession turned its attention to medical education. Following the AMA-funded Flexner Report,[1] organized medicine essentially gained the power to certify medical schools, and it became the unofficial regulator of the number of medical students allowed to receive training and enter the profession each year. County medical societies acquired the power to sanction doctors who engaged in such "unethical" practices as undercutting approved fee schedules, advertising for patients, making unflattering quality comparisons with other doctors, and in other ways competing too aggressively. Among the sanctions that could be imposed were a denial of hospital privileges, and this was enforced by medical committees that dominated hospital management decisions. The hospitals themselves also adopted a code of ethics that saw price cutting, quality competition, and quality comparisons as violations of professional ethics.

Then attention turned to the matter of health insurance. BlueCross was essentially created by the hospitals, and BlueShield was created by the doctors. In both cases, the objective was the same: drive the commercial insurers out of the market and establish health insurance that saw its purpose as (1) making sure everyone was insured and (2) making sure providers were paid enough to cover the costs of their services. (You can think of this as *private-sector socialism.*) To achieve the first goal, the typical BlueCross plan practiced community rating (charging everyone the same premium regardless of health condition) and accepted all applicants, regardless of pre-existing conditions. To achieve the second goal, BlueCross insurers adopted the principle of cost-plus finance.[2] Basically, if BlueCross patients constituted 50 percent of the patient bed-days for a hospital, BlueCross agreed to pay 50 percent of the hospital's annual expenses. Other insurers were expected to pay in the same way.

By the 1950s, BlueCross was the dominant insurer in just about every state—helped along by state legislation that favored these entities over their competitors. If some other insurer refused to pay hospitals the way BlueCross was paying, hospitals could simply refuse to do business with it and would bill their patients directly. Since all the other insurers were a small part of the market, none could afford to buck the system.

Throughout the 1950s, 1960s, and 1970s, the AMA vision was largely in place. Yet astute readers will be aware that much has changed in the last four decades to cause that vision to erode. A challenge by the Federal Trade Commission led to a consent decree, which effectively eliminated all the prohibitions on competition.[3] Today, doctors can cut prices. They can advertise. They can make quality comparisons with their rivals. Hospitals can do all these things as well.

Many of the original BlueCross ideas about how health insurance should be priced and sold have been legislated—both nationally and at the state level—however. One idea in particular tends to dominate: the idea of managed competition.

Managing Competition[4]

Employees of the federal government,[5] as well as many state and local governments,[6] make an annual choice among a dozen or more competing health plans. Some private employers have erected a similar system for their employees.[7] In most cases, the employer makes a fixed contribution to the premium, and employees who choose richer plans must pay any additional premium themselves.

Where the plans are independent organizations, they effectively compete against each other to enroll members. The competition that exists, however, is not the same as one would find in a free market. It takes place under artificial rules managed by the employer or some other sponsoring organization. Such a system is called managed competition. Its adherents, including Stanford University professor Alain Enthoven, who is known as the "father of managed competition," think this is the answer to the nation's healthcare woes.[8]

During its first term, the Clinton administration proposed a system of managed competition nationwide. Subsequently, it became the guiding principle behind the Massachusetts health reform (RomneyCare) and national health reform (ACA).

Under managed competition, health plans do indeed compete, but in a way that is artificially constrained. For example, each health plan is required to charge the same premium to every applicant (community rating) or to every applicant of the same age and sex (modified community rating) and to accept all applicants regardless of health conditions (guaranteed issue). In the federal employees program, an 80-year-old retiree pays the same premium to join a health plan as a 20-year-old employee.[9] As a result, insurers are precluded from competing on their ability to price and manage risk. Instead, they must compete on their ability to provide healthcare and manage its cost. Such competition is not really competition among firms in the business of insurance; instead, it is competition in the delivery of healthcare.

The artificial market changes the nature of the product not only for the sellers, but also for the buyers. Buyers are not purchasing protection against the loss of their assets when they select one of these health plans. The system as a whole provides protection against the loss of assets due to an expensive illness. What customers are selecting is the right to particular healthcare services, such as access to one doctor network rather than another. This is comparable to choosing an auto insurer so you can have your car repaired at a particular auto repair shop, or choosing a casualty insurer so you can get hail damage repair from a particular roofer.

The benefits of competition flow principally from the fact that sellers find it in their self-interest to compete for the trade of potential customers. To do so, they make buyer-pleasing adjustments in their competitive strategies. However, none of the valuable benefits of competition can be expected to emerge if sellers find it in their self-interest not to sell to some buyers and if they compete with each other to avoid such customers. Yet, these are the perverse incentives that managed competition creates.

People who know before they select an insurer that they need expensive medical treatment will use this knowledge to select a health plan. Since insurers understand this, they can structure their products so as to discourage the most expensive customers. Let's look at some ways this might happen.

How Perverse Incentives Affect the Behavior of Buyers

Imagine a system in which health plans offer networks of doctors and hospitals in return for fixed premiums. People who are seriously ill and need specific, expensive medical treatment will select in a very different way from other people. Take a heart patient in need of cardiovascular surgery. The individual has a self-interest in finding the best cardiologist and the best heart clinic. Armed with this knowledge, the patient will try to learn which health plan employs that cardiologist or has a contract with that clinic. The premium is of secondary importance, since the value to the patient of receiving the best cardiovascular care will far exceed any premium payment.

The incentives facing healthy people are different. Since their probability of needing any particular service in the near future is small, they are unlikely to spend much time investigating particular doctors and clinics. To the degree that they do investigate, they are likely to inquire only about the primary care services they are likely to receive.

Thus, the people who carefully compare the acute care services offered by competing health plans are likely to be the people who intend to use them. These are the very people health plans want to avoid. By contrast, those who choose a plan based on the quality and accessibility of nonacute services are more likely to be healthy.

As Alain Enthoven has noted (disapprovingly), "A good way to avoid enrolling diabetics is to have no endocrinologists on staff. . . . A good way to avoid cancer patients is to have a poor oncology department."[10]

How Perverse Incentives Affect the Behavior of Sellers

To see how managed competition affects the incentives of insurers, imagine two competing HMOs. In the first, enrollees can see a primary care physician at any time, but there are cumbersome screening mechanisms and waiting periods for knee and hip replacements, heart surgery, and other expensive procedures. In the second, joint replacements and heart surgery are available when needed, but primary care facilities are limited. Given a choice, most of us would enroll in the first HMO if we were healthy and switch to the second if we had a serious health problem. But if everyone acted in this way, the second HMO would attract only expensive-to-treat patients. It might seem that the second HMO could compete successfully by offering more primary care services. But to be truly competitive, it would have to change its strategy completely. To cover its costs, it would have to charge a premium many times higher than the first HMO. The premium would have to equal the cost of the expensive procedures, but few people could afford the premium, and they might be better off to simply buy their medical care directly. In any event, the HMO would face financial ruin.[11]

A survey by the Kaiser Family Foundation discovered how HMOs were competing for seniors on Medicare. The HMO ads in print and on television showed seniors snorkeling, biking, and swimming but did not feature the sick or disabled. In addition, nearly one-third of HMO marketing seminars were held at sites that were not wheelchair accessible.[12] The following are just a few other examples of how managed competition works, uncovered by *The Washington Post*:[13]

- When a Minnesota network began offering direct access to an obstetrician while rivals required referrals from a gatekeeper, it attracted disproportionate numbers of pregnant women, lost millions of dollars, and soon ended the practice.
- When Aetna offered unusually generous coverage for in vitro fertilization, people with fertility problems flocked to the HMO, and Aetna had to end the practice.
- In another case, a California health plan severed its relationship with a university hospital known for practicing high-tech medicine and tackling complicated cases.
- Other HMOs avoided contracting with doctors' groups known for expertise with high-risk patients.

The term *medlining* is sometimes used to describe the practice of avoiding the sick. It is healthcare's version of redlining, the banking and insurance practice of avoiding deteriorating neighborhoods. The other side of the coin, of course, is attracting the healthy. In addition to health club memberships, health plans also have offered dental benefits and vision care. The theory is that anyone who will switch health plans to get a free pair of eyeglasses cannot be very sick.[14]

The Results of Competition

In Figure 8.1, patients are arrayed along the horizontal axis from most to least costly (left to right). The cost-of-care line shows what would be spent on each patient, given current standards of medical practice. This line is highly skewed, reflecting the fact that in a typical pool about 5 percent of the group spends about half of the healthcare dollars, 10 percent spends almost two-thirds, and the majority have very small expenses in any given year.[15] The premium is based on the average cost of care for all patients under community rating. It is the premium that must be charged all plan members if the plan is to cover its costs.[16] The figure also illustrates how healthy people subsidize sick people: most enrollees have costs well below the premium they pay, and a few have costs

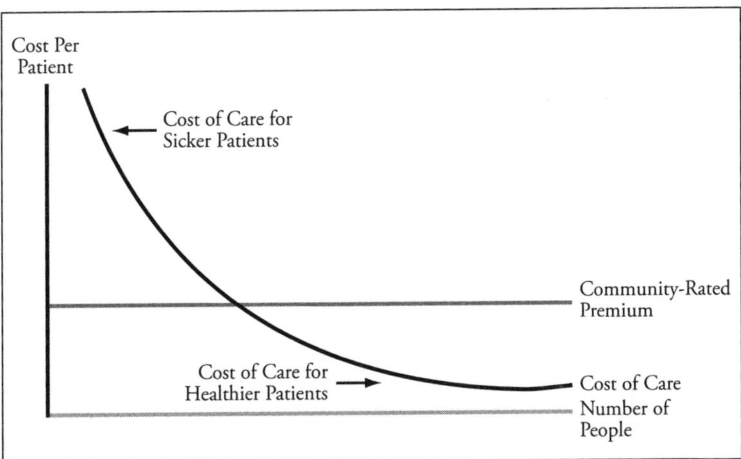

Figure 8.1. Disequilibrium for a Health Plan Under Managed Competition

well above it. Clearly, this is what many proponents of managed competition believe equilibrium would look like for each health plan under their scheme. But simple analysis shows this cannot be the case.

Roughly speaking, an equilibrium exists if no health plan can adjust to become more profitable.[17] However, the plan represented in the figure can easily become more profitable if it can lower the cost of caring for its sicker members. As long as these members stay in the plan, it will have the same premium income and lower costs. If sicker members shift to another plan, this is even better from the plan's point of view—since the sick are unprofitable by definition. On the other hand, healthier customers are being overcharged, since the cost of care they are receiving is below the premium they are paying. This means that other health plans can lure away these customers by providing higher benefits for the same premium. Thus, to retain profitable customers and attract even more, the health plan represented in the figure should increase the amount it spends on healthy members and reduce the amount it spends on the sick.

In free markets, competition tends to cause the price to change until it equals marginal cost. The same tendencies exist under artificial competition. Yet, because community-rated premiums are constrained to be the same for all members, competition will cause cost to change until it equals price. If premiums could rise for unprofitable members, health plans would compete for them up to the level of the cost of those people's care. But if the premiums are artificially constrained, the plans will compete the cost of care down to the level of the artificial premium.[18] The reverse pressures exist for profitable members. If the artificial premiums cannot be competed down to the level of average cost, the tendency will be to compete cost up to the level of the artificial premium.

These conclusions follow from well-known principles of the economics of regulation. In the United States, we have had decades of experience with regulated markets. Under regulations imposed by the Civil Aeronautics Board (CAB) for most of the post-World War II period, the federal government established minimum airfares higher than those that would have prevailed in a free market. Unable to compete on price, the airlines competed by offering more frequent flights, more convenient departures, more spacious seating, and other in-flight amenities. The CAB's price regulation potentially allowed the airlines to earn supranormal profits, but those profits were competed away on passenger-pleasing adjustments.[19] (Note that, since deregulation in 1976, the real price of airline travel has fallen by 33 percent.)[20]

The reverse tendency emerges when prices are kept artificially low. Under rent control laws, landlords are prohibited from raising their rents to the level of average cost. Since rents cannot rise, landlords tend to allow housing quality to deteriorate until housing costs equal the government-controlled rent.[21]

Consider this result in terms of a basic principle taught in all introductory economics courses: when firms are maximizing profits, marginal revenue must equal marginal cost. Under artificial competition, marginal revenue (the amount of premium each additional enrollee brings to a plan) must be the same for every enrollee. Thus, if health plans are maximizing profits, marginal cost (the amount the plan spends on the healthcare of each additional enrollee) also must be the same for every enrollee.

Health plans, therefore, face competitive pressures to adjust the delivery of healthcare until the cost-of-care line coincides with the (community-rated) premium line. (See Figure 8.2.) This means that health plans have a strong financial self-interest in underproviding services to the sick and overproviding services to the healthy. Left unchecked, the end result of this process is a condition under

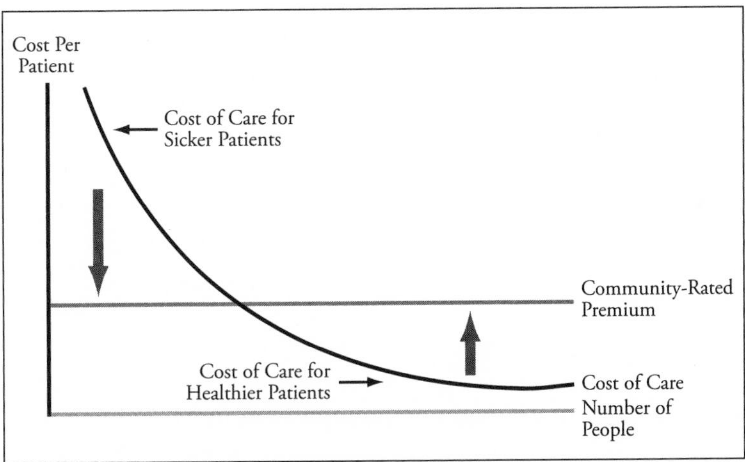

Figure 8.2. Competitive Pressures Under Managed Competition

which each person receives health services whose cost is exactly equal to the premium he or she pays.

The Effect of Limited Open Seasons

The analysis presented here assumes that patients make choices among insurers based solely on the value of medical services those patients consume. This assumption would be justified to the degree that patients can easily shift back and forth among insurers as their health needs change. However, the federal employee program and most other managed competition programs allow plan changes only during "open season," which occurs once a year.

To the degree that people's choices are constrained by limited open seasons, they must consider the insurance value of the plan they select as well as its direct consumption value. Consider an expectant mother choosing among competing health plans. She expects to need well-baby delivery services. However, she might experience complications in pregnancy or childbirth, or her child might be premature and require sophisticated medical treatment. In those cases, the woman would benefit from highly skilled medical personnel. Thus, in selecting a plan, she will be interested in purchasing real insurance as well as specific medical services.

For such potential problems as heart disease, cancer, and AIDS, it seems unlikely that people will willingly pay much to insure for expensive treatment while they are healthy—if they can switch insurers at least every twelve months. The tendency will be to select a plan that is strong on preventive and diagnostic services, secure in the knowledge that one can eventually switch to a plan that is best at treating a particular disease should the affliction occur.

Periodic open seasons cause us to modify our prediction in recognition of an insurance component to people's choices. Yet, even with this modification, we are left with the prediction that artificial competition will ultimately result in a radical deterioration in the quality of care sick people receive.

The Effect of Risk Adjustment

To thwart these perverse incentives, some proponents of managed competition favor risk adjustment mechanisms that take income away from plans that attract healthier people and give it to plans that attract sicker people.

Many methods of risk adjustment have been suggested. None of them work very well.[22] It might seem that the logical way to start constructing a risk adjustment mechanism would be to tax or subsidize health plans based on the health of people at the time they joined a plan. Thus, sicker people would have a subsidy added to their premium payments, and healthier people would have a tax deducted from theirs. Although enrollees would pay the same community-rated premium, health plans would receive a risk-adjusted premium. In theory, this would make the health plans indifferent in addressing potential enrollees.

The problem with this approach is that it does not work very well. Health economist Joseph Newhouse notes that in the RAND Health Insurance Experiment, 1 percent of the patients accounted for 28 percent of the total costs, but most of the high-cost patients could not have been identified in advance. In fact, Newhouse found that only 15 percent of the variation in healthcare costs among individuals could be predicted in advance, even when researchers had full knowledge of the patients' demographic characteristics.[23]

Subsequently, Newhouse and his colleagues concluded that as much as 25 percent of the variation in health expenditures for individuals can be predicted by such observable factors as health status and prior health expenditure.[24] That leaves 75 percent unexplained. More recently, the American Academy of Actuaries has examined a dozen claims-based, risk-adjustment models and concluded the models are able to explain only 15 percent to 28 percent of the variation in medical claims among individuals.[25]

Some health economists argue that it doesn't matter whether a risk-adjustment mechanism is perfect. As long as the adjuster predicts as well as the health plans themselves, the adjuster can remove any financial incentives a plan has to encourage or avoid a person at the time of enrollment. Yet, this does not solve the problem for two reasons. First, after an initial enrollment, everyone will be a member of a health plan. Therefore, at least one plan can probably predict that member's future health costs better than an impersonal risk adjuster, who relies only on statistical data. Second, the perverse incentives of health plans do not end at the point of enrollment. To the contrary, health plans do not have to be able to predict which enrollees will get heart attacks to know that it doesn't pay to invest too much in cardiology. The incentive to underprovide to the sick is ongoing, 365 days a year.

If adjustments cannot solve the problem based on prior knowledge of patients, the only alternative is to base them on knowledge of the experiences of patients after they enroll.[26] But if we do that, how much should the plan be paid? Consider again the cost-of-care line in Figure 8.2. If the net amount insurers receive for each applicant were based on this line rather than on the artificial premium line, insurers would have no reason to overprovide or underprovide care to any enrollee. The problem is that we never get to observe what the efficient cost-of-care line looks like. All an outside observer can see is the actual amount spent. And if we reimbursed health plans for actual expenditures, health plans would have no incentive to provide efficient care. Indeed, the practice of paying providers based on their costs was what led to so much healthcare inefficiency before the managed care revolution. Whatever the defects of managed care, a return to cost-plus finance is not the answer.

An alternative to paying health plans based on actual costs is to pay fixed fees determined by the patient's diagnosis. This is the way Medicare currently reimburses hospitals, and it has produced perverse results: costs have been high and quality lower, in response to the government's prospective payment formulas.[27] One positive aspect is that hospitals get to keep the diagnosis-related payment, regardless of actual costs. Since the lower their actual costs, the higher their profit or the lower their losses, this encourages hospitals to be more efficient. The disadvantage of this approach is that fixed payment is almost always based on expected average cost for patients with a particular condition. By definition, the sum fails to cover the treatment costs of the sickest patients. The more competitive the market, the greater the pressure is to underprovide to the patients whose cost of care is above average.[28]

Regardless of how risk adjustment is carried out, it can at best ameliorate the problem of quality. It cannot solve it. Even if premiums vary with changes in expected costs, the underlying economics are the same. Health plans will have an incentive to adjust the quality of care they deliver until they are spending an amount on each enrollee equal to that enrollee's risk-adjusted premium.

Of course, just because health plans have an economic incentive to let treatment costs fall until they are no greater than the premium payments made on behalf of the sickest patients does not mean they will do so. Fear of tort liability lawsuits is one obstacle to quality deterioration. Doctors' fear of censure or loss of a license to practice is another. But these obstacles are somewhat crude instruments for combating incentives that affect every decision providers make.

What Is the Alternative to Managed Competition?

The alternative is a market in which risk is priced as accurately as possible. Instead of trying to set premiums that ignore risk, consider a world in which each insurer tries to charge each new enrollee a premium that reflects the expected cost and risk that enrollee brings to the plan. Wouldn't that disadvantage people who happen to become sick? It would under the current system. However, if individuals could buy "change of health status" insurance or, even better—if that were part of their normal health insurance contract—their original health plan would pay the extra premium being charged by the new health plan, reflecting the deterioration in health condition. In this way, people would be insured against the economic consequences of developing a pre-existing condition.

Employer-Based Insurance and Managed Competition

In the conventional history, health insurance as an employee fringe benefit is an accident of World War II wage and price controls. Employers were not allowed to raise wages. So in competition for scarce labor, they offered fringe benefits instead. This practice was helped along by a favorable Treasury Department ruling: unlike wages, employer-paid health insurance was not taxable to the employer.

Although there is nothing wrong with calling this evolution an accident, something else had to happen that was very deliberate: Congress denied individuals purchasing insurance on their own the same tax advantages enjoyed by those who got insurance at work. Instead of paying taxable wages, employers can pay premiums with pre-tax dollars. Although the tax law governing individual purchase has changed from time to time, for the most part, people today must pay premiums for individually owned insurance with after-tax dollars. For a middle-income family, this can effectively double the after-tax cost of health insurance.

Individually purchased insurance and employer-provided insurance do not compete on a level playing field. That is why more than 90 percent of all private health insurance is employer-provided insurance. It's also why regulations that affect employer-provided health insurance are so encompassing.

Three other legal changes, in particular, are worth noting.

The Employee Retirement Income Security Act of 1974 (ERISA) was mainly focused on imposing federal regulations on employer-created pension plans, and that is still the way it is often thought of today. Yet, the very same act liberated employer-provided health insurance. Under the act, employers can self-insure—essentially becoming a health insurance company for their employees—and most large employers do this.

Self-insured employers, moreover, are largely unregulated insurance companies. Since they completely escape all state insurance regulations and since there were very few pre-ACA federal mandated benefits, for the last thirty-five years or so employers have had enormous discretion over what health benefits they offer their employees and over the terms and conditions surrounding those benefits. They can choose provider networks as narrow or wide as they like. There is no requirement to hold cash reserves. They can charge their employees any share of the premium they like, and they can include or exclude almost any specific healthcare service.

The second important legislative change was the Health Insurance Portability and Accountability Act of 1996 (HIPAA). This act requires insurers who sell group insurance to offer coverage to every member of the group (guarantee issue). It limits the waiting period for coverage of pre-existing conditions, and it requires insurers to credit prior coverage toward the waiting period.[29] An insurer may set premiums according to a group's experience but may not vary premiums for individuals within the group based on health status.[30] These same rules also apply to self-insured employers.

Although HIPAA has the word *portability* in its title, it does nothing to create real portability. In fact, it actually outlaws it. Prior to its passage, some employers bought individual insurance for their employees (a practice called *list billing*). But most states interpret HIPAA to say that the only health insurance that employers can purchase with pre-tax dollars is group insurance. As a result, when individuals leave their jobs, they ultimately lose whatever coverage the employer was providing.

The third piece of legislation was the Consolidated Omnibus Budget Reconciliation Act (COBRA). Under this act, former employees have the right to stay in an employer's health insurance group for up to 18 months, but they have to pay 102 percent of the actual cost.[31] As a practical matter, the typical employee is directly paying only about 25 percent of the actual cost of health insurance. So when the price of insurance quadruples for departing employees, they experience real sticker shock. Due to the high premium, people who take up COBRA continuation coverage tend to be those who expect substantial medical bills. Almost all employers believe they lose money because of this behavior.

COBRA has the benefit of allowing people searching for a new job to maintain coverage even if they have a serious health problem. HIPAA guarantees that, if their new employer offers health insurance, they will be able to enroll for the same premium healthy people pay.

So where does that leave us? Astute readers may have noticed that the entire employer-based system has a lot in common with our description of managed competition. When people choose employment, they are also choosing health plans. The premium they pay is unrelated to the expected cost of their health care. All the perverse incentives for buyers of health insurance under managed competition are there for the new employee. All the perverse incentives for sellers of health insurance under managed competition are there for the new employer.

In a very real sense, the employer-based health insurance system, therefore, is managed competition writ large.

PART III

Letting People Out of the Trap

9

Empowering Patients

FUNDAMENTALLY, WE CANNOT get off the current spending path unless someone is forced to choose between healthcare and other uses of money. Someone must be willing to say that one more MRI scan or one more blood test or one more physician visit is not worth the cost—that the money is better spent meeting other needs.

Who will that someone be? We could assign responsibility to employers, insurance companies, or even government bodies. How will they make those decisions? There are a number of ways of deciding who gets what: decide by lottery, ration by waiting, allocate by triage, etc.

I like to remind people, however, that no one cares about you more than you care about you. If you control more of your own healthcare dollars and make more of your own decisions, at the end of the day, the system is likely to work better for you than if those decisions are made by impersonal bureaucracies.

Something else to keep in mind: if the system is working better for you, it is probably also working better for me and everyone else as well.

How Patients Make Their Own Choices Between Healthcare and Other Uses of Money

The classic investigation of this issue was conducted by the RAND Corporation about 30 years ago.[1] In that study:[2]

- People with a deductible of about $2,500 (in today's prices) cut back on spending by about 30 percent relative to people who faced no out-of-pocket costs.

- Aside from some minor quibbling, there was no negative impact on health from the higher deductible.
- People with high deductibles were as likely to cut back on useful health services as they were to cut back on unnecessary care.

Latter-day critics seized on the last finding to argue that patient choices appear to be random, and therefore the experiment in consumer-directed care showed it to be a failure. In fact, the patients' behavior is exactly what you would expect from a rational consumer of any product. When something is free, the temptation is to take everything that is offered. The incentive to distinguish between what is "necessary" or "useful" and "unnecessary" or "unuseful" is largely nonexistent. When you have to pay market prices, however, you have an incentive to pay more attention—figuring out what's unnecessary and dropping that, as well as those necessary items whose value is less than their price.

In the 30-year period since the RAND experiment was conducted, a number of experiments—both within this country and abroad—have explored ways to create greater patient cost-sharing without encouraging people to forgo needed care. These include Medisave Accounts in Singapore[3] (dating from 1984), Medical Savings Accounts in South Africa[4] (dating from 1993); and in the United States, an MSA pilot program[5] (dating from 1996), the current Health Savings Account program[6] (dating from 2004), Health Reimbursement Arrangements[7] (dating from 2002), and even cash accounts in Medicaid.[8] Many of these experiments have been subjected to considerable academic scrutiny.

Virtually every serious study of consumer-directed healthcare has reached conclusions similar to the original RAND research. One of the most comprehensive of these (but not as comprehensive as the original) was conducted by RAND itself. The new study concludes that people with high-deductible plans and HSAs spend about 30 percent less on healthcare than those with conventional coverage, with no apparent adverse effects on health.[9]

One thing that distinguishes the latest RAND study is the special attention the researchers gave to the plight of "vulnerable families" (low-income and/or high-risk). The finding: These patients are not disadvantaged by the spending reductions. The researchers report:

> There are no statistically significant differences between non-vulnerable families and low-income or high-risk families in terms of dollar

> reductions in total spending that result from benefit designs and few differences in the components of spending. However, since high-risk families have higher levels of spending, the proportional reductions in total annual spending are generally smaller for those at high risk.

RAND researchers were particularly concerned about whether vulnerable families would fail to receive recommended preventive care services. They found:

> As with spending, there are few significant differences between low-income and non-vulnerable families regarding the effect of plan design on receipt of the cancer screening. However, there are significant differences for those at high risk. For them, a high deductible is not associated with reductions in receipt of two of the three recommended procedures, and the reduction for the third is significantly less than for the non-vulnerable population, though this latter is not significant when we adjust for multiple comparisons.

In other words, people at high risk are not deterred by the plan design from getting needed screening.

Saving for Healthcare

In general, there are two types of insurance: third-party insurance and self-insurance. When we contract with an insurance company, we are shifting risk from ourselves to a third party. Any risks that we don't transfer continue to be ours, and we are self-insured for those risks by default. It is almost never a good idea to shift all the risks to an insurance company. One complaint often heard about the US healthcare system is that too many people are underinsured. In fact, a far greater number are overinsured. That is, too many people are paying insurance companies to pay medical expenses that they could more economically pay themselves.

I will show below that some people are paying insurance companies more than a dollar to assume a dollar's worth of risk, at the margin. Obviously, such people would be better off by lowering their premium payments and assuming more risk themselves. But even paying 40, 50, or 60 cents to transfer a dollar of risk is rarely a good idea. Insurance that expensive is simply not worth what it costs.

The Mechanics of Self-Insurance

One problem with self-insuring for medical expenses is that the expenses tend to be irregular, while most family incomes are produced by a steady stream of paychecks. Adequate self-insurance requires putting money aside during periods when people are healthy to be able to pay the bills in time of medical need. Since most families are not used to thinking about self-insurance in this way, my colleagues and I at the National Center for Policy Analysis proposed to formalize the process, by having individuals or their employers make monthly payments to an actual account. More often than not these days, the account has its own credit or debit card so that it can be easily accessed.

Opportunities for Self-Insurance

The idea behind a formal Health Savings Account is actually a simple one. Instead of giving all of your health dollars to an employer or insurance company, you put some of those dollars into an account that you own and control. Instead of leaving the third-party payer with the burden of managing all of your care, you are in a position to pay for some of your care directly and manage it yourself. The question then becomes: which risks should people self-insure for and which risks should be transferred to third-party insurers? From the beginning, Congress has been unwilling to leave these decisions fully to individuals and the marketplace—even when they involve small amounts of money.

Types of Accounts

Two very popular accounts are the Health Savings Account and the Health Reimbursement Arrangement, which are sometimes confused with the Flexible Spending Account (FSA). However, the FSA really is a spending account rather than a savings account. Because all three accounts involve allowing individuals to purchase healthcare with pre-tax dollars, all three are subject to provisions of the tax code that in some ways are much too restrictive.

Roughly speaking, an HSA plan is required to have an across-the-board deductible, covering all expenses other than preventive care. For 2012, for example, the minimum deductible is $1,200 (individual) and $2,400 (family), and both the employer and the employee can make deposits. In general, people pay expenses up to the deductible from their HSA or out of pocket, and the insurer begins paying after that point. However, employees and their employers can deposit more than the deductible amount in an HSA. For 2012, the statutory maximum contribution is $3,100 per individual and $6,250 per family, regardless of deductible.[10] Money that is not spent rolls over and grows, tax-free. At age 65, the funds may be withdrawn without penalty, but they are subject to normal income taxes.

The advantage of this design is that it gives individuals direct control over the first few thousand dollars of medical expenses; and, as we have seen, when that happens healthcare spending tends to decrease substantially. A disadvantage is that this design treats all healthcare spending the same way without distinguishing between care for which discretion is appropriate and desirable (say, for a routine doctor visit) and care for which it is much less so (say, for diabetes).

In contrast to HSA plans, HRA plans are in principle completely flexible. There is no minimum deductible and no requirement that all health spending be treated the same way. Special accounts can be created for diabetics, asthmatics, and those with other chronic conditions. The disadvantage is that the individual is not entitled to withdraw unspent money in future years. All the money that flows through these accounts comes from employers, and employees really have no property right in the accounts the way they have a property right in an HSA account. This means that owners of HRA accounts may not regard the funds in the account as their own.

Why the Tax Law Is Important

Under an interpretation of the tax law that began in World War II, employer payments for employee healthcare, unlike wages, are not counted as taxable income to the employees. Until recently, however, employers could not make tax-free deposits to a health account that the employee owns and controls. This means that for most of the postwar period, third parties could pay medical bills with pre-tax dollars, while patients had to pay their share of the expenses with after-tax dollars. In this way, the federal tax law favored third-party insurance and discriminated against individual self-insurance. The ability of employers to create HRA accounts for their employees in 2002 and HSA accounts in 2004 was a major step toward leveling the playing field. Although much more needs to be done, self-insurance for medical expenses is treated much more equally under the current tax law.

Advantages of Self-Insurance

What difference does self-insurance make? To the degree that people regard the money in HSA and HRA accounts as their own, they will be more careful, prudent shoppers when they enter the medical marketplace. They will not spend a dollar on care unless they get a dollar's worth of value from the expense. That is in contrast to first-dollar, third-party insurance, which gives people an incentive to consume care until its value approaches zero. In addition, third-party insurance is not free. The administrative expenses alone mean that it rarely makes financial sense for insurers to pay small medical bills.

There are also supply-side effects. When patients are paying for their care with their own money, providers are free to be unrestricted agents of their patients, rather than agents of a third-party payer bureaucracy. In addition, to attract patients spending their own money, providers come under pressure to make prices transparent and to compete on price. Moreover, price competition normally leads to quality competition as well.

Some Criticisms of Individual Self-Insurance

A frequently heard objection is that many people cannot afford to fund their HSAs. If that's true, they cannot afford to pay premiums either. The issue is: Whatever people can afford, how should it be divided between third-party insurance and individual self-insurance? Another complaint is that individuals on their own cannot get the price discounts a large employer or insurance company can get. Actually, they can often get better deals, but that is largely beside the point. In almost all HSA plans, the patient is able to pay the discounted rate the third-party insurer has negotiated, whether the payment is made from the HSA account or by the insurer.

What about the claim that these accounts favor the healthy? That turns out not to be true of HSAs, according to RAND and other studies.[11] What is true, however, is that in the legislation that made HSAs possible, Congress passed up a huge opportunity to encourage the use of such accounts in treating chronic illness. Fortunately, HRAs can be specifically designed for people with chronic conditions. What about the claim that these accounts favor the wealthy? Again, this is disproved by the evidence,[12] but on the surface, this complaint seems off base.[12]

Do Bill Gates and Warren Buffett care about whether they can put $3,100 a year into a tax-free savings account? These accounts are self-evidently paternalistic devices designed to nudge middle-income employees into managing their own healthcare dollars. Remember, every dollar the employer deposits into an HSA is a dollar the employer could have used to pay the employee additional wages or make a deposit to the employee's 401(k) account.

The History of Health Savings Accounts[13]

Although I am often called the father of HSAs, I have never claimed that it was my original idea. My colleague, Jesse Hixson, brought the concept to my attention in the 1980s, and then Gerald Musgrave and I wrote about it in *Patient Power*.[14] Our work at the National Center for Policy Analysis was important because Pat Rooney, chairman of Golden Rule Insurance Company, was on our board of directors. Pat became so convinced that the idea was workable and practical that he tried it out on the Golden Rule employees, and I helped him. Following that success, Golden Rule began marketing what we then called Medical Savings Account plans to the general public. Along the way, we took the idea to Capitol Hill, and under the leadership of House Ways and Means Chairman Bill Archer and Speaker Newt Gingrich, we were successful in getting a MSA pilot program started in 1996. Then, in 2003, House Ways and Means Chairman Bill Thomas successfully made HSAs part of the Medicare prescription drug bill, with the support of the Bush White House. Since that time, HSA plans have been the fastest-growing product in the health insurance marketplace.

In the early days, we went to great lengths to ensure that the effort was bipartisan. Democratic Sen. Tom Daschle, for example, was a co-sponsor of an early MSA bill, as was Democratic Sen. John Breaux. The original House bill was sponsored by Republican Bill Archer and Democrat Andy Jacob. Only with the passage of time did the concept become identified with the Republican Party, and that has been a matter of regret for me. Good ideas should stand or fall on their own merits. They should not be adopted or disowned, depending on the party of their advocates and opponents.

Inconsistent Public Policy

As Table 9.1 shows, today we have an array of account options—each with advantages and disadvantages when compared to each other. This reflects the complete lack of a public policy purpose. Why should the contribution limit be $3,100 for an HSA, $2,500 for an FSA, and unlimited for an HRA? Why should people be able to withdraw cash from the HSA, but not from the FSA or HRA? Why are FSAs and HRAs flexible, while HSAs are not?

Market Prices for Health Insurance

Some opportunities to reduce third-party insurance premiums by increasing the amount of self-insurance are reflected in Table 9.2, which shows the

Table 9.1. Types of Health Savings Accounts

	Is It Flexible?[1]	Reasonable Deposit Allowed?	Permits Cash Withdrawals?	Use It or Lose It?	Employees Can Contribute?
Flexible Spending Account (FSA)	Yes	No	No	Yes	Yes
Health Saving Account (HSA)	No	No	After Taxes & Penalties	No	Yes
Health Reimbursement Arrangement (HRA)	Yes	Yes	No[3]	Ultimately Yes[4]	No
Proposed Roth HSA	Yes	Yes[2]	Yes	No	Yes

1. Can it wrap around any health plan?
2. Allows deposit up to half of the cost of the health plan?
3. Personal income taxes apply plus 20 percent penalty before age 65.
4. Since funds can never be withdrawn in cash, this is a long-term use-it-or-lose-it account.

Table 9.2. UnitedHealthcare Premiums

Middle-Age Family of Four, Dallas, Texas	
$35 per Office Visit Plan	
Deductible	**Monthly Premium**
$1,000	$1,450
$2,500	$1,037
$5,000	$797
Across-the-Board Deductible Plans	
Deductible	**Monthly Premium**
$1,500	$1,067
$2,500	$773
$5,000	$705

Source: http://www.eHealthInsurance.com.

premiums charged by UnitedHealthcare for a middle-aged family of four in Dallas. Consider the first group of plans, with a $35 co-pay per office visit. The monthly premium for a family of four with a $1,000 per person deducible ($2,000 per family) is $1,450—or $17,400 per year.

In moving from a $1,000 annual deductible to a $2,500 deductible, the family is exposed to an additional risk of $1,500 per individual ($3,000 per family).[15] In return, they can save almost $5,000 a year in reduced premiums. In moving from a $1,000 to a $5,000 deductible, the family takes on an additional $4,000 of risk per individual (but no more than $8,000 per family). But the premium savings is nearly $8,000.

If you think about it, why would anyone buy the $1,000 deductible plan? Note: Dallas is a high-cost city, and the savings from higher deductibles may not be as large in other areas. Also, the savings from higher deductibles are generally smaller for group insurance.

The Ideal Medical Savings Account

As good as Health Savings Accounts are, the current structure is not ideal. Consider people in the 25 percent income tax bracket. If they take a dollar out of an HSA and spend it on other goods and services, they must pay 25 cents in taxes. If they are not yet 65 years of age, there will be another 20 percent penalty, leaving them with only 55 cents for other spending. For this person, a dollar's worth of healthcare trades against 55 cents of other goods and services.

As Mark Pauly and I explained in *Health Affairs* some time ago, an ideal account is one that does not distort incentives.[16] In the current period, people must choose between spending on healthcare and spending on other goods and services. When saving comes into play, people must choose between current and future healthcare and between future healthcare and future other goods and services. An ideal savings account is one that keeps all these choices on a level playing field with respect to the tax law.

I call this account a Roth Health Savings Account, or Roth HSA. The Roth account involves after-tax deposits and tax-free withdrawals. That means a dollar of healthcare always trades on a level playing field against every other use to which that dollar can be put—both in the current period and in future periods. This is the account that is most compatible with subsidizing health insurance with lump-sum tax credits—an approach advocated by Sen. John McCain[17] and incorporated in the Coburn/Burr/Ryan/Nunes health reform bill.[18] This type of account would be ideal for reforming Medicare.

What Both the Left and the Right Don't Understand about Health Savings Accounts

The biggest misconception among both friends and foes is that HSAs have their primary impact on the demand side of the market. The view leads to much unnecessary consternation over whether patients have the knowledge and the intelligence to make good decisions, whether they will forgo things they should have or purchase things they shouldn't have, and so on.

In fact, HSAs and their companion accounts are having their greatest impact on the supply side of the market. If everybody had first-dollar coverage, there would be no such thing as Rx.com (the first online mail order drug business) or MinuteClinic (the first walk-in clinic chain), or Teladoc (the first telephone consultation service), or Wal-Mart's $10 price for prescription drugs. Once money is in the hands of the patient, entrepreneurs on the supply side will try to compete for it by better meeting patient needs.

Needed Policy Changes

Although we will discuss a number of needed changes in public policy in this book, none is more important than giving patients more control over healthcare dollars.

A Simple Way to Control Healthcare Spending

There is something rather simple the federal government could do that would have enormous impact in controlling healthcare costs: Allow deposits to FSAs to roll over at year end and grow tax-free.[19]

Here's the backstory. Like HSAs and HRAs, Flexible Spending Accounts are set up by employers. But unlike those use-it-or-save-it accounts, FSA accounts are use-it-or-lose-it. Any account balance left at year end (or after an extra two and a half-month grace period) is forfeited.

Employers are allowed to make deposits to FSAs, and there is no limit to how much they can deposit, but few take advantage of this opportunity. Because of the use-it-or-lose-it feature, these plans are additions to, rather than integrated parts of, employer health plans. Because the deposits are tax-free, they almost certainly add to healthcare spending, as they are currently structured. They encourage employees to purchase designer eyeglasses with pre-tax dollars, for example, rather than purchase other goods and services with after-tax dollars. At year's end, employees will view almost any kind of permissible spending as preferable to forfeiting the money left in the account.

Why are these accounts use-it-or-lose-it? Apparently this feature is the result of a Treasury Department ruling, not the result of any act of Congress. So I believe the Treasury could undo this unfortunate rule without any new legislation.

What if these accounts could roll over and grow tax-free? Then employers and their employees would have a vehicle much better than any option currently available to them to control healthcare spending:

- FSAs could be combined with high deductibles, allowing employees to directly control, say, the first $2,500 of spending without all of the pointless restrictions that hamper the usefulness of HSAs.
- FSAs could be created to allow employees control of whole areas of spending, say, all preventive care and all diagnostic tests—services for which individual discretion is both possible and desirable.[20]

- FSAs could be created for the chronically ill[21]—allowing, say, diabetics or asthmatics to manage their own healthcare dollars, much as homebound, disabled Medicaid patients manage their own budgets in the Cash and Counseling Programs.[22]
- FSAs could be combined with value-based purchasing insurance plans[23]—where the insurer pays only for certain drugs, doctors, and hospitals but allows patients to add money out-of-pocket and make other choices—thus allowing the development of a real market for more expensive healthcare services.[24]

Currently, about 25 million people have an HSA or HRA account (roughly evenly split), and another 35 million people have FSAs. That means that over half the people with a health account have an incentive to spend rather than to save. If FSAs could roll over and become use-it-or-save-it accounts:

- There would be a huge immediate impact on the incentives of the 35 million current account holders if they could save for more valuable future healthcare spending.
- Employers across the country would consider integrating these accounts into their health plans, making employer contributions to them, and experimenting with some of the new health plan designs described here.
- Many of the companies that currently have HSA or HRA plans might discover the FSA approach better for controlling costs.

Another Simple Way to Control Healthcare Spending

Critics of consumer-directed healthcare often argue that patients are not knowledgeable enough and the market is not transparent enough for consumerism to work in healthcare. But a study by The Commonwealth Fund notes an international trend toward self-directed care (SDC), and it is focused on a most unlikely group of patients: the frail, the old, the disabled, and even the mentally ill.[25]

- In the United States, Medicaid Cash and Counseling Programs—under way for over a decade—allow homebound, disabled patients to manage their own budgets and choose services that meet their needs.

- In Germany and Austria, a cash payment is made to people eligible for long-term care—with few strings attached and little oversight on how the money is used.
- In England and the Netherlands, the disabled and the elderly manage budgets in a manner similar to Cash and Counseling in the United States.
- Also in this country, Florida and Texas have SDC programs for patients with serious mental illness, and the Veterans Administration has an SDC program operating in twenty states for long-term care and mental illness.

Moreover, it appears that we have barely scratched the surface in taking advantage of patient power opportunities. The greatest potential in this area is in the treatment of chronic illness.[26] Studies show that chronic patients can often manage their own care with results as good or better than traditional care; and if patients are going to manage their own care, it makes sense to allow them to manage the money that pays for that care.

The British National Health Service is already contributing to SDC budgets for muscular dystrophy, severe epilepsy, and chronic obstructive pulmonary disease. The NHS believes it is saving money in reduced hospital and nursing home costs. The NHS is also about to launch pilot programs that will include mental health, long-term chronic conditions, maternity care, substance abuse, children with complex health conditions, and end-of-life care.

Other countries are moving in a similar direction. The fastest-growing use of personal budgets in the Netherlands is for families with children who have attention-deficit hyperactivity disorder, autism, and other types of serious emotional disturbances. The advantages of empowering patients and families in this way are straightforward: lower costs, higher quality care, and higher patient satisfaction.

Lower Costs

In Germany, long-term care patients who agree to manage their own budgets spend 50 percent less than what would have been spent in a normal plan. In the Netherlands, spending is 30 percent less. In England, long-term care services purchased by individuals cost from 20 percent to 40 percent less than equivalent services purchased by local governments. In the Arkansas Cash and Counseling Program, participants were given more than what Medicaid would have spent, but an 18 percent reduction in nursing home use reduced Medicaid's overall costs.

Higher Quality

In Arkansas, Cash and Counseling patients got 100 percent of their authorized hours of personal care, compared to only 70 percent for those in traditional Medicaid. In New Jersey, "mentally ill adults with physical disabilities . . . were less likely to fall, have respiratory infections, develop bed sores, or spend a night in a hospital or a nursing home if they were directing their own personal care services."

Overall, SDC participants get more preventive care; and as a result, "make significantly less use of crisis stabilization and crisis support." One reason is that SDC gives participants access to a broader range of services. "In Texas . . . [where] Medicaid will not cover routine counseling . . . SDC is providing individuals access to counseling using funds from their individual budgets."

Higher Satisfaction

In the Netherlands, close to 80 percent of disabled and elderly participants who were eligible for long-term care services and opted for a personal budget had a positive assessment of the services they received, compared with less than 40 percent in traditional care. In England, 79 percent of those who employ a personal assistant were very satisfied with the care and support they received, compared to only 26 percent in traditional care. In the United States, satisfaction rates in the Cash and Counseling programs have hovered in the high 90 percentiles.

A Third Simple Way of Controlling Healthcare Spending

Deductibles and co-payments are inefficient tools for giving patients proper incentives with respect to healthcare spending.[27] The problem with a deductible is that although the incentives are ideal as long as spending is below it, they become completely perverse once you reach it. That is, below the deductible, every dollar you spend is yours, but above the deductible, every dollar you spend belongs to someone else, except for your co-payments.

The problem with co-payments is that the incentives are too weak. A 20 percent co-insurance requires you to spend 20 cents out of pocket every time you spend a dollar on healthcare. That means you have an incentive to spend until healthcare is worth 20 cents on the dollar to you. That's hardly a formula for prudent buying.

Here is my health insurance plan with ideal incentives, but no deductibles or co-insurance. First, I would carve out entire areas of spending that are entirely the patient's responsibility and are purchased from an HSA. This would include any area where it is both appropriate and possible for patients to assume complete control. I would include in this category almost all primary care, most diagnostic tests, and most outpatient care.

With respect to cancer, for example, when you are searching for cancer (screenings), the patient pays. After you find cancer, the plan takes over financial responsibility. This allows people to make their own decisions about all the contradictory information we seem to get daily about who should be screened, when, and how often. People would be free to make their own decisions and pay the full cost (or reap the full benefits) of the decisions they make.

Second, I would put people with chronic conditions in a separate category, along the lines suggested above.

The third important element of ideal health insurance is what I originally called the *casualty insurance model.* It is consistent with what is today more frequently called *value-based purchasing.* This idea is especially important for expensive drugs and expensive procedures. It works like this.

The health plan fixes what it will cover and how much it will pay, following established criteria and procedures. The insured is free to purchase a different drug, say, or go to an out-of-network doctor or facility. If they do so, however, they must pay the full marginal cost of the choice.

10

Liberating Institutions

TO CONFRONT AMERICA'S healthcare crisis, we do not need more spending, more regulations, or more bureaucracy. We do need to liberate all Americans, including every doctor and every patient, so that they can use their intelligence, creativity, and innovative abilities to make the changes needed to create access to low-cost, high-quality healthcare. Here are 10 steps to achieve these goals.

Freeing the Doctor

Of all the people in the healthcare system, none is more central than the physician. Fundamental reform that lowers costs, raises quality, and improves access to care is almost inconceivable without physicians leading and directing the changes. Yet of all the actors in modern healthcare, none are more trapped than our nation's doctors. Let's consider just a few of the ways your doctor is constrained, unlike any other professional.[1]

Sometime in the early part of the last century, all the other professionals in our society—lawyers, accountants, architects, engineers, and so on—discovered the telephone. It's a handy device. Ideal for communicating with clients. Yet, telephone consultations are not on Medicare's list of about 7,500 tasks it pays physicians to perform. (At least, it's not there in a way that makes telephone consultations practical.) Private insurance tends to pay the way Medicare pays. So do most employers.

Sometime toward the end of the last century, all the other professionals discovered email. In some ways, it's even better than the phone. But reading and responding to emails doesn't make Medicare's list in a practical way, either.[2]

At a time when doctors feel that third-party payers are squeezing their fees from every direction, most are going to try to minimize their non-billable time. Because patients cannot conveniently use modern media to consult with physicians, they make unnecessary office visits. The result is more rationing by waiting at the doctor's office, which imposes disproportionate costs on chronic patients who need more contact with physicians. This might be one reason why so many are not getting what they most need from primary care physicians and what is most likely to prevent more costly problems later on: prescription drugs.[3]

The ability to consult with doctors by phone or email could be a boon to chronic care. Face-to-face meetings with physicians would be less frequent, especially if patients learned how to monitor their own conditions and manage their own care.

Other doctor tasks that might be helpful—but are not compensated by Medicare and other insurers—are providing advice about the cost of brand-name drugs versus generic and therapeutic substitutes as well as over-the-counter alternatives. Information about comparative prices and how patients can save money through smart shopping would be a valuable service, and who would be in a better position to provide it than the physician? In addition, numerous studies have shown that chronic patients—people with diabetes or asthma, for example—can often manage their own care, with lower costs and as good or better health outcomes than with traditional care, reducing the number of trips they make to the emergency room. ER doctors could save themselves and future doctors a lot of additional time and trouble if they took the time to educate the mother of a diabetic or asthmatic child about how to monitor and manage the child's healthcare. But time spent on such education is generally not billable.

Escaping the Trap

What is the common denominator for all of these problems? Unlike other professionals, doctors are not free to repackage and reprice their services in ways they believe will best help their patients. Instead, third-party payer bureaucracies tell them what tasks they will get paid for performing and how much they will be paid to charge. Doctors are the least free of any professional we deal with. Yet these unfree actors are directing one-fifth of all consumer spending.

By now readers will be familiar with what I regard as the essential way out of this trap: Medicare should be willing to pay for innovative improvements that save taxpayers money. And doctors and hospitals should be able to repackage and reprice their services (the way other professionals do), provided that the total cost to government does not increase and the quality of care does not decrease. This change in Medicare would almost certainly be followed by similar changes in the private sector.

Freeing the Patient

Many patients have difficulty seeing primary care physicians. All too often, they turn to hospital emergency rooms, where there are long waits, and the cost of care is high. Part of the reason is that third-party payer bureaucracies decide what services patients can obtain from doctors and what doctors will be paid for each. To correct this problem, patients should be able to purchase services not paid for by traditional health insurance, including telephone and email consultations and patient education services. This can be done by allowing them to manage more of their own healthcare dollars in a completely flexible Health Savings Account.

The biggest change brought about by giving patients direct control over healthcare dollars is not on the demand side of the market. It's on the supply side. Here are some examples of healthcare markets dominated by patients paying out-of-pocket for services:

Cosmetic Surgery[4]

Cosmetic surgery is rarely covered by insurance. Because providers know their patients must pay out of pocket and are price-sensitive, patients can typically (1) find a package price in advance covering all services and facilities, (2) compare prices prior to surgery, and (3) pay a price that has been falling over time in real terms—despite a huge increase in volume and considerable technical innovation (which is blamed for increasing costs for every other type of surgery).

Laser Eye Surgery[5]

Competition is also holding prices in check for vision correction surgery, and laser surgeons compete on quality as well. Recent quality improvements include more accurate correction, faster healing, fewer side effects, and an expanded range of patients and conditions that can be treated. For instance, rather than traditional LASIK surgery, patients can pay slightly more per eye for the newer, Wavefront-guided LASIK.

Laboratory and Diagnostic Testing[6]

Patients can order their own blood tests without a doctor's appointment and compare prices at different diagnostic testing facilities. Prices are 50 percent to 80 percent lower than identical tests performed in a hospital setting. These services lower patients' time costs as well as money costs. In many cases, the results are available online within 24 to 48 hours.

Price Competition for Drugs[7]

Wal-Mart became the first nationwide retailer to compete aggressively for buyers of generic drugs by charging a low, uniform price—$10 for a ninety-day supply. In many cases, patients with drug coverage have found the cash price at Wal-Mart is lower than their health plan's co-pay at conventional pharmacies. Other chain drugstores have responded with their own pricing strategies.

Price Competition for Drugs over the Internet[8]

Rx.com was the first mail-order pharmacy to compete online in a national market for drugs. To compete with local pharmacies, they offer lower costs and more convenient service, including free home delivery. They also compete on quality. For instance, high-volume mail-order pharmacies have much lower dispensing error rates than conventional pharmacies. Online mail-order pharmacies have thrived on the business model of improved quality, lower cost, and greater convenience.

Patient Education for Drugs as a Product[9]

DestinationRx.com is a pharmacy benefits management company. In addition to operating an online mail-order drug delivery service, it also offers a Web site to help patients identify low-cost therapeutic substitutes for the drugs they currently take. In addition, the firm is partnering with Safeway supermarkets to install drug comparison kiosks in store pharmacies.

Retail Clinics[10]

Walk-in clinics in shopping malls and drugstores offer primary care services. They compete by offering low costs in terms of both time and money. To ensure a consistent level of quality, nurse practitioners follow computerized protocols, and electronic medical records are a natural adjunct of that process. Further, once such a system is in place, electronic prescriptions are a straightforward next step, and electronic prescribing allows the use of error-reducing software. One study found MinuteClinics follow treatment guidelines better than traditional medical practices.[11]

Telephone-Based Practices[12]

Teladoc now has 2 million customers paying for a telephone consultation—access to a doctor at any time of day from any location. And because each on-call physician needs access to patients' medical histories (and the treatment decisions of previous physicians), personal and portable electronic medical records are a necessary part of the company's business model. The physicians prescribe drugs electronically—facilitating the use of safety-enhancing software that checks for harmful interactions.

Concierge Medical Practices[13]

Some innovative physicians are rebundling and repricing medical services in ways that are not possible under third-party insurance. For a fixed monthly fee, they offer same-day or next-day appointments, help in scheduling diagnostic tests and appointments with specialists, help in negotiating prices and fees, and other services. Many will meet their patients at the emergency room to ensure prompt service.

Concierge physicians tend to relate to their patients in much the same way lawyers, accountants, engineers, and other professionals interact with their clients—including phone calls, email consultations, and convenient Web- based services.

Concierge Services for Patients with High Deductibles

You don't actually have to leave your health insurance plan to take advantage of concierge doctor services. Compass of Dallas is a firm that specializes in helping people with high-deductible insurance wade through the complexities of the medical marketplace. For example, the company "will search for the least expensive hospital or facility for a given procedure, find doctors who best suit a patient's wants and needs, screen for best outcomes and the fewest lawsuits, set up appointments, make sense of bills and challenge questionable ones."

"If we find mistakes, which by the way happens quite a bit, we can go back and speak the same coding language with the doctor's office or hospital and say, 'Let's re-evaluate this and see if it needs to be coded differently and resubmitted,'" says Eric Bricker, the company's CEO. "We might find three in-network primary care physicians who take same-day or next-day appointments and are within their geographic area."[14]

Freeing the Employee

For the working age population, one of the biggest problems in the US healthcare system is that health insurance is not portable. In general, when you leave your employer, you must eventually lose the health insurance plan your employer was providing. Almost all the problems people have with pre-existing conditions arise because of a transition from employer-provided insurance to individually purchased insurance. And those problems arise because the employee doesn't own employer-purchased insurance.

So if everyone wants portable insurance, why don't we have it? First, the federal tax law generously subsidizes employer-provided insurance, but it offers very little tax relief to those who must purchase insurance on their own.

BETTER SOLUTIONS FOR PRE-EXISTING CONDITIONS

Here are ten ways to deal with the problem of pre-existing conditions that give people good incentives instead of perverse incentives.[15]

Encourage Portable Insurance. In almost every state, employers are not allowed to buy the kind of insurance employees own and can take with them from job to job and in and out of the labor market.[16] That prohibition needs to be rescinded. Most of the time, the problem of pre-existing conditions arises precisely because health insurance isn't portable.

Allow Special Health Savings Accounts for the Chronically Ill. Cash and Counseling pilot programs in Medicaid are under way in more than half the states.[17] Homebound, disabled patients manage their own budgets and hire and fire those who provide them with services. Satisfaction rates are in the mid-90 percentile (virtually unheard of in any health plan anywhere in the world).

Allow Special Needs Health Insurance. Instead of requiring insurers to be all things to all people, we should allow plans to specialize in treating one or more chronic conditions.[18] Plans could specialize, for example, in diabetic care, heart care, or cancer care, and they would be able to charge a market price (say, to employers, other insurers, and even risk pools), and price and quality competition should be encouraged.

Allow Health Status Insurance. To facilitate the market for chronic illness insurance, we should encourage two kinds of insurance: Standard insurance would cover the health needs of people during the insurance period, while health status insurance would pay future premium increases people face if they have a change in health status and then try to switch to another health plan.[19] You can think of this as a way of insuring against the emergence of a pre-existing condition.

Allow Self-Insurance for Changes in Health Status. The tax law allows employers to pay for current-period medical expenses with untaxed dollars. But there is no similar opportunity for either employers or employees to save for a future change in health status—one that will generate substantial increases in medical costs. Clearly, people need the ability to engage in contingency savings—a Health Savings Account for future, rather than current, medical costs.

Give Individual Buyers the Same Tax Break Employees Get. Most people who have a problem with pre-existing conditions are trying to buy insurance in the individual market. Yet, unless they are self-employed, they get virtually no tax relief, and even the self-employed are penalized vis-à-vis employer-provided insurance. All insurance should get the same tax relief regardless of where it is obtained, and individuals should get the same tax relief, regardless of how they obtain it. This would encourage people to be continuously insured—and increase the likelihood that they will be insured when a health condition arises.

Allow Providers to Repackage and Reprice Their Services Under Medicare and Medicaid. We should encourage providers to create innovative solutions to the care of diabetes, asthma, cancer, heart disease, and other chronic health issues. Along these lines, providers should be able to offer a different bundle of services and be paid in a different way so long as they reduce the government's overall cost and provide a higher quality of care.

Allow Access to Mandate-Free Insurance. Studies show that as many as one out of four uninsured Americans—most of them healthy—have been priced out of the market for health insurance by cost-increasing, mandated benefits.[20] At the same time, however, these mandates raise premiums for the chronically ill and divert dollars away from their care. There is no reason a diabetic should have to pay for other peoples' in vitro fertilization, naturopathy, acupuncture, or marriage counseling, in order to obtain diabetic care.

Create a National Market for Health Insurance. More competition, especially among the special needs insurers, would be a huge benefit for the chronically ill. Being able to buy insurance across state lines would encourage that competition.

Encourage Post-Retirement Health Insurance. If the past is a guide, more than 80 percent of the 78 million baby boomers will retire before they become eligible for Medicare. This group has the greatest potential for denial of health insurance because of pre-existing conditions. Fortunately, one out of every three baby boomers has a promise of post-retirement healthcare. However, two out of three do not, and even for those who have a commitment, almost none of the promises are funded. A solution: give post-retirement health insurance the same tax encouragement as active-worker insurance and allow pre-retirement insurance to be portable.

Employer-paid premiums avoid federal income taxes, federal payroll taxes (FICA), and state and local income taxes as well. But individuals tend to get none of these tax benefits when they pay premiums out of their own pockets.

Even with these discriminatory tax subsidies, insurance could still be portable if employers bought individually owned insurance rather than group insurance for their employees. But here is the second problem. It is illegal in almost every state for employers to use pre-tax dollars to purchase individually owned insurance that travels with the employee from job to job, as well as in and out of the labor market.

Clearly, both state and federal laws need to change. We need to move in the opposite direction—making it as easy as possible for employees to obtain portable health insurance.

The case for portability is strong and goes far beyond the fact that most people want it. First, portability allows a long-lasting relationship with a health plan, which in turn allows a long-lasting relationship with providers of care. This means that people who switch jobs frequently can still have continuity of care—which is usually a prerequisite for high-quality care. Second, people who have portable insurance (as well as portable retirement plans and other benefits) will not be locked into jobs solely because of the nonportable nature of their benefits. Portable benefits are consistent with a mobile labor market, which is a necessary component of a dynamic, competitive economy. Finally, a system of portable benefits is one in which the employer's role is financial, rather than administrative. Employers, therefore, can specialize in what they do best, leaving health insurance to the insurance firms.

Freeing the Employer

When health insurance is company-specific, the employer is necessarily involved in the management and administration of every employee's healthcare. Manufacturers of automobiles, for example, find that they are in the health insurance business as well as the car manufacturing business. Ditto for the makers of home appliances, electronic equipment, and every other good or service in our economy. Most employers, and certainly all small-business owners, would prefer not to be in the health insurance business, however. In a world of portable insurance, they would not have to be.

Rather than offering health insurance as a defined benefit, employers should be able to offer health insurance as a defined contribution. They would make a monetary contribution to the health insurance premiums of each employee, each pay period. The 401(k) retirement plan is a model. New employees would know not only their salary, but also how much the employer is willing to pay toward the cost of insurance. In this way, the employer's role in health insurance is purely financial. In fact, employers would have no more involvement in the employee's health plans than they have in their employee's 401(k) portfolio.

Freeing the Nontraditional Workplace

If a new employee has coverage under a spouse's health plan, he or she doesn't need duplicate coverage. But the laws governing the workplace do not allow the employer to pay higher wages instead.[21] On the other hand, a part-time employee might be willing to accept lower wages in return for the opportunity to enroll in the employer's health plan. Yet, the law does not allow that either.

The institutional structure of our tax system and our employee benefits system were formed decades ago when lawmakers had a simple view of how life would be lived: There would be a full-time worker husband and a homemaker wife who, if she entered the labor market at all, would do so only temporarily. If this is the way you live your life, these institutions will still work pretty well for you. But many people don't these days.

To bring our labor market institutions into the 21st century, employers should be free to give employees the option to choose between nontaxed benefits and taxable wages, where appropriate.

Freeing the Uninsured

Most uninsured people do not have access to employer-provided health insurance, purchased with pre-tax dollars. If they obtain insurance at all, they must buy it with after-tax dollars, effectively doubling the after-tax price for middle-income families. The answer: people who must purchase their own insurance should receive the same tax relief as employees who obtain insurance at work.

Freeing the Kids

During the first year of the Obama administration, Congress voted to expand the state Children's Health Insurance Plan to cover 4 million additional children. Yet, in doing so, Congress caused up to half of those children to lose their private coverage, as parents stopped paying premiums for private coverage to take advantage of insurance they could get for free, according to the Congressional Budget Office.[22]

Why does that matter? One reason is that on their private insurance plan, these children could see almost any doctor in their community and go to almost any healthcare facility. However, under CHIP, children have access to fewer doctors and medical facilities than children in private plans. Also, doctors spend more time with privately insured children.[23]

These incentives should be reversed. CHIP money should be used to encourage parents to enroll their children in their employer's plan or other private plans of the parents' choosing.

Freeing the Parents

Under the current system, a child could be enrolled in CHIP, a mother could be enrolled in Medicaid, and a father could be enrolled in an employer's plan. However, medical outcomes are likely to be better with a single insurer with a single network of providers. The answer: if Medicaid and CHIP funds were available to subsidize private health insurance, all family members could enroll in the same health plan. They would be able to see the same doctors and enter the same facilities.

Freeing the Chronically Ill

By some estimates, more than three-quarters of US healthcare spending is for patients with chronic conditions.[24] Care is often delivered in discrete, disjointed, and disconnected ways that waste money. The most efficient form of therapy (drugs) is substantially underutilized.[25] And many chronic patients are not receiving care at all.[26]

In a normal market, entrepreneurs would regard this situation as a huge opportunity. If the market for medical care were allowed to operate like other markets, providers would find it in their self-interest to solve other people's problems. The more problems they solved and the more thoroughly they solved them, the more take-home pay they would realize. Without in any way discouraging altruism, an unfettered market for care would harness the pursuit of financial self-interest in the cause of lower cost, higher quality, more accessible care.

The problem with the current system is that neither employers nor sellers of group insurance are allowed to adjust an individual's premiums to reflect higher expected healthcare costs. This encourages insurers to seek the healthy and avoid the sick before enrollment. After enrollment, insurers have an incentive to overprovide care to the healthy and underprovide to the sick.

These incentives need to be reversed. In the Medicare Advantage program, the government pays higher premiums for seniors with more expensive health needs. This encourages insurance companies to create specialized plans—especially for chronic illnesses—that compete with each other.

Chronic patients also need to be able to manage more of their healthcare dollars directly. For example, Cash and Counsel programs in many states allow homebound, disabled Medicaid patients to hire and fire the vendors who provide them with services.[27] Patient satisfaction in these programs is above 90 percent.

Freeing the Retirees

There are 78 million baby boomers, and a very large number of them have retirement on their minds. If the past is a guide, more than 80 percent of them will retire before they become eligible for Medicare (at age 65). Although about one-third of US workers have a promise of postretirement healthcare from an employer, almost none of these promises are funded, and as in the case of the automobile companies, they may not be completely honored.

As a result, millions of retirees will find themselves buying their own insurance in the individual market. There they will face some unpleasant realities, which for many of them may come as a shock:

- Whereas employers typically pay about 75 percent of the premium at work, these retirees will have to pay 100 percent of the premium out of their own pockets.

- Whereas the share of premium paid by employees tends to be the same—regardless of age—individual insurance premiums for, say, a 60 year old are often five or six times higher than for a 20 year old.
- Whereas employers are forced to accept employees into their health plans and charge the same premiums regardless of health status, people in the individual market typically face medical underwriting. They may be charged higher premiums because of a health condition; they may face exclusions or be denied coverage altogether. If they are forced into a risk pool, they may face waiting periods as well as higher premiums.

In general, tax law, labor law, and employee benefits law favor the active employee and discriminate against the retiree. For example, here are three public policy barriers that will stand between early retirees and affordable health insurance:

- Employers cannot make premium contributions to the individually owned insurance of their retirees with untaxed dollars.
- Retirees must pay their premiums with after-tax dollars.
- There is no easy way for employers and employees to save (tax-free) for future medical expenses—including postretirement expenses.

Employer promises of postretirement healthcare are usually an all-or-nothing proposition. That is, employers can keep their retirees in their group insurance plan—paying expenses with pre-tax dollars—or they can do nothing. It's hard to be in between. If an employer cannot afford, say, $12,000 for family coverage for a retiree, the employer cannot split the difference and contribute $6,000 to the employee's individually owned insurance. Such a contribution would be treated as taxable income.

The obvious solutions to these problems are:[28] (1) allow employers to make contributions (say, to a retiree's Health Savings Account); (2) allow retirees to pay their share of premiums with pre-tax dollars; and (3) allow active employees and their employers to save tax-free—knowing that they will face the problem of postretirement care.

11

Designing Ideal Health Insurance

THE MODERN ERA has inherited two models of health insurance: the fee-for-service model and the HMO model. Both models create perverse incentives for patients and their doctors.

Virtually all recent variations on these two models are attempts to ameliorate and control those perverse incentives—usually by introducing features that have a new set of perverse incentives. It is probably no exaggeration to say that the evolution of health insurance is one of cascading perversions, with each new wave of design trying to overcome the bad outcomes of the previous designs.

Under the fee-for-service model, insurance is designed to pay a separate fee for each service rendered, with patients responsible for some portion of the fee—in the form of a deductible, coinsurance or co-payment amount. Under the HMO model, providers receive a fixed fee, irrespective of the amount of service rendered.

When healthcare is perceived as free (the HMO model), patients will have an incentive to consume it until its value at the margin approaches zero. Since the cost of care is well above zero, this implies that unconstrained patients will consume healthcare resources very wastefully. The deductibles and co-insurance that are features of a typical fee-for-service plan are only a small improvement on these distorted incentives. If patients pay 20 percent of the bill, for example, their incentive is to consume care until its value at the margin is worth only 20 cents on the dollar.

On the provider side, the fee-for-service model encourages overprovision—since more service results in higher income for the doctor, hospital or other supplier of care. The HMO model, by contrast, encourages underprovision, since any portion of the fixed fee that is not spent on medical care is available to the providers as take home pay or some other form of compensation.

Readers may wonder why either model was ever found appealing to anyone in the past. The short answer is that both models are the product of the technocratic approach to healthcare I discussed in Chapter 3. Both, in other words, ignore economic incentives.

Both models, for example, implicitly assume that (1) the amount of sickness is limited and largely outside the control of the insured, (2) methods of treating illness are limited and well defined, and (3) because of patient ignorance and asymmetry of information, treatment decisions will always be filtered by physicians, who will make decisions based on their own knowledge and experience or clinical practice guidelines. In this way, both models implicitly assume—one way or another—that economic incentives can be ignored.

Although the HMO model is often viewed as the more contemporary, it is actually less compatible with the changes the medical marketplace is undergoing. The traditional HMO model is fundamentally based on patient ignorance. The basic idea is a simple one: make healthcare free at the point of consumption and control costs by having physicians ration care, eliminating options that are judged "unnecessary" or at least not "cost effective."

But this model works only as long as patients are willing to accept their doctor's opinion. And that only works as long as patients are unaware of other (possibly more expensive) options.

However, an explosion of technological innovation and the rapid diffusion of knowledge about the potential of medical science to diagnose and treat disease have rendered these assumptions obsolete.

We could spend our entire gross domestic product on healthcare in useful ways. In fact, we could probably spend the entire GDP on diagnostic tests alone—without ever treating a real disease. The new reality is that patients are becoming as informed as their doctors—not about how to practice medicine, but about how the practice of medicine can benefit them. Combine the potential of modern medicine to benefit patients with a general awareness of these benefits and zero out-of-pocket payments, and the HMO model is simply courting disaster. The fee-for-service model is only a slight improvement.

Some believe that managed care and practice guidelines can solve these problems. Imagine grocery insurance that allows you to buy all the groceries you need; but as you stroll down the supermarket aisle, you are confronted with a team of bureaucrats, prepared to argue over your every purchase. Would anyone want to buy such a policy? Traditional health insurance isn't designed to work much better.

Accordingly, I propose a new approach. It combines an old concept, casualty insurance, with two relatively new concepts: universal Health Savings Accounts (to control demand) and a proliferation of centers of excellence or "focused factories" (to control supply). I believe this is the approach that would naturally emerge if we relied on markets, rather than regulators, to solve our problems.

Designing an Ideal Health Insurance Plan[1]

Let's begin by wiping the slate clean. Imagine you could get together with 999 other people and create an insurance plan just for 1,000 people. The 1,000 people are not alike. Some are old; some are young. Some are male; some are female. Some are in good health; some are not. Given these and other differences, how can you design a plan that all would want to join?

In answering this question, forget the normal insurance industry bureaucracy. Forget state and federal regulations. Forget federal tax law. Forget everything else that would pose an artificial impediment to achieving a unanimous agreement. You're on your own. You must design a plan that will come closest to meeting your needs and those of your colleagues. What follows is a discussion of some inevitable problems and some proposed solutions. I hope this thought experiment will point to how insurance markets would evolve if left free to do so.[2]

Terms of Entry

One of the first decisions you must make is what premiums should be charged to people when they join the insurance pool. No matter what benefits you decide to include in the plan, you have to collect enough premiums to cover all the costs. So how much should each person pay? I have a suggestion that not only will solve this problem, but also will avoid many others. In fact, failure to follow my suggestion on this issue will virtually guarantee that your group will not agree on anything else. My suggestion is this: Each person should pay a premium equal to the expected healthcare costs he or she adds to the 1,000-person pool. If individual A will add $1,000, the right premium for A is $1,000. If B's expected costs are $5,000, B should pay $5,000. If C's expected costs are $10,000, C should pay $10,000.[3]

What if the premium is so high for some people that they cannot afford to pay it? Then either they will be left out of the pool, or others must make a charitable contribution on their behalf. Since all agreements are voluntary in this imagined scenario, coercion is not an option. As we have seen, politicians usually try to solve the problem by keeping the premium artificially low for people with high healthcare costs. If some people are undercharged, however, others must be overcharged.

People who are overcharged will want less coverage than they otherwise would, and those who are undercharged will want more. If we want people to make economically rational decisions, they must be charged a premium that makes the expected benefit of their additional coverage equal to its expected cost.

Terms of Renewal

At the end of an insurance period of, say, one year, on what terms should people be allowed to renew? Should those whose health has deteriorated be charged more? Should people whose health has improved be charged less?

Insurance can be compared to gambling. Our decision to charge each entrant in the pool a premium equal to his or her expected costs makes the gamble a fair bet for all. But changing premiums based on changes in health status would be like changing the rules after throwing the dice. It would defeat the purpose of insurance, which is to transfer risk to others. Therefore, a reasonable rule is to raise or lower everyone's premium at renewal time, based on whether the whole group's costs have been more or less than expected. Those who got sick and generated high medical costs after joining the pool would not be penalized and would get the full value of the insurance.

Such a rule is broadly characteristic of the market for individual insurance. At the time of initial enrollment, people may be charged different premiums, based on age, sex, and perhaps health status. But once in a plan, no one can be expelled from it or charged an extra premium because their health deteriorates.

Renewal is guaranteed, and if premiums are increased, they must be increased proportionately for everyone.

The small-group market now operates quite differently in most states. A firm's premiums are readjusted annually, based not on the experience of the larger group with which the firm's employees have been pooled, but on the firm's employees' own experience over the previous year. In effect, it's as though every firm's employees were kicked out of the pool at the end of the year and allowed to reenter only if they pay new premiums based on the changes in their expected health costs. Subject to regulatory constraints, in the small-group market people can buy insurance only one year at a time. If this practice applied to life insurance, everyone's premium would be reassessed annually, and rates for those diagnosed with cancer or AIDS during the previous year would be astronomical. Such a practice would virtually destroy the market for life insurance.[4] Small wonder that small group health insurance markets are in perpetual crisis.

Third-Party Insurance Versus Self-Insurance

The next decision for our hypothetical group of 1,000 is how to allocate financial responsibility. Federal law now allows deposits to Health Savings Accounts to receive the same tax advantage as employer-paid premiums. But current law is not nearly as flexible as it needs to be.

In our hypothetical exercise, let us imagine that federal tax law is completely neutral between payments for insurance premiums (third-party insurance) and deposits to Health Savings Accounts (self-insurance). Which services would we want people to pay for directly from their HSA accounts, and which ones would we want to cover out of the general insurance pool? That is, what medical costs would we want the group as a whole to pay for, and which ones would we want people to cover from their own resources?

Any time people transfer their resources to an insurance pool, there are two negative consequences (increased cost, at least for the group as a whole, and decreased autonomy) and one positive (reduced risk). The problem is to assure that the reduction in risk is worth the extra premium we must pay to obtain it. Our imaginary insurance pool faces the same problems as every other insurance scheme. Any time insurance pays a medical bill, the incentives of the patient are distorted. All of us tend to overconsume when someone else is paying the bill, and this tendency raises costs. To counteract the tendency, we could consider some of the techniques of managed care, but that will restrict our choices, reduce our autonomy, and perhaps reduce the quality of the care we get. Even if the quality is not diminished, administering the restrictions will be costly.

Thus, no matter how well the plan is designed, medical care for the group as a whole will cost more than the sum of everyone's bills if individuals simply purchased the same care on their own. Presumably, the higher costs are worthwhile if we enjoy enough reduction in risk. But at what point does the price we're paying for risk reduction become too high? Specifically, when is it worthwhile to transfer risk to a pool, and when does it make better sense to self-insure by putting funds into an account we own and control? Three general questions can help us arrive at an answer:

1. Is the medical service to be purchased prompted by a risky event or by an individual preference?
2. Is the price of transferring risk to a third party high or low?
3. Does the failure to obtain a service or the purchase of an inappropriate service potentially create costs for others in the pool?

The first question relates to the terms under which people obtain healthcare services. People differ in their attitudes toward medical care. They also differ in their levels of aversion to risk. Take diagnostic tests for the detection of cancer. As noted, the more frequent the tests, the higher the cost. But medical science offers varying evidence on how frequent such exams should be, making this a subject of continuing controversy.[5] That means that decisions about diagnostic tests often reflect a personal value judgment, and people's values differ. In general, when a test is not prompted by a risky event or some other indication, it should be a matter of individual preference.

As a general rule, the more that expenditures depend on personal choices rather than external events, the more appropriate self-insurance becomes. This consideration suggests we should encourage individuals to purchase directly most diagnostic tests, most forms of preventive medicine and most primary care.

The second question reinforces this conclusion. Transferring the risk of cancer treatment to an insurance pool is relatively low-cost. For each dollar of exposure transferred, the extra premium is only a few pennies. On the other hand, transferring diagnostic testing to an insurance pool is relatively high-cost. For each dollar of exposure transferred, the extra premium is a large part of a dollar. So the payoff for using insurance to cover cancer treatment is high, while the payoff for covering cancer detection is low.

The third question is whether the medical consequences of one's decision will generate costs for other members of the pool. Take immunization for childhood diseases. Studies show that these procedures pay for themselves by avoiding future healthcare costs that are greater than the costs of the vaccinations.[6] This implies that members of an insurance pool have an economic self-interest in seeing that all children covered by the pool are vaccinated. It may make economic sense for the pool to pay for vaccinations, thereby incurring more cost than self-pay would generate, or to require that members obtain them, thereby reducing autonomy.

Closely related to the problem created by the failure to obtain a desirable service is the problem created by the purchase of the wrong service. Suppose our plan has a $3,000 deductible, and a member is diagnosed with cancer. Under this arrangement, the patient would pay the first $3,000 of treatment costs and presumably would make his or her own decisions about how to spend that sum. But that $3,000 of decision making could have a large impact on later treatment costs, and bad decisions early on could generate larger subsequent costs for the group. Such considerations may create a presumption in favor of paying for all treatment costs from the pool in cases where the entire treatment regime promises to be expensive.[7]

Table 11.1 summarizes the case for a division between individual payment for medical services and third-party payment. Third-party payment for every medical service is potentially very wasteful. Such waste can be controlled only by invasive, expensive third-party oversight of individual medical care consumption. Such control necessarily interferes in the doctor-patient relationship. Some people may prefer this sacrifice of autonomy, and that may explain why there has always been a market for the traditional HMO. But many people will prefer self-pay and self-control, especially where no real reduction in financial risk is achieved by transferring control to a third-party payer.

Figure 11.1 shows that even after taking into account each of the general rules in Table 11.1, some health services may not neatly fit into unambiguous "self-pay" or "third-party pay" categories. Ideal health plans might have considerable

Table 11.1. General Rules

Individual Choice	Collective Choice
1. No risky medical event.	1. Risky medical event.
2. Price of third-party insurance is high.	2. Price of third-party insurance is low.
3. Exercise of choice creates no externalities.	3. Exercise of choice creates risks for others.

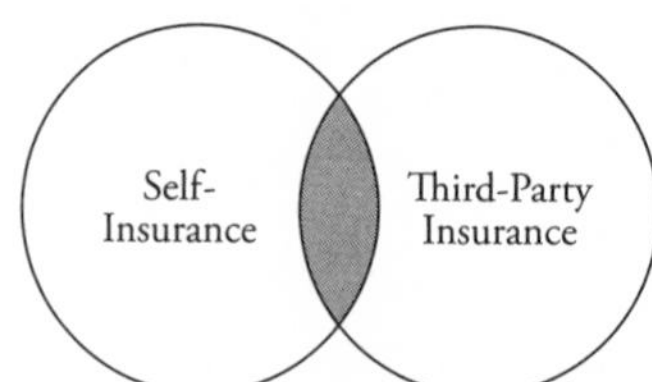

Figure 11.1. Appropriate Division of Financial Responsibility

discretion, therefore, and how they exercise it would depend on their members' preferences. What is important is to recognize that in the ideal insurance arrangement, some decisions will be individual while others will be collective.

Financing Mechanism for Self-Insurance: HSAs

A common objection to individual control is that people will not always make wise decisions. But in our imaginary pool, everyone must voluntarily agree to the design of the plan, so we cannot entirely escape individual choice and preference. In addition, even with the most comprehensive coverage, individuals must make decisions about when to see a doctor and whether to purchase a nonprescription drug. So even if a patient wanted to turn all decisions over to someone else, that would be impossible. A more sophisticated objection to self-paid healthcare is that most medical expenditures are unexpected and are hard for people living from paycheck-to-paycheck to incorporate into a budget.

One answer to this objection is the Health Savings Account. Under a standard practice, many employers make monthly deposits to accounts from which their employees can pay expenses not covered by the employer's health plan. Money not spent for medical care must remain in the account until the end of the insurance period, usually one year, after which the employee can withdraw it and use it for other purposes—after payment of taxes and (before age 65) a 20 percent penalty.[8] HSAs make individual self-insurance workable for families who otherwise might find direct payment too burdensome. But how should such accounts be designed in conjunction with third-party insurance coverage?

Implications for HSA Design

The left side of Figure 11.2 illustrates the design of HSAs in employer plans as mandated by federal law.[9] In this example, the plan pays all costs above a deductible of, say, $3,000. The HSA deposit in this example is $2,000. Thus, the employee pays the first $2,000 of medical expenses from the HSA and the next $1,000 is paid out of pocket. Any remaining costs are paid by the plan.

(Note that with freedom comes added responsibility. In current employer plans, individuals are usually free to use their HSA funds to purchase noncovered services. So, an employee might spend all of his or her HSA account on chiropractor services—even if these services are not covered by the plan, and

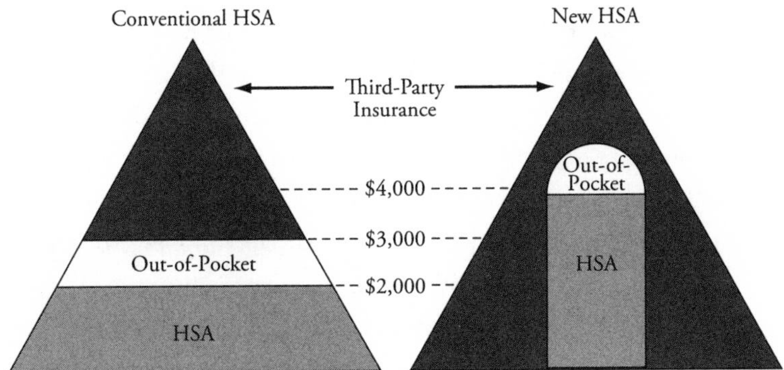

Figure 11.2

the payments do not count toward the deductible. A careless employee could exhaust the HSA funds on noncovered services and risk having to pay the entire deductible out of pocket.)

However, HSAs designed in this way are not necessarily ideal. The design pictured on the right side of Figure 11.2 is preferable. Under this design, the plan pays first dollar for some treatments, while leaving the insured free to pay even higher amounts for other services. The diagram on the right has a further advantage: It can fit into existing managed care plans. One problem these plans have in maintaining member satisfaction was summarized by Stanford University professor Alain Enthoven in a well-publicized letter to then-governor Pete Wilson of California.[10] Enthoven described a woman who was angry at her HMO doctor because he refused her a "medically unnecessary" sonogram. Enthoven surmised that if she'd had to pay fifty dollars out of her own pocket for the service, she would have thanked her doctor for saving her the expense. This and other incidents have convinced Enthoven that having patients pay out-of-pocket is essential to make managed care work.

The diagram on the right has become a reality in South Africa. In 1993, virtually all major forms of insurance in that country began competing on a level playing field (HMOs, PPOs, etc.), partly due to liberal insurance regulations and partly due to a favorable ruling from the South African equivalent of our Internal Revenue Service. Anyone with an idea on how to design a better health insurance plan was free to try. And during the decade of the 1990s, Medical Savings Account plans captured more than half of the market for private health insurance.[11]

Under US law, a tax-free HSA for Americans must have at least a $1,200 deductible for individuals and $2,400 for families, and the deductible applies to all services other than preventive care. South African MSAs are more flexible. The typical plan has first-dollar insurance coverage for most hospital procedures—on the theory that within hospitals, patients have little opportunity to exercise choices. On the other hand, a high deductible applies to discretionary expenses, including most services delivered in doctors' offices.[12]

South Africa's more flexible approach also allows more sensible drug coverage. While the high deductible applies to most drugs for ordinary patients, a typical plan pays from the first dollar for drugs that treat diabetes, asthma, and other chronic conditions. The theory: it's not smart to encourage patients to skimp on drugs that prevent more-expensive-to-treat conditions from developing.[13]

The Design of Third-Party Payment

Most employer plans these days allow employees to seek care "out of network" by paying a higher co-payment. This option has been popular because employees complained about the restrictiveness of closed networks. Yet, analysts say such options can raise the cost of health insurance substantially.[14] It seems that people flock to managed care plans to take advantage of their low premiums, then demand options that undermine the ability of the plans to keep costs down.

The approach summarized in Table 11.1 points to a partial solution. The reason out-of-network doctors cost more, even when paid the same fees as in-network physicians, is that they are likely to order more tests and generate the use of more ancillary services. But this would be of much less concern if third-party payments were restricted largely to treatment or curative services and patients paid with their HSA funds for diagnostic services.

The problem of how to control curative costs without unduly restricting patient choice or endangering quality remains. A possible solution is a variant on an old idea: a fee schedule. From time to time, the insurance industry has flirted with plans that pay doctors a set fee for various services. If patients selected doctors who charge more, they paid the difference out of pocket. In modern medicine, we know that the doctor's fee is only one part of a complex array of costs a doctor can generate. So controlling the physician's fee isn't enough. But why not fix the plan's cost for an entire treatment regimen?

Some commentators refer to insurance designed in this way as "value-based" health insurance.[15] However, it is also consistent with some of the characteristics of traditional casualty insurance.

Suppose a patient is diagnosed with cancer, and the health plan normally would contract to pay a fixed fee to a medical facility to cover all costs. If the plan could be assured that this fixed fee were its maximum exposure, the plan would have no economic interest in restricting the patient's choices. It could, for example, allow the patient to go to an alternative provider and pay more, if needed, out of pocket or from an HSA. In this way, the plan controls its costs, and patients still exercise choice; the exercise of choice puts pressure on the plan to maintain quality in its own preferred medical facility.

The decision to take the plan's money and seek treatment elsewhere need not be made once and for all. For chronic conditions, it could be reaffirmed annually. Take diabetes. Because traditional care for diabetes has been less than optimal, many patients and doctors have long maintained that patients (with the help of a physician) can manage diabetes more efficiently than managed care can.[16] Why not let them try? The health plan might make an annual deposit to the patient's HSA and shift the entire year's financial responsibility to the patient. If there was concern that the funds might be wasted, the health plan could hold the account and monitor it.

An example of the range of possibilities is again provided by South Africa. Discovery Health (one of the largest sellers of MSA plans there) allows its diabetic patients the opportunity to enroll in a special diabetes management program. Under the arrangement, Discovery pays the program about $75 per month, while patients pay another $25 from their MSA accounts. Discovery is considering handling many other chronic diseases in the same way.[17]

The Casualty Insurance Model

To appreciate where this line of thinking might lead, compare casualty insurance with traditional health insurance. After an automobile accident, a claims adjuster inspects the damage, agrees on a price, and writes the car owner a check. Hail damage to a home's roof is handled in the same way under a homeowner's policy. In both cases, the insured is free to make decisions about paying for damage repair. In contrast, traditional health insurance is based on the idea that insurers should pay not for conditions, but for medical care. That health insurers rejected the casualty model is not surprising. BlueCross was started by hospitals for the purpose of insuring that hospital bills would be paid. BlueShield was started by doctors to ensure that doctor fees would be paid.[18] Had auto insurance been developed by auto repair shops, they also would have rejected the casualty model.

I am not suggesting that we give the insured complete freedom of choice. Paying people for a condition and allowing them to forgo healthcare and spend the money on pleasure may not be in the self-interest of a health insurance pool because an untreated condition today could develop into a new and more expensive-to-treat condition later on.[19] I am suggesting that if people were largely free to make their own treatment choices and the market were free to meet their needs, health insurance would take a major step in the direction of the casualty model.

Covered Services

One of the most contentious issues in health policy today concerns the services health insurers must cover. Special interests have persuaded state legislatures to require insurers to cover a vast array of costly services, whether or not those buying the insurance want to pay for the coverage.[20]

In our hypothetical plan, these special interests get no voice. Only the 1,000 enrollees count. That said, traditional insurance has made a lot of arbitrary distinctions that an ideal plan need not make. For example, traditional insurance pays for treatment of back problems by a doctor of medicine, but not a chiropractor. It pays for mental health services provided by a psychiatrist, but not a psychologist. The rationale was partly a misplaced attempt to save money, but it also reflected the physicians' interest in promoting insurance that pays for the services of doctors rather than the individual's interest in protecting against catastrophic costs.

The casualty model of insurance helps solve this problem. Health plans could control costs and give patients greater freedom to choose among competing providers at the same time. Coupled with the idea that people should pay their full cost when entering a health plan and that medical consumption decisions not arising from a risky event should be paid by the individual from an HSA, our ideal health plan should make coverage decisions a lot easier.

Terms of Exit

Recall that insurance contracts in the individual market are almost always guaranteed renewable. Once in an insurance pool, people are entitled to remain there indefinitely and pay the same premiums others pay, regardless of changes in their health status. That commitment is completely one-sided, however. The insurer makes an indefinite commitment to the members, but the members are free to leave the pool at any time.

This one-way commitment creates the following problem. New insurance pools attract mainly healthy people because insurers tend to deny coverage to, or attach exclusions and riders limiting the coverage of people who are already sick (the result of a process known as *medical underwriting*). As time passes, some enrollees get sick, and the premium paid by all must be increased to cover the cost of their care. Thus, mature insurance pools will almost always charge higher premiums than young pools. This gives healthy people an incentive to leave the mature pool. By switching to a young pool, healthy people can escape high premiums. But this option is not open to the sick members of the mature pool. If they try to switch, the new pool will either deny them coverage or charge them a higher premium because of their medical condition. As a result, it is not unusual in the individual market to find an insurer providing the same coverage, but charging vastly different premiums, depending on the age of the pool. Members of a mature pool, for example, might pay $1,000 a month or more for their coverage, while entrants into a young pool might pay only a few hundred dollars. Clearly, these are not the features of an ideal insurance system.

A possible solution is to make the long-term commitment apply both ways. In return for an indefinite commitment on the part of the insurer, members would commit to the pool for a period of, say, three, four, or five years. This does not mean that people would remain stuck in a plan they wished to leave. It does mean that leaving the pool would require the consent of the pool. For example, if a healthy member left high-cost plan A to join low-cost plan B, B would compensate A for its loss. Conversely, if a sick member left A to join B, A would compensate B to take the member and pay for the higher expected cost of care.[21] In this model, recontracting is always possible, but only the type of recontracting that leaves everybody better off.[22]

Moreover, in the ideal system described here, people would have far less reason to switch insurers because their pool would be providing mainly financial (insurance) services rather than healthcare. A member would not need to switch from plan A to plan B to see a particular doctor or gain a higher quality of care.

Can Markets Develop Ideal Health Insurance Plans?

The ideas outlined here are merely suggestive. We do not expect individuals to develop their own health plans. That's what competition and markets are supposed to do. Entrepreneurs are supposed to innovate and experiment to find the products people want to buy. But intrusive regulations aside, can we rely on the market to achieve the best result?

Patients as Buyers of Healthcare

One objection to individuals paying directly for most diagnostic and preventive services is that they would not get the lowest price or find the highest quality. But anecdotal evidence suggests that uninsured individuals, spending their own money, get as good a discount as do large buyers.[23] Even if this were not true, there's no reason why the health plan itself cannot negotiate discounts for its members, even if the members spend their own money when they receive the services.

The issue of quality is a bit more difficult. But the solution is not first-dollar managed care for every service. Suppose that as part of its HMO network, BlueCross set up primary care clinics for its members. BlueCross asserts that these clinics deliver high-quality, cost-effective care. If the assertion is true, why limit the care to the HMO members? Why not allow anyone to enter the clinic and pay out of pocket for the same services? There's no reason why a health plan should object to patients directly contracting for their healthcare, as long as the plan's own costs do not go up. Indeed, the plan itself could provide consulting and other buying services to help patients make wise choices.

Centers of Excellence and Focused Factories

Can there be a workable market for expensive curative services—with patients paying the bill? In some places, there already is. Managed care advocates often point to the Mayo Clinic as an example of cost-effective medicine. They ignore the fact that most of Mayo's customers are fee-for-service patients. What Harvard University professor Regina Herzlinger calls *focused factories,* providing highly efficient, specialized care, are becoming a reality.[24] These healthcare businesses deliver lower prices, lower mortality rates, shorter stays, and higher patient satisfaction.

The Johns Hopkins Breast Center is a focused factory for mastectomies. The M.D. Anderson Cancer Center in Houston, Texas, is a focused factory for cancer. The Pediatrix Medical Group, which manages neonatal units and provides pediatric services in thirty-three states, is another example.[25] Focused factories also are cropping up around the country to provide cancer, gynecological, and orthopedic services.[26] One spectacular success story is Dr. Bernard Salick, a kidney specialist who has become a millionaire by pioneering a national chain of round-the-clock cancer clinics.

Patients on their own can already take advantage of these emerging markets. Indeed, some focused factories are advertising directly to patients. In a television advertisement, Cancer Treatment Centers of America profiled Roger Stump, a patient who survived pancreatic cancer after doctors at another hospital had given up hope.[27]

The Benefits of Ideal Health Insurance

Three features of ideal health insurance would make it especially superior to the health insurance arrangements that prevail today.

Ideal Health Insurance Is Patient Centered

A large portion of our healthcare dollars would be placed in accounts that we individually own and control. Patients would pay for the vast majority of medical services from these accounts, and doctors would be free to act as agents for their patients rather than for third-party payers. Because patients would be spending their own money in the medical marketplace, physicians would be encouraged to become financial advisers as well as health advisers. Doctors would compete not just on the basis of price and quality, but also on the basis of delivering value for money.

Ideal health insurance in the treatment of expensive conditions would be patient-centered. Rather than have a third party pay every medical bill, insurers would make regular deposits to the HSAs of patients with chronic conditions, leaving them free to choose among competing focused factories for ongoing treatment. Rather than have a third party dictate terms and conditions for the delivery of expensive acute care, patients would be able to draw on a fixed sum of money and get their health needs met at a center of excellence or a focused factory of their own choosing.

Ideal Health Insurance Allows Insurers to Specialize in the Business of Insurance

One of the consequences of the managed care revolution is that insurers have been turned into providers of care. Often the entity that pays our medical bills is the same entity that delivers our medical care. This development has had three negative consequences.

First, when the businesses of insurance and healthcare merge, health plans have perverse incentives to deny care. The rash of news stories reporting on the tragic consequences of underprovision of care is testimony to what can go wrong.[28]

Second, when the choice of insurer is also effectively a choice of provider networks, consumers must make decisions that are humanly impossible. Ideally, one should not have to choose a cardiologist until one has a heart problem. One should not have to choose an oncologist until one gets cancer. But in today's market, when you choose your insurer you are at the same time choosing your heart specialist and your cancer specialist, whether you are aware of it or not.

Third, the managed care revolution has delegated to those on the buyers' side of the market (insurers) the responsibility of forcing those on the sellers' side of the market (doctors, hospital administrators, etc.) to deliver care efficiently. In no other market do we depend upon buyers to tell sellers how to produce their product. Undoubtedly, there are good reasons why other markets are not organized this way.

Ideal health insurance, by contrast, allows insurers to specialize in what they do best: price and manage risk. The supply side of the market would be encouraged to organize into focused factories and adopt other efficient techniques to produce high-quality care for a low cost. The market would still be free to combine insurance and healthcare delivery where the combination makes sense. It may turn out that for such specialized services as cancer care, efficiency warrants specialized insurance products. Ideal health insurance would allow those market developments by providing a mechanism for people to leave one insurance pool and join another (without extra cost) when their health condition changes.

Ideal Health Insurance Is Improved by the Free Flow of Information

Under the current system, consumer information is a threat to the stability and peace of mind of typical third-party payer personnel. The more patients learn, the more they are likely to demand. Under ideal health insurance, by contrast, accurate consumer information is a positive. The reason is that the insurer and the insured are on the same team, with a similar interest and objective: acquiring good value in a competitive market.

Needless to say, the changes outlined here will require appropriate changes in public policy. Of these, three are particularly important.[29]

First, federal tax law must create a level playing field between third-party insurance and individual self-insurance through HSAs. As noted, we have already made major steps in that direction. Individual preference and market competition, not the peculiarities of the tax law, should determine the appropriate division.

Second, federal tax law must create a level playing field between employer purchase and individual purchase of health insurance. Although employers can purchase employee health insurance with before-tax dollars, people who purchase their own insurance get virtually no tax relief and must pay with after-tax dollars. (An exception to this generalization is the self-employed, who get partial tax relief.) Employers may have an important role to play in helping people obtain health insurance, but this role should be determined by the marketplace, not by tax law.

A third important change needs to be implemented at the state level. Many employers would like to move to a defined-contribution approach for employee health insurance. As a result, employees could enter a health insurance pool and stay there—taking their insurance coverage with them as they travel from job to job. Personal and portable health insurance is an idea whose time has come.

These changes will not solve our most important health insurance problems. They will create a legal environment in which individuals, their employers, and their insurers—pursuing their own interests—are likely to create the institutions they need.

12

Solving the Problem of Patient Safety

RECALL THAT HOSPITALS are dangerous places to be. Doctors' offices aren't very safe either. By one estimate, as many as 187,000 patients die every year for some reason other than the medical condition that caused them to seek care. By another estimate, there are 6.1 million injuries caused by the healthcare system, including hospital acquired infections that afflict one in every twenty hospital patients.

Although some have questioned whether these estimates err on the high side, even the most optimistic estimates of hospital safety are unacceptably high.

Adverse medical events (also known as iatrogenic events) are typically divided into three categories: preventable and negligent; preventable but not negligent; and other adverse events. Events in the first category, also called malpractice errors, are injuries or deaths resulting from medical misconduct or lack of adherence to minimum standards of care. Examples are performing surgery on the wrong site, or leaving a sponge in a patient after an operation. Events in the second category are considered avoidable, although they are not the result of negligence. Most hospital-acquired infections are examples of this sort of medical error. The third category is "other" events. These are events that we do not know how to prevent with our current knowledge and technology.

As it stands, malpractice lawsuits are the only recourse patients have to adverse events. Yet as Figure 12.1 shows, only about one in four adverse events falls into the category of malpractice. Even if the malpractice system worked perfectly—and even if patients are prepared to go forward with the expense and stress of a lawsuit—we are basically unprotected against three-fourths of all the things that can go wrong in hospitals.

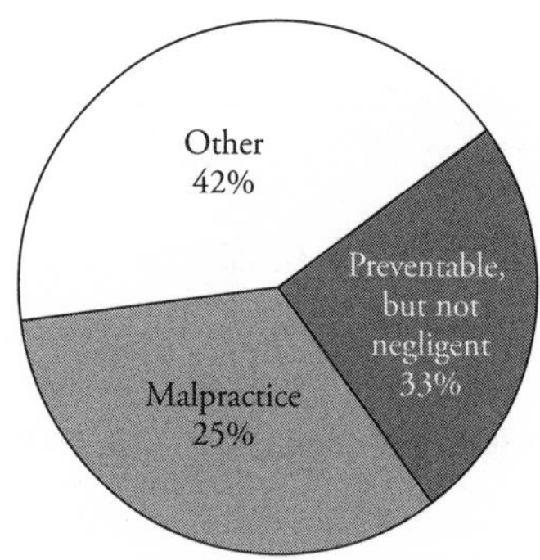

Figure 12.1. Adverse Medical Events
Source: National Center for Policy Analysis.

Our system for dealing with these events is highly imperfect. Only 2 percent of victims of malpractice ever file a lawsuit,[1] and fewer still ever receive any compensation. On the other hand, 37 percent of lawsuits filed involve no real malpractice.[2] To add insult to injury, more than half the money spent on malpractice litigation goes to someone other than the victims and their families.[3]

What can be done to make the healthcare system safer for patients?

How the Current System Is Trapping Us

Despite this poor track record, the malpractice system imposes a heavy social cost—as much as $2,500 per household per year, including defensive medicine, at today's prices.[4] And it may be making hospitals less safe than they otherwise would be.

The malpractice system distorts the incentives of doctors and hospitals by encouraging them to make malpractice events as rare as possible, even if in doing so, they *increase* the number of other adverse events. As explained in our *Health Affairs* study,[5] the system encourages doctors to order more blood tests and other procedures in order to reduce the risk of malpractice litigation, even though these procedures may put patients at additional risk.

A Better Way

For the money we are now spending on a wasteful, dysfunctional malpractice system, we could afford to give the families $200,000 for every hospital-

MALPRACTICE REFORM: TEN PRINCIPLES OF A RATIONAL TORT SYSTEM

Principle No. 1 Victims of torts should be fully compensated—no more, and no less.

Principle No. 2 Those who commit torts should pay the full cost of their harmful acts—no more, no less.

Principle No. 3 Whenever possible, damages should be determined in the marketplace (e.g., the market price to repair the damage).

Principle No. 4 Structured awards are generally preferable to lump sum awards.

Principle No. 5 Parties should always be free to alter by contract a court-determined award.

Principle No. 6 Reasonable limits should be set on damages for pain and suffering, subject to market-based rebuttable evidence.

Principle No. 7 Punitive damages are justified only if there are social costs over and above the victim's private costs.

Principle No. 8 Contingency fees should be paid entirely by the defendants, with meritorious exceptions.

Principle No. 9 Attorney's fees should be awarded in cases of bad faith.

Principle No. 10 The first nine principles do not apply to settlements.

Source: John C. Goodman et al., "Malpractice Reform: Ten Principles of a Rational Tort System," in *Handbook on State Healthcare Reform* (Dallas, Texas: National Center for Policy Analysis, 2007), 153–165.

caused death. We could give every injury victim an average of $20,000—with the actual amount varying, depending on the severity of the harm.

How exactly could this work? What I propose is to provide a voluntary, contractual, no-fault alternative to the malpractice system. In return for forgoing their common law rights to litigate, patients entering the healthcare system would be assured that if they experience an adverse outcome, the provider institution will write them a check—without lawyers, without depositions, without judges and juries—no questions asked.

This proposal would take quality-of-care issues out of the hands of the legal system and put it in the hands of people who are best able to do something about it. Providers would soon realize that every time they avoid an adverse death, they will save, say, $200,000. They would come to view every life as equally valuable—regardless of whether the cause of harm is negligence, preventive steps not taken, or an "act of God."

To pay off the claims, hospitals would probably purchase insurance just as they purchase malpractice insurance today. Insurers would become outside monitors of hospital quality, and their premiums would reflect doctor and hospital experience. Those with higher adverse-event rates would pay more. Those with lower rates would pay less. Further, if patients desired to pay an additional premium and top up their potential compensation—doubling or quadrupling the amount—they would have that option as well.

Under this proposal, state legislators would establish a commission to set the minimum compensation patients must receive for various adverse events. An independent commission (with patients, doctors, and hospitals all represented) would regularly review hospital records and determine whether an adverse event has occurred in marginal cases. The decision to opt out of the malpractice system is a decision to accept these nonjudicial parameters.

About three decades ago, University of Chicago law professor Richard Epstein proposed a similar idea. He called it "liability by contract."[6] The idea: let patients and doctors voluntarily agree in advance how to resolve things if something goes wrong.

In nonmedical fields, Epstein's idea is actually quite commonplace. Contracts for performance often have provisions detailing what the parties will do if something goes awry. If the parties disagree, contracts often spell out dispute resolution procedures (such as binding arbitration). My colleagues and I at the National Center for Policy Analysis propose to make this idea the cornerstone of more general reform.[7]

By voluntary, we really mean voluntary. If doctors and hospitals choose not to opt out of the tort system, they can practice under the rules of existing law.

What follows are some steps to achieve these reforms.

Reform the Tort System

A reformed tort system is one that is governed by the ten principles of a rational tort system.[8] This is the default system, and all cases of malpractice will be tried in this system unless patients and providers contract out prior to the occurrence of the alleged malpractice. The following is how liability by contract might work.[9]

Free the Patients

Under the traditional system, most hospitals and doctors ask their patients to sign a form at the time of treatment releasing the provider from any legal liability in case of negligence. In malpractice suits, the defendants point to the form and claim the plaintiff (victim) has waived the right to sue by contract, as a condition of treatment. Courts have routinely dismissed such arguments, however, on the grounds that they do not really constitute informed consent. After all, how can a patient who is ill, frightened, and intimidated by the healthcare system make rational decisions about complex legal liability issues?

The position of the courts is understandable, but it has had an unfortunate side effect: doctors and patients are unable to avoid the costs of the malpractice system through any contract whatsoever.

How can the system give patients and doctors other options, while at the same time protecting patients from making unwise decisions when they are least able to negotiate contracts? One answer is for the legislature (or a body designated by the legislature) to decide in advance what will constitute an enforceable contract. Let the state legislature decide on the minimum elements (including the amount of monetary compensation) that must be in such contracts in order to make sure patients are fairly protected, then widely publicize these elements so that people generally understand (before they get sick) what will happen if they opt out of the malpractice system and waive their common law rights to litigate.

Patients would not be required to agree to such contracts as a condition of treatment; however, if they voluntarily signed the agreement, it would be binding.

Here are some provisions that should be considered for inclusion in such contracts.

Compensation Without Fault

This provision obligates the provider to compensate the patient (or family of the patient) in the case of unexpected death or disability. In the case of an unexpected death, the amount could be set in advance and generally known to all patients. In the case of an unexpected disability, the contract might use the provisions of the state workers' compensation system.

How much compensation should be paid in the case of an unexpected death? Any number would be somewhat arbitrary. The amount could be varied by patient characteristics, including the patient's age, the age of any surviving spouse and children, the patient's income, and so forth. In other words, the amount could be based on some of the same criteria the current malpractice system uses.

Adjustments for Risk

Not all medical cases are the same. Even if the probability of an unexpected death is low, complications in one patient may create risks twice as high as for another. There must be a way of adjusting for this, or providers would try to avoid all the harder cases. One possibility is to reduce the amount of compensation for riskier patients.

Full Disclosure

As a condition of waiving the patient's legal rights to pursue liability claims under traditional tort law, providers should be required to make certain quality information public. For routine surgeries, for example, hospitals and doctors should post (case-adjusted) mortality rates, readmission rates, hospital-acquired infection rates, and so forth. Providers should also be required to disclose the use of safety measures, including electronic medical records, computer software designed to reduce errors, and procedures designed to prevent hospital-acquired infections.

In addition, in the case of death or disability, providers should be required to fully disclose all facts to appropriate investigative bodies so that steps can be taken to prevent future recurrences. The patient should also be required to provide full disclosure. The time of the last meal or the ingestion of other drugs, if undisclosed at the time of treatment, can lead to adverse medical outcomes.

Patient Compliance

Even for simple surgery, patients must comply with certain provider directives, including diet restrictions, full disclosure of medications being taken, and so forth. For maternity cases, compliance in the form of prenatal care is more involved and extends over a longer period of time. Failure to comply in all these cases would result in a reduction in the amount of compensation and perhaps no compensation at all.

Additional Insurance Options

As explained above, legislatures will set minimum requirements for liability contracts. In most cases, insurance companies will then insure those contracts. However, once premiums for a doctor, patient, and procedure are set, patients could increase the coverage by paying an additional out-of-pocket premium. For example, if the legislature requires a minimum payout of $200,000 for an unexpected death, and the providers have to pay $x of premium for the insurance, patients should be able to pay an additional $x to obtain $400,000 of insurance coverage (or any other multiple).

Free the Doctors

A system of liability by contract will not work in all cases. Many patients have a high probability of death or disability at the time they enter a hospital. Doctors are unlikely to want to pay the cost of those outcomes, should they be ruled "adverse," and it would be unreasonable to expect them to do so. Further, when patients seek care at emergency rooms, no one has time to evaluate the likelihood of death or permanent injury prior to the delivery of care. Even in these cases, however, an alternative to the current system would seem to be desirable.

Accordingly, medical providers who offer their patients the opportunity to escape the current malpractice system by contract should have the chance to escape the system themselves in cases where contracts are impossible or impractical. In particular, these providers would be able to insist as a condition of treatment that all malpractice claims must be submitted to binding, unappealable arbitration. (The exception would be cases of gross negligence.)

Two questions immediately arise: Who would the arbitrators be? What criteria would they use to make decisions?

Many people already serve as arbitrators, including former judges. They are selected and agreed upon by plaintiff lawyers and defense lawyers in cases where the parties want to avoid the costs, burdens, and risks of trial by subjecting their cases to a respected, impartial third party. Since these arbitrators are already in the business and have reputations for integrity and good judgment, they are an ideal source for malpractice arbitration.

If there is a shortage of suitable arbitrators, other options exist. For example, a case could have two arbitrators—one with a history of representing plaintiffs, the other with a history of representing defendants. The two arbitrators must agree on a final resolution; if they cannot agree, neither gets paid, and two more arbitrators replace them.

What criteria should arbitrators use in deciding cases? Basically, the same criteria that would be relevant in a reformed tort system. However, unlike the liability-by-contract system, here the paramount issue is one of fault. Doctors (and their insurers) pay nothing unless they are found to be at fault, and the amount they would pay would be based on the degree to which they are at fault.

As in the case of liability by contract, doctors would be freed from the burden of the traditional malpractice system, provided they do certain things. For example, they must make their quality data available to all patients; they must cooperate with all safety bodies; and they must (in arbitration cases) make all relevant data available to the patient without costly discovery.

Free the Experts

All too often, expert witnesses in tort cases appear time and again for one side or the other. They are selected as witnesses precisely because their testimony can be counted on to be overly generous to one of the two sides. Further, these witnesses are often handsomely paid, which gives them an incentive to continue the practice and become "professional witnesses."

These witnesses would have no role in a properly run system of arbitration. The arbitrators would be free to call on real experts who would be agents of the arbitrator rather than agents of one of the two parties.

A model for the arbitrators is the so-called "vaccine court," a branch of the US Court of Federal Claims in Washington.[10] The vaccine court was created in 1986 as Congress's response to a liability crisis. In rare cases, vaccines were being blamed for catastrophic injuries and even death. Manufacturers were threatening to quit the business, which in turn threatened the vaccine supply. The National Vaccine Injury Compensation Act shielded the industry from civil litigation by instituting a system of no-fault compensation. Under the law, aggrieved families file petitions, which are heard by special masters in the vaccine court. Successful claims are paid from a trust fund fed by a 75-cent surcharge per vaccine dose. The US Department of Health and Human Services oversees the fund, with the Justice Department acting as its lawyer.

Free the Courts

The reformed system described above should be available in all cases except gross negligence. Medical practitioners should be able to contract away responsibility for mistakes. They should also be able to insure against the consequences of their mistakes. There seems to be no socially defensible reason, however, to allow them to contract out of the consequences of gross negligence.

Advantages of Reform

A liability-by-contract system along these lines would have a number of compelling advantages, including the following:

Insurers rather than patients would become the primary monitors of healthcare quality

Under this proposal, a great deal of quality information—currently unavailable—would now be provided to patients. However, patients would not be the primary monitors of quality. That role would fall to insurers. If doctors could escape the costs and burdens of the liability system by compensating patients for unexpected outcomes, they would naturally want to insure against such payments.

So instead of buying malpractice insurance, they would be purchasing what amounts to episode-specific insurance on all patients, say, undergoing surgery.

In the current system, there are no life and disability insurance products specifically tied to episodes of medical care. However, if the contract system becomes widely used, such products are likely to emerge.

As noted above, under the current system, there is very little relationship between actual malpractice and malpractice lawsuits. As a result, malpractice premiums do not reflect the likelihood that doctors will commit malpractice. Instead, premiums reflect the likelihood that doctors will be sued. Under the liability-by-contract system, however, compensation would be based on objective phenomenon, that is, death and disability. In pricing these policies, insurers would have a strong interest in monitoring how doctors practice medicine. The market, rather than bureaucratic bodies, would determine who is a good surgeon and who is a bad one, and those determinations would be reflected in insurance premiums.

Medical providers would face strong financial incentives to improve quality

In addition to the fact that malpractice premiums are not closely related to the actual incidence of malpractice, premiums charged to doctors rarely reflect the quality of medicine being practiced. In the reformed system, insurance premiums should be closely related to actual outcomes. Surgeons with high mortality rates will pay higher premiums to insure against unexpected outcomes, other things being equal. These higher premiums, in turn, will constitute a strong financial incentive to find safer ways to perform surgery.

Multiple parties on the medical side would have strong incentives to cooperate in improving quality

Under the current system, a patient undergoing surgery typically is not dealing with a single doctor who is responsible for the entire procedure. Instead, the patient is (implicitly) contracting with several doctors, each as an independent contractor. For example, there is the surgeon, the anesthesiologist, the radiologist, the pathologist, and the hospital itself. Because each of these entities is independent of the other, none bears the full cost of his or her bad behavior, and none reaps the full benefits of good behavior.

Some have proposed making the hospital fully responsible for all malpractice claims, but that doesn't work very well when none of the other parties to the medical incident are hospital employees. Under the proposal envisioned here, all parties to a surgical event, for instance, would have strong incentives to contract with each other and cooperate with each other on error-reducing, quality-improving changes (including electronic medical records and hospital infection reduction procedures). The incentives would be to avoid the current tort system, to offer the patient a contract insured by a single insurer and to minimize the cost of that insurance.

Patients will receive cash compensation for unexpected outcomes without the stress or expense of a lawsuit

The loss of a loved one is a traumatic event. The prospect of filing a malpractice lawsuit is also inherently stressful and traumatic. The compensation system envisioned here would put doctors and patients on the same side, with only one obligation—completing the paperwork needed to collect from an insurance company.

Patients and their families could self-insure for additional compensation

How much should a surviving spouse receive for the death of a loved one? The decision will, to a certain extent, be arbitrary—especially if made by a legislative body. However, if the amount is publicized in advance and broadly known, families can make adjustments to meet their expected needs. If the amount is too low, for example, families could buy additional life or disability insurance on their own—including (as described above) insurance under the provider's insurance contract.

The social cost of a liability-by-contract system is likely to be much lower than the cost of the current system

As many as 187,000 people die each year because of adverse medical events. If the surviving family members of these patients each received a check for $200,000, the total cost would be less than $37 billion. The total cost of the current malpractice system is estimated to be as much as $250 billion, or more than five times as much.

Moreover, the current system involves a huge use of real resources—lawyers, judges, courtrooms, and so forth. By contrast, the check-writing solution involves very few real resources—other than monitoring and administration costs; it primarily involves moving money from some people to others, leaving real resources to be used in more productive ways.

Further, if hospitals were required to pay $200,000 per unexpected death, on the average, the healthcare system would not continue to sustain so many deaths from adverse medical events each year. Hospitals would quickly find ways of reducing their error rates.

Healthcare costs for patients would likely be reduced

Ultimately, the cost of any compensation system will primarily be paid by patients and potential patients. Just as the cost of malpractice premiums is embedded in the patients' cost of care, the cost of a liability-by-contract system will also be passed on to patients (and their insurers) in the form of higher prices. However, if the proposed system is socially more efficient, patients will see an overall reduction in healthcare costs (as well as an increase in quality and better personal protection against untoward events).

Liability by contract is a socially better way of handling sympathetic cases

Some of the most heart-wrenching cases in malpractice law involve newborns facing the prospect of a lifetime of care. Even if the doctors and hospital personnel committed no error, the parents are confronted with an enormous burden—in terms of both time and money. The tendency on the part of jurors, therefore, is to have great sympathy for the plaintiffs.

One reason malpractice premiums for obstetrician/gynecologists are so high is that the system is inching ever closer to a system of liability without fault. But if this is the case, why not move there directly and dispense with the lawyers, judges, and juries? The reformed system would take care of the sympathetic cases in an efficient, responsible way.

13

The Do-No-Harm Approach to Public Policy[1]

"FIRST, DO NO HARM." This principle is well known to physicians as part of the Hippocratic oath. No similar oath is taken by politicians, of course. But suppose they did. Suppose that, before they passed any new health legislation, our political representatives were required to reexamine existing laws and make sure that government is not the cause of the very problems it attempts to solve. What would our healthcare system look like?

Health economists at the National Center for Policy Analysis found the answer to that question. They began by identifying five major choices people make and isolating five ways in which public policies interfere with those choices—perversely encouraging people to make socially undesirable decisions. They then sought to determine what our healthcare system would look like if government policy were at least neutral.

If people must choose between a socially desirable alternative and an undesirable one, government policy is "neutral" if it gives equal encouragement to both alternatives. Under a set of neutral policies, government is not solving any problems; on the other hand, it is also not creating them.

In what follows, I will show the reader that all the major policy recommendations previously made in this book are consistent with a neutral, do-no-harm approach to health policy.

Choice No. 1: To Insure or Not to Insure?

Why do we care whether other people have health insurance? One reason we care is that uninsured people may incur medical bills they cannot pay using their own resources. When that happens, the cost is often borne by other people, either through shifting costs to insured (paying) patients or through free-care programs subsidized by taxpayers. The choice to insure or remain uninsured often means, as a practical matter, the choice to insure or implicitly rely on the social safety net. How do government policies affect our incentives with respect to this choice?

Subsidies for Private Health Insurance

Most people who purchase private insurance take advantage of federal tax subsidies that total about $274 billion each year, nationwide.[2] How much subsidy is available to an individual, however, depends on how the insurance is purchased, as well as the family's tax bracket. If an employee works for an employer who provides health insurance (an untaxed fringe benefit) as an alternative to higher taxable wages, the employer's premium payments avoid federal, state, and local income taxes as well as payroll (FICA) taxes. For a middle-income family facing a 25 percent federal income tax rate, a 15.3 percent Federal Insurance Contributions Act (FICA) tax, and a 5 percent state income tax rate, the subsidy is 45.3 percent—with government paying almost half the cost of the insurance.

To see the financial implications of these subsidies, consider a family health insurance plan that costs $12,000 a year. The employer's choice is to spend $12,000 on (untaxed) premiums or to forgo the fringe benefit altogether and pay the employee $12,000 in wages. In the latter, however, the employee will receive only $6,564 in take-home pay. A different way of looking at the same issue is to ask: how much would the worker have to earn in taxable wages in order to be able to buy the same insurance after the payment of taxes? Answer: almost $22,000. So, for sacrificing $6,564 in take-home pay, the worker is able to get a benefit that he would have to earn almost $22,000 to be able to purchase on his own!

Generous tax subsidies, therefore, undoubtedly encourage people who would otherwise be uninsured to obtain employer-provided insurance. There are two problems with the way these subsidies are structured, however. First, the largest subsidies are given to people who need them least. Second, the subsidies generally are not available to most of the uninsured.

Under the current system, families who obtain insurance through an employer obtain a tax subsidy worth about $2,021, on the average.[3] (See Figure 13.1.) Not everyone, however, gets the average tax subsidy. Households earning more

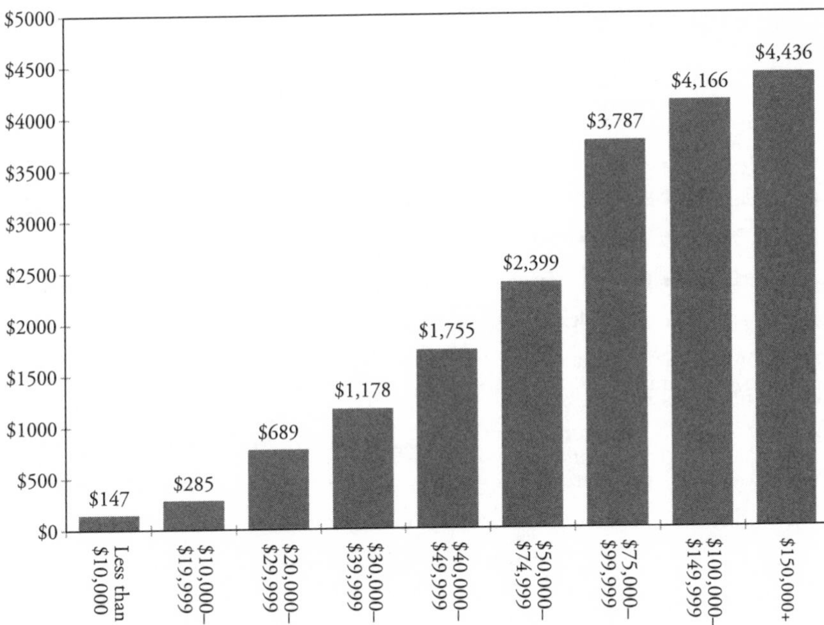

Note: Based on the Lewin Group 2011 distribution of tax subsidies.
The average tax subsidy per family is $2,021.

Figure 13.1. Average Federal Health Benefit Tax Expenditure, by Family Income Level

than $150,000 per year receive an average subsidy of $4,436. By contrast, those earning between $10,000 and $20,000 receive only about $285. One reason is that those earning higher incomes are in higher tax brackets. For example, a family in the 35 percent tax bracket gets a subsidy of 35 cents for every dollar spent on health insurance. By contrast, a family in the 15 percent bracket (paying only the FICA payroll tax) gets a subsidy of only 15 cents on the dollar.

The second problem is that people who do not obtain insurance through an employer get very little tax relief if they purchase insurance on their own. Individuals who pay premiums with their own money can deduct costs in excess of 7.5 percent of adjusted gross income (increasing to 10 percent in 2013). For instance, a family with $50,000 in income would not be able to deduct the first $3,750 in health insurance premiums. The threshold for a $100,000-a-year family is twice that amount.

Subsidies for the Uninsured

Consider now the alternative: free care, obtained through a local social safety net. What does government do to encourage this choice? Although no one knows the exact number, public and private spending on free care is considerable. The National Center for Policy Analysis has previously estimated that in the United States, we are spending about $1,500 on free (or "uncompensated") care per full-time uninsured person per year. However, I believe that in a reformed healthcare system that number could be closer to $2,000 or about $8,000 for a family of four. For expository purposes, those are the numbers I will use.

Interestingly, $8,000 is a sum adequate to purchase private health insurance for a family in many cities. Therefore, one way to look at the choice families face is that they can rely on $8,000 in free care (on the average), or they can purchase an $8,000 private insurance policy with after-tax income.

The problem with the current system of spending subsidies is that they encourage millions of people to be uninsured. Why pay for expensive private health insurance when free care provided through public programs is de facto insurance? Yet, society should not be indifferent about this decision. For one thing, the choice to rely on safety net care is a choice to be a "free rider" at the taxpayers' expense. For another thing, the two types of care are not equivalent. The privately insured patient has more choices of physicians and hospital facilities.

Further, safety net care is generally much less efficient. For instance, uninsured patients often use emergency rooms to provide care that is more economically provided in a doctor's office or at a free-standing clinic. As a result, per dollar spent, the privately insured patient typically gets more care and better care. For that reason alone, it is in society's interest to encourage people to purchase private insurance rather than rely on the public safety net.

Achieving Neutrality

Suppose the government offered every individual a uniform, fixed-dollar subsidy. If the individual obtained private insurance, the subsidy would be realized in the form of lower taxes by way of a tax credit. The credit would be refundable, so that it would be available even to those with no tax liability.

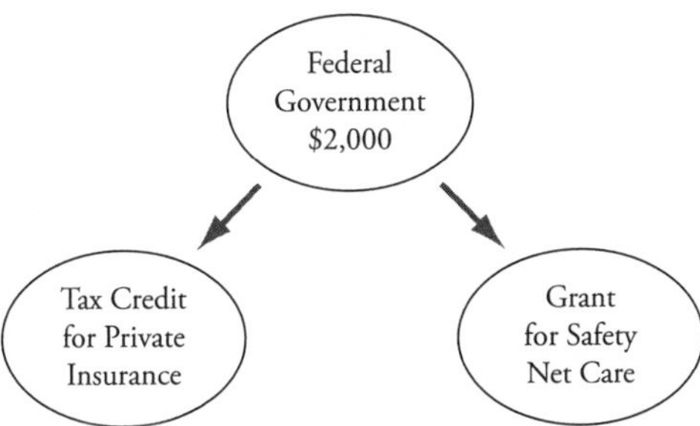

Figure 13.2. Federal Government Subsidy

If the individual chose to be uninsured, the subsidy would be sent to a safety net agency in the community where the person lives. [See Figure 13.2.] The uniform subsidy should reflect the value society places on having one more person insured. What is that value? An empirically verifiable number is at hand, so long as we are willing to accept the political system as dispositive.

It is the amount we expect to spend (from public and private sources) on free care for that person when he or she is uninsured. For example, if society is spending $2,000 per year per person on free care for the uninsured, on the average, we should be willing to offer $2,000 to everyone who obtains private insurance. Failure to subsidize private insurance as generously as we subsidize free care encourages people to choose the latter over the former.

One way to think of such an arrangement is to see it as a system under which the uninsured as a group pay for their own free care. That is, in the very act of turning down a tax credit (by choosing not to insure), uninsured individuals would pay extra taxes equal to the average amount of free care given annually to the uninsured. (See Figure 13.3.)

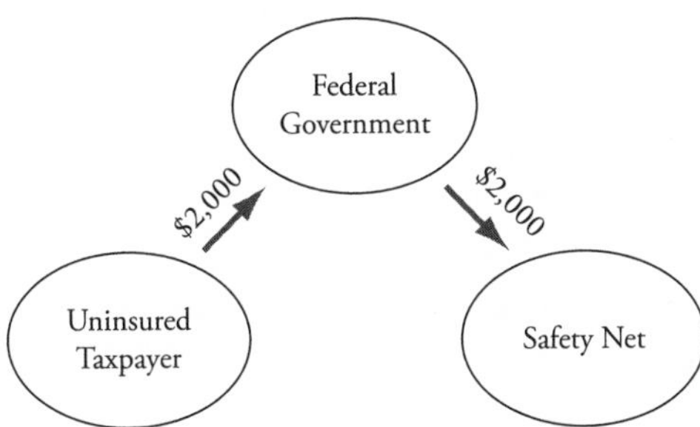

Figure 13.3. The Marginal Effect of Choosing to Be Uninsured

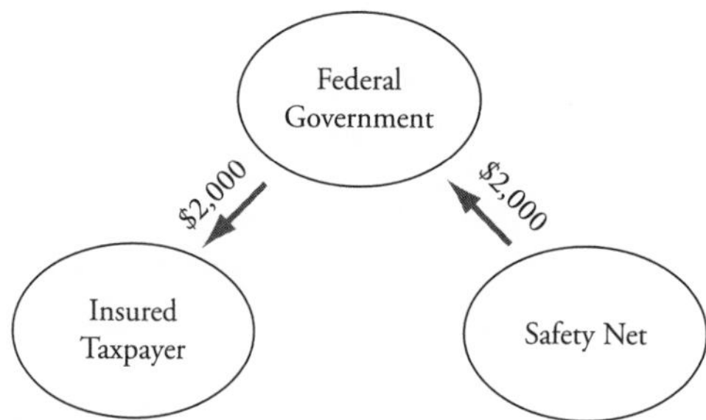

Figure 13.4. The Marginal Effect of Choosing to Be Insured

How can we fund the subsidies for those who choose to move from being uninsured to insured? We can do it by reversing the process. The subsidy should be funded by the reduction in expected free care that person would have consumed if uninsured. For example, suppose everyone in Dallas County chose to obtain private insurance, relying on a refundable $2,000 federal income tax credit to pay the premiums. As a result, Dallas County no longer would need to spend $2,000 per person on the uninsured. Thus, all of the money that previously funded safety net medical care could be used to fund the private insurance premiums. (See Figure 13.4.)

On the other hand, if everyone in Dallas County changed his mind and opted to be uninsured, the $2,000 per person in unclaimed credits would be available for safety net institutions.

Implementing Reform

To implement the program, all the federal government needs to know is how many people live in each community. In principle, it will be offering each of them an annual $2,000 tax credit. Some will claim the full credit. Some will claim a partial credit (because they will be insured for only part of a year). Others will claim no credit. What the government pledges to each community will be $2,000 times the number of people. The portion of this sum that is not claimed on tax returns should be available as block grants to be spent on indigent healthcare at the local level.

In a private insurance market, insurers will not agree to insure someone for $2,000 if the expected cost of care is, for example, $4,000. If the safety net agency expects a $4,000 savings as a result of transferring a patient to a private insurer, however, the agency should be willing to forgo up to $4,000 for such a change.

There are about 200 million people who are not on Medicare or Medicaid. At $2,000 each, potential federal spending would equal about $400 billion. Where would the federal government get the money to fund the private insurance tax credits?

We could begin with the $274 billion in tax subsidies the federal government already "spends" to subsidize private insurance. Add to that the money the federal, state, and local governments already spend on indigent care. For the remainder, the federal government could make certain tax benefits conditional on proof of insurance. For example, the $1,000 child tax credit could be made conditional on proof of insurance for a child.[4] For middle-income families, a portion of the standard deduction could be made conditional on proof of insurance for adults. For lower-income families, part of the Earned Income Tax Credit (EITC) refunds could be conditional.

How would the federal government manage to reduce safety net spending when uninsured people elected to obtain private insurance? Because much of the safety net expenditure already consists of federal funds, the federal government could use its share to fund private insurance tax credits instead. For the remainder, the federal government does not have direct control over the budgets of state and local governments. However, the federal government could reduce block grants to the states for Medicaid and other programs instead.

The Cost of Reform

A common misconception is that health insurance reform costs money. For example, if health insurance for 50 million uninsured people costs $2,000 a person, some conclude that the government would need to spend an additional $100 billion a year to get the job done. What this conclusion overlooks is that we are already spending $100 billion or more on free care for the uninsured, and if all 50 million uninsured suddenly became insured they would—in that act—free up the $100 billion from the social safety net.

At $2.5 trillion a year, there is no reason to believe our healthcare system is spending too little money. To the contrary, attempting to insure the uninsured by spending more money would have the perverse effect of contributing to healthcare inflation. Getting all the incentives right may involve shifting around a lot of money, such as reducing subsidies that are currently too large and increasing subsidies that are too small. It may also mean making some portion of people's tax liability contingent on proof of insurance. But it need not add to budgetary outlays.

Choice Number 2: Public or Private Coverage?

Many poor and near-poor families have a choice of public or private insurance. Because of their low income, they can either qualify for Medicaid or state-based Children's Health Insurance Program enrollment or obtain private insurance (typically through an employer). Clearly, we should not be indifferent about this choice. Private insurance means people are paying their own way. Further, as noted, private insurance often means better healthcare.

How does government policy affect this choice? Unfortunately, public policy overwhelmingly encourages people to drop private insurance and enroll in public programs instead. As noted, tax subsidies for private insurance are quite meager for those with near-poverty incomes (basically consisting of the avoidance of the 15.3 percent FICA tax), whereas public programs are free. Further, except for a few pilot programs underway, states do not allow Medicaid enrollees to use their Medicaid dollars to buy into an employer plan or purchase private insurance directly.

Consequences of Perverse Incentives

Many observers assume Medicaid insures people who otherwise would not have access to private insurance. However, Medicaid induces some people to turn down or drop private coverage to take advantage of free health insurance offered by the state. As a result of such crowding out, the cost of expanding public insurance programs has been high relative to the gain. For example, if for each new enrollee in a public program at least one person loses private insurance, there will be no net reduction in the number of uninsured, despite the higher taxpayer burden.

Economists David Cutler and Jonathan Gruber found that Medicaid expansions in the early 1990s were substantially offset by reductions in private coverage. For every additional dollar spent on Medicaid, private-sector healthcare spending was reduced by 50 cents to 75 cents, on the average.[5] Thus, taxpayers incurred a considerable burden, but at least half and perhaps as much as three-fourths of the expenditures replaced private-sector spending rather than buying more or better medical services.

A similar principle applies to the CHIP. Take a low-income working family covered by an employer-sponsored health plan. The employer might have covered some or all of the cost of insurance premiums for the employee and family with pre-tax dollars. However, a bigger paycheck is more attractive to actual and potential employees if coverage is provided by the state. Thus, CHIP offers some employees the opportunity to increase wages and reduce their health insurance costs.

Overall, the number of poor children without health insurance fell from 19 percent in 1997 to 11 percent in 2003. During this period, enrollment of low-income children in public programs increased from 29 percent to 49 percent. At the same time, private insurance coverage fell from 47 percent to 35 percent, although there was little change in the percentage of privately insured children in households at higher income levels. It appears that the crowd-out of private insurance because of the expansion of public programs was about 60 percent.[6]

Adopting a Policy of Neutrality

The solution here is very similar to the solution to the previous problem. If government is spending $2,000 a year per person enrolled in Medicaid, it ought to be willing to spend an identical sum on private insurance instead. (See Figure 13.5.)

On paper, Medicaid coverage often looks more generous than private insurance—covering almost all physicians, facilities, and procedures at no out-of-pocket cost to the patient, at least in principle. In practice, many physicians refuse to see Medicaid patients and, because of the low rates of reimbursement,

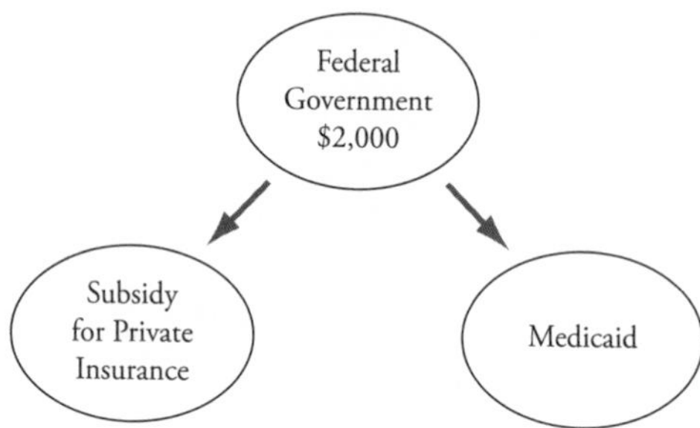

Figure 13.5. A Level Playing Field for Private and Public Insurance

there is often rationing by waiting. As a result, a policy that is financially neutral would be one that encourages private insurance.

Choice Number 3: Individual or Group Insurance?

The pros and cons of individual versus group insurance have been the subject of many discussions and debates. Employers, it is argued, are in a unique position to pool groups of people. Also, there are economies of scale in group purchase. On the other hand, employer-provided insurance is not portable. People who change jobs often must also change physicians, thus losing continuity of care. Plus, there is no guarantee that insurance at the new job will provide the same coverage for the same conditions as the original insurance.

Individual insurance has the virtue of portability. People can take their coverage with them as they move from job to job. Further, in the individual market, people have a better opportunity to purchase insurance tailored to individual and family needs. On the downside, individual insurance has higher administrative costs and subjects enrollees to individual underwriting. Why not let employers buy individual insurance for their employees the way they currently buy group insurance? Most small employers and their employees would probably jump at the chance, were it not prohibited by state laws.

This book is not the appropriate place to sort out the advantages and disadvantages of the two types of insurance. Presumably, the market could do that sorting out much better than academics. Unfortunately, the playing field is not level.

The Bias toward Group Insurance

As noted, current tax law grants very generous subsidies to employer purchase of health insurance. Yet, those same subsidies are denied to individuals who purchase their own insurance. (See Figure 13.6.) In almost everyone's estimation, this is partly the accidental result of years of tax policy rather than a methodical approach to health policy. Perhaps unintentionally, the tax-writing committees of Congress have shaped and molded our health insurance system.

Achieving Neutral Policy

In the case of individual versus group insurance, neutral policy is easy to envision and implement. A neutral government would give the same tax subsidy to every form of insurance. (See Figure 13.7.) Accordingly, individual and group coverage would compete on a level playing field. In such a world, employers would not offer insurance at all unless they had a comparative advantage in

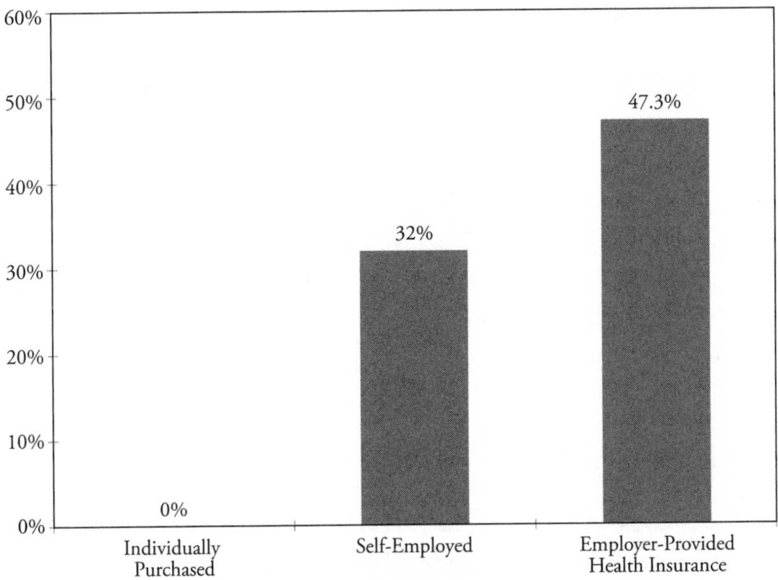

Note: Assumes taxpayer is in the 25 percent federal income tax bracket, faces a 15.3 percent payroll (FICA) tax, and a 7 percent state and local income tax.

Figure 13.6. Federal and State Tax Subsidies for Private Insurance

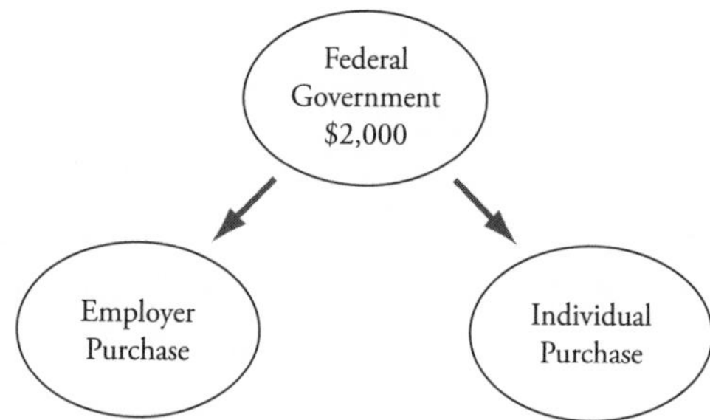

Figure 13.7. A Level Playing Field for All Insurance Purchases

doing so in their competition for labor. Undoubtedly, many large companies do have an advantage. They can do for their employees things the employees cannot do for themselves. Many small firms, however, have no such advantage and probably would be better off paying higher wages instead of paying for health insurance.

Choice Number 4: Third-Party Insurance or Individual Self-Insurance?

In every insurance field, people must decide how much risk to transfer to an insurer and how much to retain. Often, the decision focuses on the size of the deductible. There are, however, other ways to divide up responsibilities for risks. In general, risk is transferred to an insurer in return for third-party insurance. When risk is retained, the individual is said to self-insure. In a competitive market, individuals would decide how much risk to transfer to third parties based on their own attitude toward risk and insurance premiums.

Unfortunately, government policies intervene.

The Bias toward Third-Party Insurance

As noted, every dollar an employer pays in health insurance premiums avoids income and payroll taxes. For a middle-income employee, this generous tax subsidy means government is effectively paying for almost half the cost of their health insurance. On the other hand, government will tax away almost half of every dollar the employer puts into a savings account for the employee to pay medical expenses directly. The result is a tax law that lavishly subsidizes third-party insurance and severely penalizes individual self-insurance. This encourages people to use third-party bureaucracies to pay every medical bill, even though it often makes more sense for patients to manage discretionary expenses themselves.

Opportunities to Self-Insure

A number of vehicles are available to make it easier for individuals to self-insure for medical expenses. These include tax-free Health Savings Accounts, Health Reimbursement Arrangements, and Flexible Spending Accounts. Also, about half the states now have Cash and Counseling programs for the Medicaid disabled population. These are pilot programs that allow enrollees to manage their healthcare dollars.

All of these are steps in the right direction, but the restrictions on these accounts are too onerous. For example, employees cannot have an HSA unless the employer has a qualified plan, and the restrictions in such plans prevent many sensible arrangements. Moreover, unlike the Medicaid programs, employers are not allowed to put different amounts in the accounts of the chronically ill to coincide with the severity of their illnesses. Also, the law requires the same across-the-board deductible for inpatient and outpatient expenses, as if patient discretion were equally appropriate in all cases.

Achieving Neutrality

A neutral policy is one that treats third-party insurance and individual self-insurance the same. For example, if government allows third-party insurance premiums to be paid with pre-tax dollars, then deposits to an HSA account should also be made with pre-tax dollars. (See Figure 13.8.)

In the case of a lump-sum tax credit, there is another way to create neutrality. Remember, with such a credit, the marginal (extra) premium is paid with after-tax dollars. In this case, deposits to HSA accounts should also be made with after-tax dollars. The amount would grow tax-free and withdrawals would be tax-free.[7]

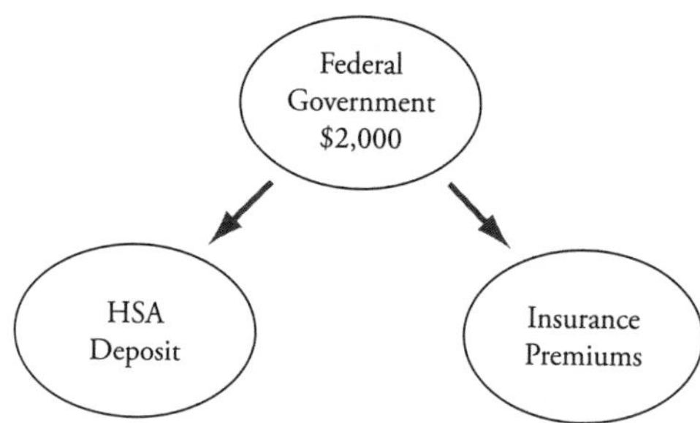

Figure 13.8. A Level Playing Field for All Types of Insurance

Choice Number 5: Decisions in the Market for Risk

In 1980, Census Bureau statistics showed that less than 1 percent of the population had been denied health insurance because of a health condition. Moreover, this was a period of time when there were few legislative remedies. Even so, this 1 percent was a politically vocal group and, in many cases, they evoked understandable sympathy. However, rather than deal with this group directly (for instance, by creating risk pools or offering direct subsidies), politicians through the years have imposed unwise restrictions on the other 99 percent of the people.

Destroying the Market for Risk

A proliferation of state laws has made it increasingly easy for people to obtain insurance after they get sick. Guaranteed issue regulations (requiring insurers to take all applicants, regardless of health status) and community rating regulations (requiring insurers to charge the same premium to all enrollees, regardless of health status) are a free rider's heaven.

They encourage everyone to remain uninsured while healthy, confident they will always be able to obtain insurance once they get sick. Moreover, as healthy people respond to these incentives by electing to be uninsured, the premium that must be charged to cover costs for those who remain in insurance pools rises. These higher premiums, in turn, encourage even more healthy people to drop their coverage.

Federal legislation has also made it increasingly easy to obtain insurance after one gets sick. The Health Insurance Portability and Accountability Act (HIPAA) of 1996 had a noble intent: to guarantee that people who have been paying premiums into the private insurance system do not lose coverage simply because they change jobs. However, a side effect of pursuing this desirable goal is a provision that allows any small business to obtain insurance regardless of the health status of its employees. This means that a small mom-and-pop operation can save money by remaining uninsured until a family member gets sick.

Individuals also can opt out of an employer's plan and re-enroll after they get sick. They are entitled to full coverage for a pre-existing condition after an 18-month waiting period. A group health plan can apply pre-existing condition exclusions for no more than 12 months, except in the case of late enrollees, to whom exclusions can apply for 18 months.

Under ACA, the perverse incentives to remain uninsured until you get sick will intensify. Basically, anyone who is uninsured will be able to obtain insurance for the same premium as a healthy individual, regardless of how long or why the person is uninsured. As in Massachusetts today, there will be fines for being uninsured, but the tax penalty will be small compared to the cost of insurance. And it may be weakly enforced, even at that.

Consequences of Unwise Regulation

By far, the worst consequence of government regulation of the market for risk is the unintended harm done to the very people the laws were intended to help. Precisely because the premium attached to high-risk individuals is much lower than their expected healthcare costs, insurers seek to avoid enrolling them in the first place. Precisely because payments to providers also do not reflect expected costs, they, too, have an incentive to avoid attracting the hard cases, especially among the chronically ill.

If healthcare markets worked the way normal markets do, health insurers and providers would vigorously compete for the business of the sick. In normal markets, entrepreneurs make profits by figuring out how to better solve other people's problems. In healthcare, by contrast, entrepreneurs run from other people's problems.

The Need for a Market for Risk

Current policy toward risk encourages all of us to remain uninsured while we are healthy. The consequences are unfortunate. People cannot make rational choices about risk if risk avoidance is not available at market prices.

A neutral policy would allow risk to be freely priced in the marketplace, with government intervening to help specific individuals only in special cases.

Consequences of a Policy of "Do No Harm"

This chapter has two objectives: first, to identify ways in which government policies create perverse incentives and lead to problems that many turn to government to solve; and second, to identify what policy changes would be needed to make government a neutral player in the healthcare system.

Under a policy of neutrality, government no longer would be a cause of the problems so many people complain about. Further, if government were removed as a source of problems, the resulting system would have some remarkably attractive features. The following is a summary.

Form of Universal Coverage

Under the neutrality reforms envisioned here, government would promise every citizen a fixed sum of money. Those who choose private insurance would get a tax credit against premiums. For those who are uninsured, the sum would be used to fund a healthcare safety net in their locality. Further, because money follows people, there would always be a minimum amount of funding regardless of how many people are uninsured.

A Level Playing Field for Public and Private Insurance

Low-income families would no longer be trapped in public systems where the quality of care is frequently suspect and there is often rationing of care, especially rationing by waiting. Instead, people would be able to apply funds spent on their behalf to enroll in an employer's plan or purchase health insurance directly.

A Level Playing Field for Individual and Group Insurance

No longer would tax policy be biased in favor of an employer-based system in which people lose their insurance whenever they leave or change jobs. Instead, tax law would grant the same subsidy to all forms of insurance, regardless of how it is purchased. Further, employers would be able to purchase individually owned, portable insurance for their employees in the same way they purchase group insurance today.

A Level Playing Field for Third-Party Insurance and Individual Self-Insurance

No longer would the tax law encourage the HMO form of insurance by subsidizing third-party insurance while penalizing self-insurance. Instead, all forms of insurance would compete against each other on a level playing field. The expected outcome is an evolving system under which people manage more of their own healthcare dollars, especially for those expenditures for which patients can exercise discretion and where it is appropriate for them to exercise discretion.

A Genuine Market for Risk

No longer would governments require insurers to charge prices for risk that are totally unrelated to an individual's real health costs. Instead, healthy people would be able to buy into the system at prices that reflect their expected costs. The insurance they buy would most likely be portable insurance, making possible a long-term relationship with their insurer and their physicians. In case of a serious illness, people would be able to transfer to other health plans at market prices (not artificially low prices) paid mainly by their current insurer. As a result, insurers would actively compete for sick people, including the chronically ill, and providers would compete to deliver that care.

Conclusion

The system described above would not be perfect. Far from it. It would, though, be a considerable improvement over the system we have today. The bottom line is that much good can come from undoing the harm that unwise government policies routinely cause to the nation's healthcare system.

PART IV

Letting Government Out of the Trap

14

Reforming Medicare

AT THE FEDERAL LEVEL, healthcare is the most serious domestic policy problem we have, and Medicare is the most important component of that problem. Every federal agency that has examined the issue has affirmed that we are on a dangerous, unsustainable spending path.

Medicare's Funding Problem

Take a look at the first column of numbers in Table 14.1. In 2009, the Social Security and Medicare Trustees calculated the unfunded liability in the two programs at $107 trillion—a figure about six-and-a-half times the size of the entire US economy (see Table 14.1). For both Social Security and Medicare to be financially secure, we need $107 trillion in the bank right now, earning interest, and it's not there.

How ACA Affects Medicare's Unfunded Liability

Now for some good news. Look at the second column in Table 14.1. It shows that by 2010, the unfunded liability had been almost cut in half. The reason: ACA. The very minute that President Obama signed the Affordable Care Act, he cut Medicare's unfunded liability by more than $50 trillion.[1] You would think this accomplishment would be an occasion for great joy—a time for dancing and celebration in the streets. Yet if you are like most Americans, you probably haven't heard about it. Certainly the Obama administration isn't talking about it.

Table 14.1. Unfunded Obligations of Social Security and Medicare (Infinite Time Horizon)

	2009	2010
Social Security	**$ 17.5 trillion**	**$ 18.6 trillion**
Medicare Part A	$36.7 trillion	–$0.3 trillion
Medicare Part B	$37.0 trillion	$21.2 trillion
Medicare Part D	$15.6 trillion	$15.8 trillion
Total Medicare	**$89.3 trillion**	**$36.7 trillion**
Total Medicare and Social Security	**$106.8 trillion**	**$55.3 trillion**

Sources: "The 2009 Annual Report of the Board of Trustees of the Federal Old-Age and Survivors Insurance and Federal Disability Insurance Trust Funds," Social Security Administration, Office of the Chief Actuary, May 12, 2009.
"The 2010 Annual Report of The Board of Trustees of The Federal Old-Age And Survivors Insurance and Federal Disability Insurance Trust Funds," Social Security Administration, August 15, 2010.

As we have seen, the Affordable Care Act uses cuts in Medicare to pay for more than half the cost of expanding health insurance for young people, but it contains no serious plan for making Medicare more efficient. All it really proposes to do is pay less to doctors and hospitals. That's why the Medicare actuaries are predicting greatly reduced access to care for the elderly and the disabled.

Most serious people inside the Washington, DC, beltway believe these cuts will never take place. The reason: our experience with similar cuts in Medicare under previous legislation. If Congress has been unwilling to allow reductions in doctor fees for nine straight years under previous legislation, how likely is it to allow the even greater spending reductions called for under ACA?

Impact on People at Different Ages

If the spending cuts do take place, however, what does that mean for individual retirees? It's much easier to say how much Medicare spending will change than it is to say what these changes will mean in terms of access to care. Table 14.2 shows the changes in Medicare spending for individuals of different ages:

Table 14.2. Value of Lifetime Medicare Benefits Compared to Taxes and Premiums, Before and After ACA

		65 Today	65 in 2020	65 in 2030
2009	Before ACA Benefits	$192,421	$254,900	$345,237
	Taxes and Premiums	−132,305	−200,651	−298,362
	Net Benefits	$ 60,116	$ 54,249	$ 46,875
2010	After ACA Benefits	$156,833	$192,585	$240,233
	Taxes and Premiums	−124,027	−181,358	−251,660
	Net Benefits	$ 32,806	$ 11,227	−$ 11,427
Reduction in Net Benefits due to ACA		$ 27,310	$ 43,022	$ 58,302

Source: Courtney Collins and Andrew J. Rettenmaier, "How Health Reform Affects Current and Future Retirees," National Center for Policy Analysis, Policy Report 333, May 2011.

- For someone turning age 65 and enrolling in Medicare in 2011, the present value of projected Medicare spending was reduced by $35,588 the day Barack Obama signed the health reform bill.
- For a 55 year old, the projected reduction in Medicare spending is $62,315.
- For a 45 year old, the loss totals $105,004.

One way to think about these changes is to compare them to the average amount Medicare currently spends on enrollees each year. For 65 year olds, the forecasted reduction in spending is roughly equal to three years of average Medicare spending. For 55 year olds, the loss expected is the rough equivalent of five years of benefits; and for 45 year olds, it's almost nine years.

Consider other reforms that would have reduced Medicare spending by an equivalent amount of money. The Medicare spending reduction called for in the health reform bill is the rough equivalent of raising the age of eligibility for 65 year olds from age 65 to 68. It is the equivalent of making 55 year olds wait until they reach age 70 and 45 year olds wait all the way to age 74!

Fortunately for beneficiaries, there are two offsetting benefits from lower Medicare spending. When spending declines, so do the required premiums and taxes needed to support those benefits. As a result, beneficiaries will have more disposable income than otherwise.

What the Medicare Payment Reductions Might Mean for Beneficiaries.

What will these reductions do in terms of out-of-pocket payments and access to care? A reasonable assumption is that seniors will need to offset some or all of Medicare's spending reductions with additional spending of their own, if they want the same level of care. Under current law, seniors are not allowed to top up what Medicare pays to match what other payers are paying for care. This inability will make them increasingly unattractive to providers. They may be able to circumvent this restriction by paying money to concierge doctors, however. That is, seniors may be able to pay doctors for non-Medicare services as a backdoor way of paying more for covered services. Another possibility is that the law may be changed.

If seniors are allowed to make up for the cuts in Medicare spending with out-of-pocket payments, they will need to spend 10 percent of the average Social Security check by 2017. Fifty years from now, they will need to spend half of their Social Security income to offset the decline in Medicare spending.

Is Medicare a Good Deal?

Think about everything you will pay to support Medicare: the payroll taxes while you are working, the premiums during retirement, and your share of the income taxes that subsidize the system. Then compare that to the benefits of Medicare insurance, say, from age 65 until the day you die.

Are you likely to come out ahead? That depends in part on how old you are. If you are a typical 85 year old, you can expect about $55,000 of insurance benefits over and above everything you have been paying into the system. If you're a typical 25 year old, however, you will pay an extra $111,000 into the system, over and above any benefits you can expect to receive.

In terms of dollars in and dollars out, a typical 85 year old is going to get back $2.69 in benefits for every dollar paid into the system in the form of premiums and taxes over his or her lifetime—a good deal by any measure. Almost everyone under the age of 50 will pay in more than they get back, however. For

Table 14.3. Medicare Benefits per Dollar Contributed*

Age	Benefits/Cost
85	$2.69
75	$1.80
65	$1.26
50	$1.06
45	$0.95
35	$0.88
25	$0.75

*payroll taxes + premiums + income taxes

Source: Courtney Collins and Andrew J. Rettenmaier, "How Health Reform Affects Current and Future Retirees," National Center for Policy Analysis, Policy Report 333, May 2011.

example, 25 year olds can expect to get back only 75 cents for every dollar they contribute. (See Table 14.3.)

Cash Flow Deficits

Medicare's more immediate problem is cash flow. Until recently, the effect of Social Security and Medicare on the rest of the federal government was relatively small. As the baby boomers retire, however, the burden will soar. Without the politically difficult Medicare spending cuts called for under ACA, it will be increasingly difficult for the federal government to continue spending on other activities: although no one expects the federal government to balance its budget anytime soon, if it does so in 2020 the federal government will require about one out of every four dollars of general income tax revenues to cover the cash flow deficits in Social Security and Medicare.[2] Education, national defense, housing, energy, Social Security—all of these activities of government will have to be put aside, if healthcare promises to the elderly are to be met.

And we haven't said anything about Medicaid. According to the Congressional Budget Office, if Medicare and Medicaid spending continue to grow at their historical growth rates relative to national income, healthcare spending will consume nearly the entire federal budget by midcentury.[3]

OTHER MEDICARE REFORM PROPOSALS

Any plan to reduce the growth rate of federal spending on healthcare without doing something about healthcare spending as a whole will necessarily shift costs—to the elderly, to the poor, to state governments, and to anybody other than the federal government.

ACA Reforms. Let's start with President Obama, since his plan is already law. The numbers you see in newspapers are almost always produced by the Congressional Budget Office (CBO), the bean-counting agency of Congress. These forecasts show a dramatic slowing of Medicare spending—about in line with other reform proposals discussed below.[4] If you are elderly or disabled, however, pay attention to a more ominous document—the Medicare Trustees report.[5] (Since the Medicare Trustees are appointed by the president, this document appears to reflect the Obama administration's view of its own health plan.) As Figure 14.2 shows, according to the Medicare Trustees, ACA will cut the rate of growth of Medicare spending in half and allow it to grow no faster than our national income.

The Ryan/Rivlin Plan. Congressman Paul Ryan (R-WI) and Alice Rivlin, former director of the CBO, have proposed an entitlement spending reform plan that is striking both for its boldness and its left-right-coming-together origins.[6] The three most important parts are:

- For the first time, Medicare would be transformed into rational insurance. Beginning in 2013, all enrollees would be protected by a $6,000 cap on out-of-pocket expenses; in return, they would pay for more small expenses on their own.
- After a decade, people newly eligible for Medicare would receive a voucher (also called "premium support") to purchase private insurance instead. The value of the voucher would grow at the rate of growth of gross domestic product (GDP) *plus 1 percent* (note: for the past four decades, healthcare spending per capita nationwide has been growing at about *GDP growth plus 2 percent*).
- Medicaid would be turned into annual block grants to the states. The value of the block grants would also grow at GDP growth plus 1 percent.

Congressman Ryan has been attacked by columnist Paul Krugman and others on the left for proposing to spend too little on the elderly.[7] Yet the Ryan/Rivlin proposal reduces government spending on Medicare by less than the ACA does—a bill supported by Krugman and other Ryan critics.

Also, Ryan's concept of "premium support," criticized by those on the left, originates with left-of-center economists Henry Aaron and Bob Reischauer, and we already have it in the Medicare Advantage programs, serving about one-fourth of all Medicare enrollees.[8] In addition, the subsidies for private plans sold in ACA health insurance exchanges will also morph into premium support.[9]

The Ryan/Rivlin proposal and others that are similar try to limit federal spending to the growth rate of GDP plus 1 percent, and all involve a premium support approach, under which the federal government makes available a fixed number of dollars (or voucher), beneficiaries add to that amount from their own resources, and health plans compete against each other. The ACA, by contrast, limits spending to the growth rate of GDP and has no premium support.

The Paul Ryan/Republican House Budget Proposal. This proposal is similar with one important exception: Medicare spending follows the ACA cuts for the next 10 years and then calls for more severe cuts. There is no difference between ACA and the House Republican plan for anyone over 55 years of age, however.

The major problem with all of these proposals is that they do not change incentives—or they do not change them enough. There is no reason to expect overall healthcare spending to change, which means the federal government would be committed to spend less and less on the elderly and the disabled.

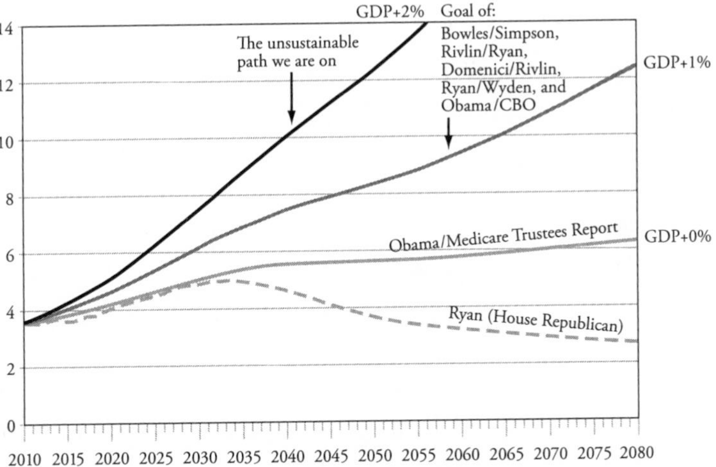

Figure 14.2. Medicare Spending Relative to GDP

Sources: Social Security Trustees, Congressional Budget Office, and House Budget Committee Chairman Paul Ryan.

What about the Trust Funds?

Although workers have been repeatedly told that their payroll taxes are being securely held in trust funds, they are actually being spent—the very day, the very hour, the very minute they arrive in the Treasury's bank account.

No money has been saved. No investments have been made. No cash has been stashed away in bank vaults. Today's payroll tax payments are being spent to pay medical bills for today's retirees. And if any surplus materializes, it's spent on other government programs. As a result, when today's workers reach the eligibility age of 65, they will be able to get benefits only if future taxpayers pay (even higher) taxes to support them.

Bottom line: For the Treasury to write a check, it cannot look to the trust funds. It must first tax or borrow.

Causes of the Problem

Why are we having these problems in the first place? Here are some of the major reasons:

- Since Medicare beneficiaries are participating in a use-it-or-lose-it system, patients can realize benefits only by consuming more care; they receive no personal benefit from consuming care prudently, and they bear no personal cost if they are wasteful.
- Since Medicare providers are trapped in a system in which they are paid predetermined fees for prescribed tasks, they have no financial incentives to improve outcomes; and physicians often receive less take-home pay if they provide low-cost, high-quality care.
- Since Medicare won't pay for lower-cost, higher-quality services produced outside the Medicare system, most seniors do not have access to walk-in clinics, freestanding emergency rooms, and other services available to non-seniors.
- Insurers are also seriously constrained; for example, they cannot offer seniors many of the same insurance arrangements that employees getting health insurance at work take for granted.
- Since Medicare is funded on a pay-as-you-go basis, many of today's taxpayers are not saving and investing to fund their own postretirement

care; thus, today's young workers will receive benefits only if future workers are willing to pay exorbitantly high tax rates.

Finding a Solution

To address these defects in the current system, my colleagues and I at the National Center for Policy Analysis propose five fundamental Medicare reforms:[10]

- Using a special type of Health Savings Account, beneficiaries would be able to manage at least one-fifth of their healthcare dollars—thus keeping each dollar of wasteful spending they avoid and bearing the full cost of each dollar of waste they generate.
- Physicians would be free to repackage and reprice their services—thus profiting from innovations that lower costs and raise the quality of care.
- Medicare beneficiaries would have immediate access to walk-in clinics and a raft of other services, where prices are being set in a real marketplace.
- Insurers would have complete freedom to provide seniors with the full range of products non-seniors have access to.
- Workers (along with their employers) would save and invest 4 percent of payroll—eventually reaching the point where each generation of retirees pays for the bulk of its own postretirement medical care.

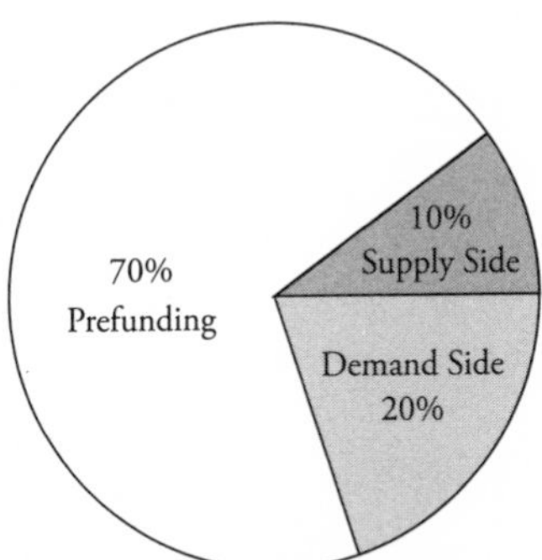

Figure 14.1. Closing the Gap on Medicare Funding (as of 2050)
Source: John C. Goodman, "A Framework for Medicare Reform," National Center for Policy Analysis, Policy Report No. 315, September 2008.

These reforms would dramatically change incentives. Whether patient, provider, or worker/saver, people would reap the benefits of socially beneficial behavior and incur the costs of socially undesirable behavior. Specifically, Medicare patients would have a direct financial interest in seeking out low-cost, high-quality care. Providers would have a direct financial interest in producing it. And young people would have a financial interest in a long-term financing system that promotes efficient, high-quality care for generations to come.

With assistance from NCPA Senior Fellow Andrew J. Rettenmaier, we have been able to simulate the long-term impact of some of these reforms. The bottom line: Under reasonable assumptions, we can reach the mid-21st century with seniors paying no more (as a share of the cost of the program) than the premiums they pay today and with a taxpayer burden (relative to national income) no greater than the burden today.[11]

How is this achieved? As Figure 14.1 (previous page) shows, about 70 percent of the reduction in projected Medicare spending is due to pre-funding of benefits through private accounts; 20 percent is the result of changes in consumption behavior because of the higher deductibles; and 10 percent is the result of supply-side changes (using very conservative assumptions).

In what follows, we will take an in-depth look at this proposal.

A Detailed Reform Plan

New Opportunities for Patients

Under the current structure, seniors pay as many as three premiums to three plans (Medicare Part B, Medigap, and Medicare Part D) and often still do not have the coverage nonseniors typically have. We propose to replace this structure with a new, simplified structure—meant to mimic the health insurance benefits the rest of Americans enjoy.

Standard Comprehensive Plan (SCP)

This provides across-the-board comprehensive coverage above the $2,500 deductible. Only one premium is needed to enroll, and it costs about 15 percent of Medicare's average member cost. All current Medicare beneficiaries will have the opportunity to enroll in a SCP as an alternative to traditional

Medicare. For all future Medicare enrollees, the SCP will be the only government plan offered.

Roth-Type Health Savings Accounts

All seniors enrolled in a SCP may deposit up to $2,500 in a Roth-type HSA. These deposits are after-tax, they grow tax-free, and they may be withdrawn for any purpose tax-free. Most seniors who enroll in SCPs will be able to fund their HSA deposits with money that would otherwise be spent out of pocket, plus the savings on premium expenses. Those who elect some of the options described below may be able to have larger accounts—funded by third-party insurers or out-of-pocket contributions. In all cases, seniors will use their HSAs to pay for expenses not paid by third-party insurance.

Risk-Adjusted Premiums

People who are already enrolled in Medicare will continue to pay premiums equal to about 15 percent of Medicare's actual cost. For those who enroll in private plans, the government will add to this amount a risk-adjusted premium reflecting the enrollee's expected health costs to a private plan selected by the enrollee. The government's goal is to ensure that the total premium will always be sufficient to purchase the SCP package of benefits, although for private plans this premium will be determined by competition in the marketplace. (The current method of making risk-rated premium payments can serve as a guide.)

Other Insurance Options

Seniors will have other insurance options. Following the method described above, we will be able to fix the government's liability. Once the government (taxpayer) contribution has been set, insurers will be able to offer different benefit packages, with higher or lower overall premiums. These options would include HMOs, PPOs, HSA plans with higher deductibles, and Special Needs Plans with HSAs. Also, retirees could remain in their previous employer's plan (if the employer is willing) by directing the government's contribution to that plan.

Seniors who choose one of the private options may have other HSA opportunities. For example, a senior choosing a $5,000 deductible plan will be able to make a $5,000 annual HSA deposit, with the extra $2,500, say, covered by a $1,250 deposit by the insurer and $1,250 from the enrollee.

New Health Savings Account Design

Private insurers offering HSA plans will not be required to have an across-the-board deductible. They will instead be allowed to reduce the deductible to zero for services they want to encourage (such as medications for schizophrenia) and maintain high deductibles for services where patient discretion is appropriate and desirable (for example, choice of drugs for arthritis or allergies). In addition, plans will be able to carve out whole categories of care (such as primary care or diagnostic tests), which patients will pay entirely from their HSAs without any deductible or co-payment.[12]

Insurers will also be able to create special HSA accounts for the chronically ill, allowing them to manage more of their own healthcare dollars. The Cash and Counsel experiment provides a model to follow. In these programs, disabled Medicaid patients manage their own healthcare budgets and can hire and fire those who provide them with custodial and even medical services.[13] The insurer's incentives to improve plan design will be enhanced by long-term contracts.

New Opportunities for Doctors

Physicians participating in Medicare today must practice medicine under an outmoded, wasteful payment system, where they typically receive no financial reward for talking to patients by telephone, communicating by email, teaching patients how to manage their own care, or helping them be better consumers in the market for drugs.

Consider the sidebar on the next page on how doctors are paid. As you read it, imagine that instead of prices next to goods at Wal-Mart, you encountered a sign that read like this sidebar. How much you pay for an item would depend on which Wal-Mart employee helped you find it, how many other employees helped you, what you intend to do with the item after you purchase it, etc. There is a reason why Wal-Mart doesn't price its goods the way Medicare does.

To make matters worse, as Medicare suppresses reimbursement fees, doctors are increasingly unable to perform any task that is inadequately reimbursed. Other healthcare providers face the same perverse incentives. All too often, Medicare's payment rules get in the way of providers working together to improve healthcare.

HOW DOCTORS GET PAID BY MEDICARE[14]

- For many procedures, Medicare pays providers for the professional and technical component. The professional component is the physician's work and expertise; the technical component provides reimbursement for equipment and supplemental staff needed to perform the procedure. If another entity performed the technical component, then the physician is only paid for the professional component. For instance, for lab tests, the lab may run the test (technical component) but the physician would be the one interpreting the test (professional component).
- If you assist in a surgery, you receive 16 percent of the fee the primary surgeon does. Under some circumstances, the individual skills of two surgeons are required to perform surgery on the same patient during the same operative session. If you are a co-surgeon (rather than an assistant at surgery), you receive 62.5 percent of the typical reimbursement for that surgery.
- If you perform a bilateral surgery—a surgery done on both sides of the body (e.g., right arm and left arm)—then you receive 150 percent of the payment you would have received from doing a unilateral surgery.
- When multiple procedures are performed through the same endoscope, payment will be made for the highest valued endoscopy (100 percent of the allowance) plus the difference between the next highest and the base endoscopy.
- If you perform multiple surgeries in the same day on the same patient, you do not get paid the same amount as if these were performed on multiple days. The highest valued procedure is paid 100 percent of the allowance. For the second through the fifth highest valued procedures, the physician receives 50 percent of the typical payment amount.
- If you are a physician assistant, nurse practitioner, or a registered dietitian or nutritionists, you receive 85 percent of the payment an MD would receive for performing the same service.
- If you are a clinical social worker, you receive 75 percent of the payment an MD would receive for performing the same service.
- If you are a certified nurse midwife, you receive 85 percent of the payment an MD would receive for performing the same service. If you are a midwife, you only receive 65 percent.

How can we produce high-quality care for a cost that is well below the price we are paying today? There are hundreds of examples of efficient, high-quality care, and many of them have been studied and described in the academic literature. For example, studies by researchers at the Dartmouth Institute for Health Policy and Clinical Practice imply that if everyone in America went to the Mayo Clinic for healthcare, the nation could reduce its annual healthcare bill by one-fourth.[15] If everyone went to Intermountain Healthcare in Salt Lake City, the nation could reduce its healthcare spending by one-third.[16] Studies by Dartmouth[17] and the National Center for Policy Analysis[18] imply that if every region of the country practiced medicine the way the most "efficient" or low-cost regions do, we could cut Medicare spending by one-third to one-fourth from its current level.

How do we get from here to there? Here are four case studies describing what's already happening.

Case Study: Geisinger Health System in Central Pennsylvania

Geisinger offers a ninety-day warranty on heart surgery. If the patient returns with complications during that period, Geisinger promises to provide treatment without sending the patient or the insurer another bill.[19]

Geisinger incurs financial losses under this practice, even as it saves money for Medicare overall, because healthcare organizations are paid more when patients have complications that lead to more visits, more tests, and more readmissions. What is needed is a willingness to pay for such guarantees. Medicare should be willing to pay more for the initial surgery if taxpayers save money overall.

Case Study: Virginia Mason Medical Center in Seattle

In another innovative example, Virginia Mason offers a new approach to the treatment of back pain.[20] Under the old system, a patient would often first receive an MRI scan or specialty consultation and other tests before referral to a physical therapist. Under the new system—which cuts the cost of treatment in half—patients are first seen by a physical therapist unless additional diagnostic measures are clearly indicated. An MRI scan is ordered only if the therapy doesn't work and symptoms persist.

The new system improves efficiency and saves money for payers but leaves the providers financially worse off. As in the case of Geisinger, Medicare should permit a new payment arrangement—one that is win-win for Medicare and Virginia Mason.

Case Study: Pharmacists Delivering Care

In a highly successful experiment in Asheville, North Carolina, pharmacists counsel diabetic patients and encourage them to take appropriate medications.[21] In this case, the provider is offering a new package of services—one that reduces trips to emergency rooms and to the offices of primary care physicians and lowers overall costs. Unless Medicare offers pharmacists in other cities the opportunity to make money by rebundling in this way, however, the potential for savings will be missed.

Case Study: American Physician Housecalls in Dallas[22]

For over a decade, this company has provided integrated care, coordinated care, medical homes, electronic medical records, electronic prescribing, and other items on the ACA "pilot project" wish list. Essentially, American Physician Housecalls (APH) treats special needs seniors who usually cost Medicare about $60,000 a year. By successfully treating them on an outpatient basis, APH cuts Medicare's cost in half.

Under the APH model, physicians and nurse practitioners visit the patients and treat them in their own homes. Among the services: portable X-ray imaging, echocardiograms, phlebotomy and other lab procedures, and podiatry and geriatric consultations. Because each patient receives care from multiple physicians, the physicians coordinate their activities by means of electronic medical records.

So how much does Medicare pay APH for saving it all that money? Not a dime, beyond the normal Medicare fee schedule. The APH management team has spent many fruitless hours trying to get Medicare to pay them in a different way. APH is considering becoming an ACO, but a full-blown ACO handles all of a patient's care (inpatient and outpatient). Were APH to attempt to do that, it would have to master a completely different skill set.

A Better Way

In general, we should be willing to reward doctors who raise quality and lower costs—who improve patient access to care, improve communication, and teach patients how to be better managers of their own care. Any provider should be able to propose and obtain a different reimbursement arrangement, provided that (1) the total cost to government does not increase, (2) patient quality of care does not decrease, and (3) the provider proposes a method of measuring and assuring that (1) and (2) have been satisfied.

Liberating the Marketplace

As noted, Medicare has a list of about 7,500 separate tasks that it pays physicians to perform. For each task there is a price that varies by location and other factors. Of the 800,000 practicing physicians in this country, not all are in Medicare and no doctor will be a candidate to perform every task on Medicare's list.

Still, Medicare is potentially setting about 6 billion prices at any one time all over the United States of America, as well as in Guam, Puerto Rico, the Mariana Islands, American Samoa and the Virgin Islands.

Each price Medicare pays is tied to a patient with a condition, and surrounding each separate fee are innumerable technical questions. Of the 7,500 things doctors could possibly do to treat a condition, Medicare has to be just as diligent in not paying for inappropriate care as it is paying for procedures that should be done. Medicare isn't just setting prices. It is regulating whole transactions.

Let's say that the 50 million or so Medicare enrollees average about ten doctor visits per year and let's conservatively assume that each visit gives rise to only one procedure. Then considering all of the ways a procedure can be correctly and incorrectly coded, Medicare is regulating 3 quadrillion potential transactions over the course of a year! (A quadrillion is a one followed by fifteen zeroes.)

Is there any chance that Medicare can make the right decisions for all these transactions? Not likely.

Things are about to get much worse. A new version of the federally mandated codebook, called ICD-10,[23] will expand the number of medical classifications to around 155,000 or more.[24] For example, there will be ninety-six different codes for bites—including three different codes for getting bitten by a squirrel (i.e. initial encounter, subsequent encounter and sequel). There will be six different codes depending on whether you are bitten by a rat or a mouse.

The level of detail is astounding. According to *The Wall Street Journal*:[25]

> [H]ealth plans may never again wonder where a patient got hurt. There are codes for injuries in opera houses..., art galleries..., squash courts... and nine locations in and around a mobile home..., from the bathroom to the bedroom.

For instance, there will be 240 different codes for injuries incurred by being "hit" or "struck," about one-quarter of which pertain only to injuries sustained while on a watercraft. There are separate codes to describe injuries on a watercraft, including different codes for whether the injury occurred on a merchant ship, passenger ship, fishing boat, sail boat, canoe, unpowered inflatable boat, etc.

Thankfully, there is an alternative to all this: Let's begin the process of allowing medical fees to be determined the way prices are determined everywhere else in our economy—in the marketplace.

In trying to do that, we face two problems. First, we have completely suppressed normal market forces in medical care for many years. How can you have market prices where no real market exists? Second, many people believe that Medicare is using monopsony (single buyer) power to push provider fees below market levels. Without government acting as a monopsony buyer, patients might end up paying more for the services they currently get. Former Medicare Trustee Thomas R. Saving and I have proposed ten important policy changes that can circumvent these two problems and free the marketplace in the process.[26]

Retail Outlets

All over the country, retail establishments offer primary care services to cash-paying patients.[27] Because these services arose outside of the third-party payment system, their prices are free market prices. Walk-in clinics, doc-in-the-box clinics, and freestanding emergency care clinics post prices and usually deliver high quality care. Many follow evidence-based protocols, keep records electronically and order prescriptions electronically.

Medicare should immediately allow enrollees to obtain care at almost all of these places—paying posted, market prices, not Medicare's prices. And since these fees are below what Medicare would have paid at a physician's office or hospital emergency room, this reform would lower Medicare's costs, even as it makes primary care more accessible.

Telephone and Email Services

Medicare should allow enrollees to take advantage of commercial telephone and email services,[28] such as Teladoc physician consultations.

Concierge Doctors

Medicare should encourage physicians to repackage and reprice their services in ways that are good for the doctor, good for the patient, and good for Medicare. For example, Medicare should encourage—rather than discourage—the emergence of concierge doctor arrangements.[29] If patients and doctors are willing, Medicare should be willing to throw its 7,500-item price list away, pay some portion of the concierge fee, and let the medical marketplace handle everything else.

Billing by Time, Rather than Task

Most professionals are not paid by task—the way doctors are paid. They are paid by the time it takes to deliver their services. As an alternative, we should allow doctors to change the mix of services they offer and pay them for their time. If the change in practice is substantial enough, we should allow patient co-payments and let them be determined in the marketplace. The test of whether the new set of services has added value is whether seniors are willing to pay more out of pocket to get them.

Paramedical Personnel

One way to expand the supply of low-cost medical care is through the increased use of nurses and physician assistants to perform tasks that do not require a physician's level of expertise. The current system discourages this: When a task is performed by a nurse rather than a physician, Medicare automatically reduces its fee.[30]

Bundling

One of the obstacles to offering patients a package price covering all services is that surgery typically involves several independent entities. In a normal market, independent entities come together all the time to jointly produce a good or service and divide the profit. The Stark amendment makes such arrangements illegal in the medical field.[31] Clearly this impediment to efficiency must be removed.

Medical Tourism

Increasingly, cash-paying patients are traveling outside the United States for surgery offering package prices that are one-fifth to one-third of the cost in the United States.[32] Moreover, a new company, Colorado-based BridgeHealth Medical offers US employer plans a specialty network with flat fees for surgeries paid in advance that are 15 percent to 50 percent less than a typical network.[33]

Since the international medical tourism market is a real market where providers routinely compete for patients based on price and quality, Medicare should take advantage of it. Further, if a patient saves money for Medicare by traveling, the patient should share in the savings. As in the case of doctors, patients should be encouraged to make money by saving Medicare money.

Domestic Medical Tourism. You don't actually have to go off shore to participate in the market for medical tourism. There is an emerging market for it on shore. As discussed in Chapter II, Canadians routinely come to the United States for surgical procedures and they usually face a package price for all services agreed to in advance. North American Surgery, Inc., has negotiated deep discounts with twenty-two surgery centers, hospitals and clinics across the United States as an alternative to foreign travel for low-cost surgeries.[34] Seniors too could be in this market and they would be if Medicare allowed the senior to share in the savings created by traveling to a higher-quality, lower-cost facility.

Selective Relaxation of Price Controls

There is substantial evidence that Medicare fees are well below normal fees paid by the private sector. There is very little evidence to show us what difference this makes, however. One way to find out is to let a few doctors in a given area charge anything they like for Medicare-covered services. Medicare would continue to pay its list price, but the patient would have to pay any remaining extra charge out of pocket.

Patients then would have a choice. They could go to doctors who charge the regulated Medicare fee. Or they could go to doctors who charge a market-determined fee. Here's the test: Can doctors who are free to do so attract patients even though those patients have to pay more than they would pay elsewhere? If so, that means that Medicare patients under the current system are being denied convenience, amenities, and perhaps quality that they are willing to pay for in the market. In the face of such evidence, Medicare should then be willing to allow even more doctors the same option.

Healthcare Stamps

Here is a novel idea for liberating low-income seniors. The proposal would be especially ideal for the dual eligible population (qualifying for both Medicare and Medicaid) because this population has first dollar coverage anyway. Supermarkets contain thousands of individual products all with prices attached. Since food consumption is a necessity, just as healthcare, how do we ensure that food is available to all? Rather than having Foodcare, we subsidize low-income individuals by selling them "dollar value food stamps" at discounted prices. These stamps are real money to the grocery stores and to the recipients. Since individuals consume more than their food stamp limit, on the margin they are spending actual money. However, if they choose to buy pricey steak instead of hamburger using food stamps dollars, they will have less to spend on other products.

The Food Stamp program (SNAP) appears to work much better than health assistance programs for low-income seniors. Currently three Medicare savings programs are designed to make Medicare more affordable for poor and near-poor beneficiaries by paying premiums and eliminating out-of-pocket cost sharing:[35]

- The Qualified Medicare Beneficiary Program pays all Medicare premiums and out-of-pocket cost sharing for beneficiaries who have incomes at or below 100 percent of the federal poverty level and who are ineligible for full Medicaid coverage.
- The Specified Low-Income Medicare Beneficiary Program pays Part B premiums for Medicare beneficiaries with incomes of 101 to 120 percent of the federal poverty level.
- The Qualified Individual Program pays Part B premiums for beneficiaries with incomes of 121 to 135 percent of the federal poverty level.

Yet amazingly, fewer than one-third of eligible Medicare beneficiaries enroll in these programs.

The Defining Principle

In each of these cases, and in others we could think of, the principle is the same: let markets do what only markets can do well. Let the market solve problems the gigantic Medicare regulatory apparatus can never solve.

New Opportunities for Insurers

The Obama administration wants to replace fragmented decision-making by independent doctors with coordinated care delivered by doctors working in teams, connected to a medical home. It wants Medicare to purchase quality, not quantity. It wants decisions to be evidence-based. It wants electronic records in order to standardize care and reduce errors.

Although the administration plans to spend hundreds of millions of dollars on pilot programs to try these ideas out, it appears to be ignoring private sector enterprises where some of these ideas appear to be working.

IntegraNet in Houston is an example of an integrated delivery network (IDN), an organization with about 1,200 affiliated doctors.[36] Every Medicare patient has a medical home. The physicians follow evidence-based practices. Care is integrated and coordinated. Electronic records are being introduced. It appears that quality is higher and costs are lower than in conventional Medicare.

IntegraNet doesn't satisfy all the government's (ACO) requirements by a long shot. For one thing, it pays its doctors fee-for-service. For another, it intentionally pays doctors more than Medicare's standard rates. IntegraNet is not alone. In many other Medicare Advantage plans, practitioners are already doing what the Obama administration says it wants to do with Medicare as a whole—without any prodding or nudging from the federal government. That is, many of these plans are using coordinated/integrated/managed care systems to achieve fewer admissions, fewer readmissions, and fewer hospital days than conventional Medicare.[37]

Of particular interest to me is the opportunity to give money back to patients who make cost-effective choices. A number of IDNs are way ahead of me—rebating some or all of the senior's Part B premium if they will cooperate and choose a medical home. As Larry Wedekind, IntegraNet's CEO, explains:

> It is the beauty of competition in a marketplace with several competitors all bidding for additional business from seniors. The ones that we have seen in the Houston market have ranged from a full Part B premium give-back to seniors to a 20 percent portion of it. . . . I've seen as low as $20 per month give-back to full premium give-back of $96 per month. . . . The Part B premium this year is $110.50, but no one is giving more than $50 per month back this coming year. The give-backs are often related to a Medicare Advantage Special Needs Plan such as a diabetic plan to help defray the higher costs of drugs.

New Opportunities for Workers

The purpose of a Health Insurance Retirement Account (HIRA) is to allow people to prefund some of their postretirement healthcare benefits, so that they do not have to rely as heavily as currently projected on future taxpayers. Eventually, each generation will pay its own way.

Contribution Levels

We envision an initial mandatory contribution level of 4 percent of payroll—2 percent each from the employer and employee. These amounts may rise in future years if they prove inadequate to achieve sufficient prefunding.

Investment of HIRA Funds

We propose that all HIRA funds be invested in diversified, conservative, international portfolios, consisting of stocks, bonds, real estate and other assets. The investment of HIRA funds will be managed by private security agencies. As is the case in Chile's social security system, these companies will compete not so much on portfolio selection but on reporting, accounting, and other services.

Contingent Ownership

Individuals are the nominal owners of their HIRAs, but their rights to these funds are contingent on several factors. First, they must survive to the age of eligibility for Medicare. In case of an early death, a worker's HIRA funds are distributed to the accounts of all remaining workers. In this sense, an individual's property rights in a HIRA are like contractual rights under an annuity insurance contract. Second, the SCPs will receive risk-rated premiums for all their enrollees. In the early years, the risk rating can be entirely accomplished by adjusting the government's contribution. Over time, however, HIRA balances in overfunded accounts may be "taxed" to make risk-rated premium payments on behalf of individuals with underfunded accounts. At this point, HIRA owners are entitled to a "risk-rated annual withdrawal."

HIRA Retirement Health Insurance Options

Owners of HIRA accounts will be given these options: (1) they can cede their HIRA funds to the government and enroll in a conventional Medicare SCP plan, (2) they can purchase an annuity—a stream of cash for their remaining years to be used to pay private health insurance premiums and to purchase healthcare directly, or (3) they can keep the account and withdraw an amount each year for the payment of premiums—with the withdrawal percentage determined by the government.

15

Reforming Medicaid

IN 2014, THE NATION is expected to start insuring about 32 million uninsured people. About half will enroll in Medicaid directly; and if the Massachusetts precedent is followed, most of the remainder will be in heavily subsidized private plans that pay little more than Medicaid rates.[1]

That raises an important question: How good is Medicaid? Will the people who enroll in it and in private plans that function like Medicaid get more care, or better care, than they would have gotten without health reform? I will begin this chapter by evaluating the evidence to answer that question. Then, I will propose three alternatives: (1) abolish Medicaid altogether and integrate the beneficiaries into the private health insurance system; (2) allow Medicaid to be a competing health plan, rather than a plan that sequesters poor people; or (3) replace much of Medicaid outpatient spending on the nonelderly, nondisabled with a health stamp program.

The Case Against Medicaid

What Will Happen to Access to Care for Medicaid Enrollees?

The 32 million newly insured citizens may not get more healthcare. They may even get less care. Even if they do get more, odds are that low-income families as a group will get less care than if there had never been a health reform bill in the first place. The reason: As we have seen, the same bill that insures 32 million new people also will force middle- and upper-middle-income families to have more generous coverage than they now have. As these more generously insured people attempt to acquire more medical services they will almost certainly outbid people paying Medicaid rates for doctor services and hospital beds. To make matters worse, the health reform bill did nothing to increase the supply side of the market to meet the increased demand.

The Effects of Underpaying Physicians

On paper Medicaid is attractive. It promises coverage for most medical services with no premium and usually no out-of-pocket payments. But Medicaid pays physicians only about 60 percent as much as private insurers pay, and many Medicaid patients have difficulty finding doctors who will see them. Increasingly, physicians are dropping out of the Medicaid program, declining to see new Medicaid patients or limiting Medicaid patients to a small percentage of their practice.[2] As a result, the patients turn to much costlier settings, such as hospital clinics and emergency rooms.

One study found that children were denied appointments 60 percent of the time when a caller reported Medicaid-CHIP as their coverage. By contrast, only 11 percent were denied an appointment when the caller reported private insurance. Of those who were able to obtain an appointment as Medicaid patients, the average wait was twenty-two days longer than those with private insurance.[3] Another study found that even the uninsured have an easier time making doctors' appointments than Medicaid enrollees.[4]

Although Medicaid rates for physicians are typically lower than what physicians receive from the private sector in every state,[5] the payment gap varies from one state to the next. New York state pays only about $30 for a comprehensive eye exam for a new patient, while Mississippi reimburses a physician $106 for the same service. Texas and Florida pay $63.55 and $66.90, respectively.

Access to Primary Care

About 30 percent of doctors do not accept any Medicaid patients, and among those who do, many limit the number they will treat. One survey found two-thirds of Medicaid patients were unable to obtain an appointment for urgent outpatient care.[6] In three-fourths of the cases, the reason was the provider did not accept Medicaid. Among general practitioners who will accept Medicaid, the lowest figures are 30 percent (Los Angeles), 40 percent (Miami) and 50 percent (Dallas and Houston).[7]

Access to Specialists

People enrolled in Medicaid and CHIP also experience difficulty finding specialists who will treat them for the low fees Medicaid pays.[8] A Government Accountability Office (GAO) report discovered that children enrolled in Medicaid or CHIP were one-third more likely to report problems accessing specialty care than children enrolled private health plans.[9] One survey finds that:[10]

- In Dallas and Philadelphia, only 8 percent of cardiologists accept Medicaid patients; in Los Angeles, it's only 11 percent.
- In both Dallas and New York City, only 14 percent of OB/GYN specialists will see Medicaid patients; the figure is 28 percent in Miami and 33 percent in Denver.

Use of the Emergency Room

According to a recent report, between 1997 and 2007 the total number of annual hospital emergency room (ER) visits doubled, mostly due to the increased frequency of use by adults with Medicaid coverage.[11] Medicaid enrollees account for more than one-fourth of all ER visits in the United States.[12]

Quality of Care under Medicaid

The academic evidence suggests that there is a severe quality problem in Medicaid. Here are some studies identified by American Enterprise Institute scholar Scott Gottlieb:[13]

- A study published in the medical journal *Cancer* found that Medicaid patients and people lacking any health insurance were both 50 percent more likely to die when compared with privately insured patients.[14]
- A study published in the *Annals of Surgery* found that being on Med-icaid was associated with the longest length of hospital stay, the highest total hospital costs and the highest risk of death.[15]

- A study published in the *American Journal of Cardiology* found that Medicaid patients were more than twice as likely to have a major subsequent heart attack after angioplasty, compared with patients who had no health insurance at all.[16]
- A study of patients undergoing lung transplants for pulmonary diseases, published in the *Journal of Heart and Lung Transplantation*, found that Medicaid patients were 8.1 percent less likely to survive ten years after the surgery than their privately insured and uninsured counterparts.[17]

In each of these studies, researchers controlled for the factors that can increase poor health outcomes in Medicaid patients. Almost everyone agrees that Medicaid is not as good as private insurance. A more contentious issue is whether Medicaid is better than no insurance at all.

Here are some additional studies identified by *Forbes* health blogger, Avik Roy:[18]

- A University of Virginia study found that individuals enrolled in Medicaid are almost twice as likely to die after surgery as privately insured patients, and about one-eighth more likely to die than the uninsured.[19]
- A study published in the *Journal of the National Cancer Institute* found that Florida Medicaid patients were 6 percent more likely to be diagnosed with prostate cancer at less treatable, later stages than the uninsured. Medicaid enrollees were nearly one-third (31 percent) more likely to be diagnosed with late-stage breast cancer and 81 percent more likely to be diagnosed with melanoma at a late stage. (Medicaid patients did outperform the uninsured on late-stage colon cancer.)[20]
- A study in the journal *Cancer* found that the mortality rate for Medicaid patients undergoing surgery for colon cancer was more than three times as high as for the privately insured and more than one-fourth higher than for the uninsured.[21]
- A study in the *Journal of Vascular Surgery* found that Medicaid patients treated for vascular problems, including plaque in their carotid (neck) arteries that pump blood to the brain and obstructions in the blood vessels in their legs, fared worse than did the uninsured (however, the uninsured with abdominal aneurysms fared worse than Medicaid patients).[22]

With respect to cancer care, it is unclear that Medicaid matters very much.[23] After reviewing the literature, Roy concludes that Medicaid patients do no better and sometimes worse than the uninsured.[24]

Health economist Austin Frakt takes issue with these studies, claiming that Medicaid and non-Medicaid populations are fundamentally different, even after adjusting for race, income, and other socioeconomic factors.[25] That claim seems improbable—at least at the margin—however, in light of the heavy ping-pong migration of people in and out of Medicaid eligibility.[26] Put another way, people who stay enrolled in Medicaid continuously probably are different from people who never enroll. But the most interesting group is the group that migrates back and forth.

Frakt points to some studies finding that Medicaid makes a positive difference over being uninsured.[27] But the results would probably have been just as good or better if we spent the money giving free care to vulnerable populations. Moreover, even with their Medicaid cards, enrollees turn to emergency rooms for their care twice as often as the privately insured and the uninsured.[28]

A RAND report on expanding Medicaid coverage in Oregon turned up some positive effects.[29] The Oregon Health Insurance Experiment found that those with Medicaid were one-third more likely to see a doctor, 15 percent more likely to fill a prescription, and 30 percent more likely to experience a hospital stay. Very poor and sick individuals enrolled in the program also reported that having Medicaid insurance made them feel healthier. However, economist Robin Hanson points out that about two-thirds of these effects occurred after being accepted into the program, before any care was actually received.[30]

How Wasteful Is Medicaid?

Fraud and abuse have plagued Medicaid since its inception. In 1997, the GAO estimated that fraud and abuse may be as high as 10 percent of Medicaid spending.[31]

A yearlong investigation of New York Medicaid by *The New York Times* found massive provider fraud. For example, a dentist in New York's Medicaid program claimed to have performed nearly 1,000 procedures in a single day. All told, she and a colleague billed New York Medicaid $5.4 million.[32]

Common fraud problems among Medicaid providers include charging for medical, transportation, and home healthcare services that were never delivered; charging for a more expensive service or good; using ambulance transportation when it is unnecessary; and charging twice for the same treatment. Because other people are paying for their healthcare, Medicaid recipients have little reason to detect and deter fraud.

Most fraud is committed by physicians and other providers, rather than patients, but providers often turn a blind eye to unscrupulous patients abusing or defrauding the system. For instance, the *Times* reports that a Brooklyn doctor prescribed more than $11 million worth of a synthetic growth hormone used to treat AIDS patients over a three-year period. Investigators say these patients were part of an elaborate scheme to obtain a drug popular with bodybuilders on the black market.[33]

Furthermore, matching funds make fraud control less enticing for states. For example, with a 50 percent match rate, if a state spends $1 to reduce fraudulent Medicaid spending by $2, the state loses $1 of the matching federal funding and its net gain is zero.

Matching-fund finance also affects state incentives to verify the eligibility of enrollees. In response to strong evidence that states were adding illegal aliens to their Medicaid rolls, the 2006 federal Deficit Reduction Act required states to demand proof of citizenship as a condition for Medicaid enrollment. In 2007, the number of nondisabled adults and children enrolled in Medicaid declined for the first time since 1996.

How Unfair Is Medicaid Funding?

On the average, the federal government pays about two-thirds of the costs of Medicaid, and it makes funds available to the states on a matching basis. In theory, the federal funding formula is designed to redistribute money from wealthier states to poorer states by giving poorer states a higher match for every dollar they spend. However, there is no cap on the amount the federal government matches. The more a state spends, the more it receives. In practice, states with above-average per capita incomes tend to adopt more liberal eligibility requirements and cover more people. They also tend to spend more per recipient.

For example, the average total expenditure per Medicaid enrollee in 2007 was $5,163. However, New York, a high-income state, spent twice as much as low-income Alabama ($8,450 versus $3,945).[34]

As a result, the distribution of federal dollars under the program is more consistent with a policy of taking from the poor and giving to the rich:[35]

- In 2009, Texas had 9.9 percent of the nation's total poverty population, but received only 6.7 percent of federal Medicaid funds.
- New York, on the other hand, had about 6.6 percent of the national poverty population, but received 12.1 percent of federal Medicaid dollars.

A much fairer way to distribute funds would be to give each state a percent of federal Medicaid spending, based on its percent of the nation's poverty population.

Are Block Grants to States a Good Idea?

An alternative favored by many health policy analysts and some governors is to replace the current Medicaid system (and its tangle of rules and regulations) with unrestricted block grants to the states. For example, if Texas is currently getting 6.7 percent of federal Medicaid dollars, under a block grant the federal government might pledge 6.7 percent of all Medicaid spending for the next five years, leaving Texas free to decide how to spend the money. A pure unencumbered block grant would require only that Texas spend the money on indigent healthcare, and nothing more. A fairer method of distribution, as noted, would be to give Texas 9.9 percent of all federal Medicaid spending, since that is the state's share of the national poverty population.

As health economist Linda Gorman has pointed out, welfare reform is an example of a successful block grant program.[36] In 1996, the Aid to Families with Dependent Children entitlement program was replaced with the Temporary Assistance for Needy Families (TANF) block grants. The switch to TANF block grants had generally positive effects on employment, earnings, and income. As states changed the structure of benefits to reward work, funds were shifted from cash assistance to childcare, housing, transportation, and education. A million children moved out of poverty as work effort increased, and caseloads fell more than 60 percent.

Case Study: Rhode Island

In its final days, the George W. Bush administration granted Rhode Island a waiver that capped total (state and federal) Medicaid spending at $12.1 billion through 2013. There is no evidence that access to care has been reduced.[37] Yet, at the current annualized rate of spending and projected growth, it appears that actual spending will be nearly one-quarter lower—or about $9.3 billion.

Private-Sector Contracting

Like Medicare, Medicaid is a public program; but a large number of Medicaid enrollees are actually in private health plans. In fact, nearly three-quarters (71.5 percent) of all Medicaid enrollees nationwide are in health plans managed by the private sector.[38] Two of the more innovative Medicaid programs are in Florida and Indiana.

Case Study: Medicaid Reform in the Sunshine State

In 2006, Florida received a waiver to implement a reform program initiated by then-governor Jeb Bush. The reform plan began as a pilot project in two large counties and has since been expanded to five counties. The population of these five counties is nearly 3 million people, with a Medicaid population of 290,000 participating in the pilot program. The goal of the exercise was to increase choice among Medicaid providers, spur competition, and boost efficiency without reducing quality or access to care for Medicaid enrollees.

The way Florida accomplished this feat was by allowing Medicaid enrollees to choose among competing, private managed-care plans, which can vary the provider network and the benefit package as long as it covers mandatory benefits. The hope was that firms that failed to provide high-quality services or that managed the care of Medicaid enrollees poorly would be punished with fewer enrollees. Those plans that provided better services would attract enrollees. Also, enrollees in the program had a stake in managing their own health; and a system of rewards was designed to encourage and reward healthy behaviors.

Five years after the start of the program, the evidence suggests that the program has achieved patient satisfaction better than traditional Medicaid and done so at a cost that is lower and rising at a slower rate than traditional Medicaid, both in Florida and nationally. Enrollees can choose from two to eleven different plans, depending on the county in which they reside. Plans offer additional services not normally covered under the old Medicaid program. Access to specialists has improved.

One estimate is that the pilot program is saving up to $161 million per year. If this program were expanded to the remaining 49 states, state Medicaid programs would save $91 billion annually while improving health outcomes and achieving enrollee satisfaction scores of 83 percent to 100 percent.[39]

Case Study: Consumer-Directed Medicaid in Indiana

Indiana Governor Mitch Daniels presided over an innovative program to insure low-income families with incomes too high to qualify for Medicaid. The Healthy Indiana Plan began in 2007 to provide low-income families with consumer-driven health plans, coupled with personal health accounts called a Power Account. The goal was not only to boost health coverage, but also to create an incentive for enrollees to take a more active role in their healthcare decisions.[40]

Low-income individuals and families who have been uninsured for at least six months can enroll in the program but must make monthly contributions to their Power account of 2 percent to 5 percent of income (up to $92). The state of Indiana contributes $1,100 to the account, which covers nearly three-quarters of the deductible. Preventive care is covered by the health plan on a first-dollar basis. Once the deductible of $1,500 is met, there are no other cost-sharing expenses or co-payments.[41]

About 45,000 people in Indiana participate in the program, and 90 percent of enrollees made their contributions.[42] Satisfaction is reportedly around 98 percent.[43] The Obama administration has apparently decided not to renew the federal waiver, which is required to continue the program.[44]

The Case for Abolishing Medicaid

Is there any reason to partition low-income people in a separate health plan called Medicaid? Is there any reason to sequester low-income children in a separate health plan called CHIP? I can't think of a reason to do either. So I propose a radical idea: let's abolish both programs. Use the money instead to subsidize the integration of poor patients into the same healthcare system everyone else has access to.

The Mechanics of Abolition: Private Insurance

Low-income families would get the same refundable health insurance tax credit other Americans get—$2,000 per person and $8,000 for a family of four, in my example. Low-income families would not get cash. Instead, they would be able to direct their refund to any participating private insurance company. The refund, in other words, would function as a voucher.

Some may worry that the $8,000 refundable tax credit would not be sufficient to purchase adequate health insurance, and the private package could be worse than Medicaid itself. This is not something I worry about. Surely private entrepreneurs can produce a better health plan for $8,000 than what Medicaid offers. But just in case the critics are right, let's keep traditional Medicaid around as a stopgap. Let people choose between Medicaid and private insurance, and let the government's $8,000 check go to the plan they choose.

The Mechanics of Abolition: Point-of-Service Reimbursement

Getting enrolled in Medicaid is so burdensome that many people who are eligible don't bother to enroll. Perhaps it's time to ask a fundamental question: why do we care whether people have health insurance when they are healthy? Isn't the real point to make sure they get care when they are sick? Put differently, why do we care whether people have insurance when they are not seeing doctors if our only real purpose is to ensure that they have coverage once they do see them?

Instead of sending out an army of social workers to track down and enroll people in a program they may never use, why not qualify them at the point when they engage the healthcare system?

The Foundation for Health Coverage Education (CoverageForAll.org) has developed a Health Coverage Eligibility Quiz to identify people who qualify for public programs or health coverage in all 50 states.[45] This is a tool that can also help hospitals identify uninsured patients eligible for Medicaid, who have been treated in the ER. In most cases, eligible but unenrolled individuals have up to 90 days to sign up for Medicaid and receive retroactive coverage for medical services they have already received. Although the eligibility quiz cannot sign people up, it takes them along that path. The purpose is to make the process as easy as possible. This tool could be used in any community health center or any hospital emergency room. It is freely available on a website (CoverageForAll.org) for anyone with a computer and Internet connection.

But why bother with enrollment at all? If the point of the whole exercise is to determine how much the state is going to pay the hospital or the community health center, why not stop there? Point-of-service-eligibility determination would seem to be all that is needed to authorize the delivery of free care.

The paperwork associated with formal insurance would seem to be superfluous and maybe even counterproductive.

Turning Medicaid into a Competing Health Plan

If abolishing Medicaid altogether turns out to be too radical for the body politic, my second suggestion is to keep Medicaid in its current form and let everybody enroll in it, regardless of income or assets. If it is good to let low-income families choose between Medicaid and competing private health insurance plans, why isn't it even better to let every family make this choice? Put differently, why should Medicaid be only for poor people? Why not open it up to everyone?

Medicaid as a Competing Health Plan

The price of admission to Medicaid would be a refundable health insurance tax credit offered to every American. At the same time, everyone now in Medicaid could get out of it and enroll in private health insurance instead. The means of transfer would be a refundable tax credit, which for those exiting Medicaid would apply to private insurance. This idea would simply turn Medicaid into one more competing health insurance plan.

(I realize this "public option" proposal puts me in the same camp with many on the political left, but public policy sometimes creates strange bedfellows.)

The Mechanics of Reform

My reform concept envisions the government making a commitment of, say, $8,000 to a family of four in the form of a refundable tax credit. The tax credit would apply to any health plan the family chooses, including Medicaid. Federal money (federal dollars) would follow people and flow to the plans they prefer. At least for noninstitutionalized patients, there would be a level playing field on which Medicaid would compete with every qualified plan in the market.

Advantages of Reform

There are several advantages to this approach. First, with no income and asset test, we immediately solve the problem of discontinuity of care—under which people become eligible, ineligible, and eligible again as their income rises and falls. Under this proposal, they could join Medicaid and stay there, regardless of income changes.

Second, it would allow low-income families to replace non-price rationing under Medicaid with the ability to pay market prices that many private plans allow. Non-price barriers to care are a greater deterrent to care than price barriers for many low-income patients. Access to private plans should increase access to care.

Third, this reform takes us closer to the goal of genuinely universal healthcare. Instead of being segregated into an inferior heath care system, low-income families would have the opportunity to participate in the same system everyone else uses.

Reforming Medicaid with Health Stamps

If Medicaid is retained in anything like its current form, however, it needs radical reform. So the third proposal to be considered here is to get Medicaid out of the business of dictating prices and replace that activity with a health stamp program, fashioned after the food stamp (SNAP) program. Enrollees would get stamps, depending on their health condition, and they would be free to add their own money and pay any price for any service the medical marketplace has to offer. In this way, low-income families on Medicaid would be empowered patients who could compete for healthcare resources on a level playing field with other patients, at least for small dollar health purchases, which would include almost all primary care.

The idea behind health stamps is straightforward. Like food, health is generally considered a necessity. So why not treat it the same way we treat food?

We don't segregate grocery stores into those that sell to poor customers and those that do not. Grocery stores take all comers, and they charge the same price to each of them. The way we subsidize low-income families is through the food stamp program, a highly successful poverty program that now reaches 60 million people. The program allows poverty and near-poverty families to have access to the full range of food products. Because they pay market prices, food stamp families are welcome customers at every grocery outlet. Although they live with more limited budgets, food stamp families are able to make tradeoffs in grocery choices—using food stamps in a way that meets their own preferences and needs. Competition for food stamp dollars forces stores to compete on price and, unlike healthcare, the prices are transparent. Every paper contains full-page ads in which price plays a dominant role.

This proposal makes certain that the poor have the wherewithal to pay for their healthcare not by forcing them to wait or take poorer quality, but with healthcare dollars. These healthcare dollars are full dollars to providers, insuring that the poor can complete for resources with all other buyers of care.

16

Understanding the New Healthcare Law

NO ONE WILL be untouched by the Patient Protection and Affordable Care Act,[1] arguably the most radical piece of legislation ever passed by Congress. It will affect everyone with private insurance, every senior on Medicare, everyone on Medicaid. The bill will create 159 new regulatory agencies. Its ten-year cost is close to $1 trillion. It is intentionally designed to fundamentally alter the way medicine is practiced in this country.

The Patient Protection and Affordable Care Act will radically transform the US healthcare system. The most significant changes (e.g., a requirement that most people obtain health insurance) will not become law until 2014. A tax on employee "Cadillac" health plans does not take effect until 2019. This means there will be at least one presidential election before most provisions become law as well as other opportunities for voters to express their will. In the meantime, here is a brief summary.

A New Health Insurance Mandate

The most striking feature of the new law is one that Barack Obama actually opposed when he was running for the presidency: a requirement that most people obtain health insurance, whether they want to or not. At the time of this writing, the constitutionality of this requirement is being reviewed by the Supreme Court. In the meantime, here are some particulars:

- Beginning in 2014, most people will be required by law to have health insurance and to attach proof of insurance to their tax return.

- If you fail to insure, you will be fined—with the penalty rising to $695 ($2,085 per family) in 2016 or 2.5 percent of your adjusted gross income, whichever is greater.
- If your employer fails to offer health insurance, your employer can be fined as much as $2,000 per employee per year. If your employer offers insurance, and it is deemed unaffordable, the fine is $3,000 for each worker who cannot afford the coverage.
- Although some businesses have been granted waivers and others are protected by grandfather status, these exemptions from the requirements of the new law will be temporary in the vast majority of cases.
- The type of insurance most employees must have—including co-pays, deductibles, and the employee's share of the premium—will be determined by federal regulations (and, for the first two years, by state regulations as well), rather than by you and your employer.
- If you are not covered by an employer plan, Medicare, Medicaid, or other government plan, you will be required to buy insurance in a government-regulated health insurance exchange, where competing insurers will offer the government-mandated health insurance benefit package.

Some Major Benefits of the Reform

The health reform law produces winners and losers. Here are some of the most important benefits:

- You may be able to buy insurance you cannot now afford. Beginning in 2014, for example, a couple with an income of twice the poverty level (currently $29,000) will be able to buy insurance for an annual premium no higher than 6.3 percent of their income ($1,827).
- If you have a pre-existing condition, you will be able to buy insurance for the same premium as that paid by people in good health.
- In the meantime, newly created risk pools are offering subsidized insurance to some of the people who have been turned down by health insurers because of a pre-existing condition.
- If you have a very expensive and continuing health problem, there will be no annual limit and no lifetime limit on your health insurance coverage.

- By 2013 under the new law, close to 90 million Americans with employer and individual health policies will no longer have to pay a co-payment or deductible for preventive screenings recommended by the US Preventive Services Task Force.[2]
- Overall, the CBO expects 32 million otherwise uninsured people (about 60 percent of the total) to obtain health insurance,[3] and Medicare's chief actuary puts the estimate at 34 million[4] (although some outside analysts think these projections are too optimistic).[5]

Some Major Costs of the Reform

In general, for every benefit, there is an offsetting cost. More than half the costs of this reform, for example, will be borne by the elderly and disabled on Medicare:

- $523 billion of health reform's first ten-year cost will be paid for by reduced spending on Medicare enrollees, according to the CBO.[6]
- In addition, there are new taxes on drugs and on such medical devices as wheelchairs, crutches, pacemakers, artificial joints, etc.—items disproportionately used by Medicare enrollees.

Reduced spending and reduced subsidies will have an especially big impact on seniors:

- Of the 15 million people expected to enroll in Medicare Advantage programs, 7.5 million will lose their plans entirely, according to Medicare's chief actuary, and the remainder will face higher premiums and lower benefits.[7]
- Nearly 6 million retired employees will lose their employer drug coverage, according to the most recent Medicare Trustees report.[8]

Other measures will affect the more general population:

- A new tax on health insurance is likely to cost the families of employees of small businesses more than $500 a year in higher premiums.[9]
- A 40 percent tax on the extra coverage provided by expensive "Cadillac" plans will apply to about one-third of all private health insurance in 2019;

and because the tax threshold is not indexed to medical inflation, over time the tax will eventually reach every health plan.

There are also hidden costs of certain benefits:

- Health insurers will have to raise premiums for everyone in order to charge people with pre-existing conditions less than the expected cost of their care. Young people, for example, could see a doubling or tripling of their premiums, according to industry estimates.[10]
- To provide health insurance (or more generous insurance) to their employees, employers will have to reduce what they pay in wages or provide other benefits.
- The extra burden on employers could cost as many as 700,000 jobs by 2019, according to the CBO.[11]

Expected Impact of the Reform

There are three major problems in healthcare: cost, quality, and access. Yet, when all is said and done, there is no assurance that under ACA any of the three problems will get better. They may all get worse.

Costs May Rise, Rather than Fall

Although the CBO initially predicted a slight lowering of overall healthcare costs in future years, it subsequently expressed doubts.[12] Medicare's chief actuary and most private forecasts expect overall costs, as well as the government's costs, to be higher as a result of the new law. A more recent analysis by the Office of the Medicare Actuary predicts that the new law will increase, rather than decrease, healthcare spending.[13] The RAND Corporation has made a similar prediction.[14]

Quality of Care May Fall, Rather than Rise

To address the problem of quality, the new law authorizes pilot demonstration projects, allots research funds to discover "best practices," and gives Medicare new powers to try to force doctors and hospitals to change how they practice medicine. Some scholars are skeptical of how well this will work. In the meantime, new problems will arise as doctors try to deal with a surge in demand for their services. In Britain, Canada, and other developed countries, doctors often deal with these problems by creating waiting lists and reducing the amount of time they spend with each patient.[15] Also, health plans will have perverse incentives to skimp on care for their sickest enrollees.

Access to Care May Fall, Rather than Rise

Under ACA, up to 34 million additional people will be insured, and most of the rest of the population will have more generous coverage. The result: the demand for medical care is likely to greatly exceed the supply. Although there is disagreement about the size of the coming physician shortage, Medicare's chief actuary and some private sector economists are predicting major problems in access to care, including increased waiting times.[16]

How ACA Intends to Change the Practice of Medicine

Some of the supporters of the Affordable Care Act have been very explicit. Harvard Medical School professor Atul Gawande, for example, thinks that medicine should be more like engineering—with all doctors following the same script, rather than exercising their individual judgment. "We have to be more like engineers building a mechanism whose parts actually fit together, whose workings are ever more finely tuned and tweaked," he writes.[17]

Karen Davis, president of The Commonwealth Fund, envisions a complete reorganization of the practice of medicine, in which "physicians, hospitals, and other providers . . . join together to form accountable care organizations [ACOs] to gain efficiencies and improve quality of care."[18]

Peter Orszag, former director of the Office of Management and Budget and Obama administration point man on healthcare while the legislation was being written, says that under the new law, Medicare has broad authority to refuse to pay for treatments that are not evidence-based.[19] Orszag also believes the malpractice laws should be rewritten so that doctors who practice evidence-based medicine are given a safe harbor against lawsuits.[20] Former White House health advisers Nancy-Ann DeParle and Susan Sher have made a similar recommendation.[21]

Critics worry that in actual practice, reform efforts will fall very short of the goals; that practice guidelines, rather than representing the best that medicine has to offer, will become cookbook recipes; that while these recipes may work for most patients most of the time, doctors will not feel free to make exceptions for patients that don't fit the norm. Rather than resemble a finely honed machine, the healthcare system could more closely resemble the US Postal Service.

Accountable Care Organizations

Accountable Care Organizations have been described as "HMOs on steroids." On paper, it sounds as though doctors will be rewarded for providing higher quality services. In practice, ACOs may reward doctors for underproviding care, as traditional HMOs were accused of doing.[22]

Moreover, the business model of the ACO requires that patients see only the doctors that the ACO employs. If you are getting care from an ACO, therefore, your insurance may not pay for you to see doctors outside the ACO. Also, part of the ACO vision is that all doctors and nurses will practice medicine in the same way. This means that when you visit an ACO clinic, you will not necessarily see the same doctor you saw on your last visit. ACOs will probably be given a lot of freedom to limit the terms and circumstances under which you can see doctors.

Nationwide, Medicare started paying fees to ACOs in 2012. Eventually, the Obama administration would like to see everyone in an ACO.

But if no one had any previous interest in forming ACOs, let alone joining them, what is going to cause them all to change our minds? Money. Insurers won't be able to get premium increases unless they adopt ACO plans. Doctors and hospitals will be paid less if they don't join. Eventually, doctors will find they are ineligible to treat Medicare patients or patients insured in the newly created health insurance exchanges if they are not practicing in ACOs. As for the patients, there won't be any plans to join other than ACO plans.

ACOs will have capitated payments—the organization gets a fixed annual fee per patient, regardless of the costs that patient actually incurs—and, like the traditional HMO, the ACO will get to keep any money it doesn't spend. The organization will also incorporate all the latest fads in health policy: electronic medical records, pay-for-performance incentives, quality report cards, and so on.

If ACOs can reduce costs and raise quality, why don't they already exist? The results from the few demonstration projects with ACOs have been lackluster and mixed.[23] A comprehensive review of all the studies of report cards and other quality-measuring-and-reporting techniques finds they don't work and may do more harm than good.[24] Just as teachers will "teach to the test" if test results are how they are graded and rewarded, doctors will tend to "practice medicine to the test" if that is how they are paid. If you're the patient, that may not be good for you. The latest comprehensive review of all the studies of electronic medical records finds they do not live up to their promises.[25] And the most recent study of pay-for-performance from Britain finds that it doesn't work either.[26] As Scott Gottlieb, a former US Food & Drug Administration deputy commissioner and writer on health policy, has pointed out, the ACA approach will stifle innovation and entrepreneurship and is already causing venture capital to leave the healthcare market.[27]

So how do we explain the administration's commitment to ACOs? Whether they raise or lower costs, whether they raise or lower quality, there is one thing that ACOs will indisputably accomplish. They will drive doctors into organizations where their behavior can be controlled.[28] For the first time in our history, both the practice of medicine and the way money is spent on medical care will fall under federal control.

ACOs are the portal through which we will all march toward a truly nationalized healthcare system. I don't know any advocates of ACOs who are not also advocates of global budgets, under which providers are given a fixed amount of money to spend and forced to ration care if the funds prove to be inadequate—as they do in Britain and Canada.

Where Private Insurance Is Headed

Even if you are not enrolled in a traditional HMO or an ACO, you can expect a return to some of the heavy-handed health insurance industry practices that were so unpopular in the 1990s and gave rise to the "patient bill of rights" proposals. The reason? The new healthcare reform takes away just about every other tool insurers have to control costs. In response to the new law, for example, health insurers are already trying to keep premiums down by offering policies that cover, say, *only half the doctors in the area where you live.*[29] In some of these plans, you get no reimbursement whatsoever if you see a doctor outside the insurer's network.

Levers of Government Power: Medicare

Will the federal government be able to tell doctors how to practice medicine? An undisguised goal of health reform is to change what most doctors do. The Medicare payment system will be used to push doctors to use electronic medical records, join group practices, and ultimately join ACOs. Doctors who do these things will be paid more. Doctors who don't will be paid less.

A federal Coordinating Council for Comparative Effectiveness Research will study alternative ways to treat various conditions, and Medicare could refuse to pay doctors and hospitals that refuse to follow the guidelines. National guidelines will almost certainly govern who will get diagnostic tests, under what conditions, and how often. Medicare doctors are likely to have much less discretion about such diagnostic tests as mammograms, Pap smears, PSA tests, colonoscopies, and so on. Medicare doctors are also likely to have much less freedom to order CAT scans, MRI scans, PET scans, and sonograms.

Levers of Government Power: The Private Sector

The government will have less control over the way in which doctors practice medicine for patients who are privately insured. However, health plans in the exchange will face competitive pressure to limit what they spend on people with expensive health problems. Undoubtedly, federal guidelines for Medicare will give these plans permission to adopt the same payment strategies for physicians seeing the privately insured. Ultimately, whatever happens under Medicare is likely to spread to the entire private sector.

Some Questions and Answers about Reform

Where Will I Get My Insurance?

If you are like most people, you will get it the same place you get it today—through an employer, through Medicare or Medicaid, or through a private Medicare or Medicaid contractor (e.g., a Medicare Advantage plan).

If you buy your own insurance, however, you will probably have to obtain it through a health insurance exchange, in which competing insurers will offer government-mandated packages of benefits. States may have flexibility in how the exchanges operate. You may be able to obtain insurance online, for example.

If your income is below 133 percent of the poverty level (currently $14,856 for an individual and $30,657 for a family of four), you will be required to enroll in Medicaid, and you will not be allowed access to subsidized private insurance offered in the exchange.

Will I Be Able to Keep the Insurance I Now Have?

Probably not. No promise was repeated more often by Barack Obama than the pledge that, "If you like the plan you are in, you can keep it." For the vast majority of people, however, this promise almost certainly will not be kept. Here's why.

Your Employer May Be Forced to Switch to Another Plan

In general, if employers make very few changes to their current plan, that plan will be grandfathered. But most plans will be unable to qualify for grandfather status. A government memorandum predicts that:[30]

- More than half of all employees with employer-provided health insurance will have to switch to a more expensive, more regulated plan, and the number may be as high as two-thirds.
- Among those who will be required to switch plans, as many as 80 percent are employees in small businesses.
- Within three years, more than *100 million people* will be forced into a health plan more costly and more regulated than the one they have today.
- Moreover, grandfathering is only a temporary phenomenon. The memorandum suggests that eventually all plans will lose their grandfather status.

A more recent survey of employers by AonHewitt, a human resources consulting service, suggests that this prediction may have been too optimistic: 90 percent of employers expect to lose their grandfather status by 2014.[31]

Your Employer May Drop Coverage Altogether

Most employers will be required to offer health insurance or pay a fine. But since the fine will be as little as one-seventh the cost of the insurance, many employers—especially small employers—may drop their coverage. This will force you and other employees to go to a health insurance exchange for your health insurance. To a modest degree, this has already happened in Massachusetts,[32] with a similar health reform law, and the reaction is likely to be more pronounced in other states. Overall:

- The Congressional Budget Office estimates that 9 million employees will lose their employer plan.[33]
- Medicare's chief actuary estimates that 14 million employees will lose the coverage they now have and, of those, about 2 million will enroll in Medicaid.[34]
- A former CBO director is predicting a much larger employer response, with 35 million employees losing their current coverage.[35]
- Nearly one-third (30 percent) of clients surveyed by McKinsey reported they would likely drop employee health coverage.[36]

Loss of Medicare Advantage Coverage

As noted, about half of the enrollees in Medicare Advantage (MA) plans (7.5 million people) are likely to lose their coverage and will be forced to return to conventional Medicare—a figure consistent with independent analysis.[37] That process has already started. In 2011, Cigna Corp., Harvard Pilgrim Healthcare, several BlueCross BlueShield plans, and others announced they would not renew Medicare Advantage plans for 700,000 beneficiaries, who must find new policies.[38] If you are able to keep your MA plan, expect higher premiums and fewer benefits in the years ahead.

Loss of Postretirement Coverage

The health reform law removes an important employer tax subsidy. As a result, almost all retirees with employer coverage for prescription drugs (5.8 million out of 6.6 million) are expected to eventually lose it, according to the latest Medicare Trustees report. For example, 3M, with 23,000 US retirees, has announced that it will drop coverage.[39]

Loss of Independent Drug Plans

Seniors who have independently purchased Medicare Part D drug plans are also at risk. In 2007 there were 1,875 plans, while in 2012 there will be only about 1,041 plans—834 fewer than five years earlier.[40] The loss of plans will force seniors to choose a new plan, with possible changes in premiums and co-payments.

Loss of Limited Benefit Plans

More than 1 million Americans currently have a health insurance plan that features "limited benefits," sometimes called "mini-med" plans. Medical benefits in these plans are capped anywhere from a few thousand dollars to $25,000 or even $50,000 or more annually. Premiums are affordable—a family policy can be as little as $1,000 per year. Many other employees are in health plans that limit annual and lifetime benefits as a way to constrain the cost of coverage. Regulations under the new health reform law, however, ban annual and lifetime limits on medical benefits. They phase out completely by 2014.

As a temporary measure to prevent the possibility of millions of Americans losing their health coverage, the US Department of Health and Human Services has granted 1,722 waivers to more than 4 million people with limited benefit health plans. The waivers will allow these employees to keep their coverage for at least one more year. Some of the organizations that received waivers were staunch supporters of the health reform bill. More than half of the people covered by these waivers are members of labor unions, including the Service Employees International Union, the Teamsters, and United Food and Commercial Workers.[41]

How Much Will Health Insurance Cost?

Unless you qualify for an exception, beginning in 2014, the new law will require you to obtain a health insurance plan. For the first two years, state governments will have the power to dictate most of the benefits the plans must include. Beyond that point, the benefits will probably be mandated under federal law. In all likelihood, this new mandatory coverage will be more extensive and more costly than the insurance you currently have. The typical coverage in 2016, for example, will average about $5,800 (individual) and $15,200 (for a family of four), according to the Congressional Budget Office.[42]

Your Share of the Cost in the Exchange

The out-of-pocket premium you pay will be no more than 3 percent if your income is at the poverty level (currently $14,404 for an individual and $29,327 for a family of four), rising to 9.5 percent of income at 400 percent of poverty (currently $43,320 for an individual and $88,200 for a family). However, if you earn above that level, you may have to pay the full premium yourself. Your subsidy will be based on income from up to two years earlier, based on your income tax return. If it is later discovered that you received a larger subsidy than you are qualified for, you will have to reimburse the government for a portion of the subsidy received in error.

Your Share of the Premium at Work

If your income is less than 400 percent of poverty, your share of the premium will be limited to no more than 9.5 percent of your income. Otherwise, the insurance will be judged to be unaffordable, and you will be entitled to subsidized insurance in a health insurance exchange. There is a big difference between the limits in the exchange and the limits at work, however. In the exchange, your share of the premium will be kept low by a refundable tax credit—a gift from the government that will pay the remaining premium expenses. But, in general, there will be no new subsidies for employer coverage. So if your employer is required to reduce the amount of the premium you pay at work, the extra cost to your employer will have to be made up by reducing other compensation (cash wages and other benefits). In the exchange, someone else (the government) pays to keep your premium low, but at work it's likely that you will pay.

How Will the Government Enforce the Requirement to Buy Insurance?

The enforcer of health reform is the Internal Revenue Service (IRS).

On your annual tax return, you will be required to show proof that you and other members of your family have the minimum insurance the government is going to require almost everyone to have. Failure to provide proof will subject you to tax penalties that will reach $695 (individual) or $2,085 (family) or 2.5 percent of your income, whichever is greater, in 2016. Further, providing fake information (claiming you have insurance when you don't) will subject you to the same penalties that would apply to other types of false reporting to the IRS.

Some analysts estimate the IRS will need to hire 16,000 additional agents to enforce the requirement that everyone obtain individual health insurance, although the agency has not confirmed this estimate.[43]

What Will Happen to My Taxes?

You will join other Americans in paying more than $500 billion in nineteen new types of taxes and fees over the next decade to fund health reform.[44] Some of the new taxes will be indirect and will be passed on to you in the form of higher prices, higher premiums, or lower wages. You will pay other taxes directly. According to the Joint Committee on Taxation, about 73 million taxpayers earning less than $200,000 will see their taxes rise as a result of various health reform provisions.[45]

Tax on Medical Devices

These taxes will reach everything from surgical instruments and bedpans to wheelchairs and crutches. Even pacemakers and artificial hips and knees are taxed. All told, the tax on medical devices will collect nearly $20 billion over the next decade.

Tax on Insurance

A $60 billion tax on health insurance, beginning in 2014, will ultimately be reflected in higher premiums. For example, the Senate Finance Committee's Republican staff estimates the new taxes—including taxes on medical devices, taxes on drugs, taxes on insurers—could ultimately push up health insurance premiums for a typical family of four by nearly $1,000 per year.[46]

Tax on Drugs

A new tax on drugs will collect about $27 billion. In anticipation, some drug makers have already started raising their prices.[47] These taxes and the changes in the treatment of medical savings accounts have been called the "medicine cabinet tax."

Tax on Medical Savings Accounts

If you have a Flexible Spending Account, a Health Reimbursement Arrangement (HRA) or a Health Savings Account, you are no longer able to use these tax-free accounts to purchase over-the-counter drugs. That means you will have to buy such items as Claritin, aspirin, or Advil with after-tax dollars (making the cost to you 30 percent higher or more for a middle-income family). In addition, tax-free contributions to an FSA will be capped at $2,500 annually. People setting aside funds for chronic care, corrective eye surgery, or other out-of-pocket medical expenses will be limited to $2,500, regardless of medical need. Taken together, these two actions are expected to cost consumers $18 billion over the next decade.

Taxes on Indoor Tanning

If you plan to use an indoor tanning bed, expect to pay 10 percent more thanks to a new excise tax expected to raise nearly $3 billion.

Taxes on Cadillac Plans

A 40 percent excise tax will be levied on so-called "Cadillac" health plans for the amount in excess of $27,500 for families and $10,200 for single coverage. About one-third of health plans will be subject to the tax beginning in 2019. But since these thresholds are not indexed to increase as fast as medical costs, over time virtually all plans will be subject to the tax.

Taxes on Illness

If you have a lot of medical expenses, today's tax law allows you to deduct from your taxable income the amount that exceeds 7.5 percent of your adjusted gross income (AGI). Under the new law, this threshold is being raised to 10 percent of AGI—making your deduction smaller.[48] The increase is effective in 2013 for people under 65 years of age and in 2017 for those 65 years of age and older.

Additional Taxes on Wages, Investment Income, and Even Home Sales

The Medicare payroll tax will increase by almost one-third for some people—from 2.9 percent today to 3.8 percent on wages over $200,000 for an individual or $250,000 for a couple. In addition, the 3.8 percent Medicare payroll tax will be levied on investment income (capital gains, interest, and dividend income) at the same income levels. This tax is not only on the rich, however. Under some circumstances, the sale of a house could trigger the provision, making you "paper rich" for a single year and forcing you to pay a 3.8 percent levy on a portion of the appreciated value above a certain limit. Moreover, the threshold above which people must pay the higher tax is not indexed to rise with inflation. Consequently, over time more and more middle-class Americans will have to pay it.

What If I Am on Medicare?

You and others like you are probably going to be more affected by the new health reform law than any other population group.

Benefits of Reform

There are a number of new benefits, including:

- Medicare will pay for an annual checkup.
- Deductibles and co-payments for many preventive services and screenings (colonoscopies, mammograms and bone mass density tests, etc.) will be eliminated.
- If you are in the prescription drug "donut hole" and you are not getting other drug subsidies, you may qualify for a $250 rebate.
- Eventually (in 2019), the donut hole will be eliminated.

Costs of Reform: Cuts in Medicare Spending

If you are in conventional Medicare, you can expect that reduced spending will average $290 in 2014. If you are in a Medicare Advantage plan, you can expect more severe cuts: $1,267 in 2014. If you are able to retain your coverage, these cuts will lead to increases in premiums or reductions in benefits. Note that these cuts are on top of a planned 30 percent cut in doctor fees that are already part of current law, but that Congress has been postponing for the past nine years. Comparing the path we have been on to the path required under the new law:[49]

- The annual reduction in spending will reach $2,300 per beneficiary by 2020, $3,844 by 2030, and $9,413 by midcentury (all numbers at current prices).
- By the time today's teenagers reach the retirement age, one-third of Medicare will effectively be gone.

Moreover, in some cities, the combined effect of cuts in Medicare and cuts in Medicare Advantage will be especially large. By 2017, thousands of people in Dallas, Houston, and San Antonio will face more than $5,000 a year in lost healthcare benefits, according to one study. For some New York City dwellers, the figure will exceed $6,000 a year. Residents of Ascension, LA, will lose more than $9,000 in benefits.[50]

The Obama administration claims that it will target these cuts to eliminate waste—to encourage low-cost, high-quality care and discourage high-cost, low-quality practices. Critics are not hopeful. In fact, Medicare's own actuaries believe that the most likely way spending cuts will be made is through a reduction in fees paid to doctors, hospitals, and other providers. In particular:[51]

- Medicare fees will fall below Medicaid rates by 2019 and continue to fall further behind other payers in the years that follow.
- By 2050, Medicare will pay only half as much as private plans pay; by 2080, it will pay only one-third.

Costs of Reform: Reduced Coverage for Prescription Drugs

Under current law, employers who provide their employees with postretirement healthcare benefits can set up and administer retiree drug plans as an alternative to Medicare Part D. In return, employers get subsidies worth about $665 per retiree, and tax breaks make the value of the subsidy even higher. The Patient Protection and Affordable Care Act removes the tax subsidy, however, and the loss to major employers is substantial:[52]

- AT&T estimates the change will cost it $1 billion.
- John Deere estimates it stands to lose $150 million.
- Caterpillar puts the loss at $100 million.
- A Credit Suisse report estimates that S&P 500 companies face losses of $4.5 billion.

In response, many large firms will completely do away with their retiree drug plans.

In addition, 27 million seniors will pay higher premiums for the Medicare Part D Plan to allow the donut hole to be closed. Only 4 million seniors are thought to reach the donut hole annually, but fewer than 1 million will surpass the threshold and receive the full benefit of closing the donut hole. Expect your premiums to rise to pay for this benefit.[53]

How Cuts in Medicare Spending Will Be Made

The new law assumes that the federal government can make Medicare grow at about half the rate of growth of healthcare spending overall and eventually no faster than the rate of growth of national income. To achieve this goal, the law gives an Independent Payment Advisory Board (IPAB) the power to recommend spending cuts. Congress must either accept these cuts or propose its own plan to cut costs as much or more than the IPAB's proposal. If Congress fails to substitute its own plan, the IPAB's cuts will become effective. In this way, the growth rate of Medicare spending will be officially capped.

This approach gives an independent agency much more power than any similar agency has had before. However, there are two problems. First, the IPAB is barred from considering just about any cost control idea other than cutting fees to doctors, hospitals, and other suppliers. Second, this implies that Medicare fees will fall further and further behind private payments, making Medicare patients less desirable customers to the medical community. In some parts of the country, doctors are increasingly reluctant to take Medicare patients—including the Mayo Clinic in Arizona.[54]

What about the Medicare Trust Fund?

US Department of Health and Human Services Secretary Kathleen Sebelius has claimed that cuts in Medicare spending help Medicare's Trust Fund, making it easier to pay benefits in future years.[55] Yet CBO Director Douglas W. Elmendorf rejected such claims, saying that they amount to impermissible double counting.[56] The money that is saved by cuts in Medicare spending either (1) will be used to pay for health insurance for younger people or (2) will be put aside to pay Medicare benefits in the future. But you cannot use the same dollars to buy two different things. Since the bill explicitly uses cuts in Medicare spending to finance health insurance subsidies for young people, it does nothing to aid the future financial health of Medicare. Medicare's chief actuary has said the same thing.[57]

What about Andy Griffith?

At a cost to the taxpayers of about $708,000, a television ad features the TV lawyer Matlock telling you how great the new health bill will be for you. Yet, a fact-check by the Annenberg Public Policy Center finds the claim not believable:[58]

Currently, about one in every four Medicare beneficiaries is enrolled in a Medicare Advantage plan. For many of them, the words in this ad ring hollow, and the promise that "benefits will remain the same" is just as fictional as the town of Mayberry was when Griffith played the local sheriff.

What about AARP?

The organization that claims to represent seniors has been fully supportive of the new law. But the interests of AARP and the interests of seniors are not the same. For example, AARP markets its own Medigap insurance, collecting more in premiums and other revenue from other commercial ventures than it collects in member dues. With fewer seniors in Medicare Advantage plans, the market for Medigap insurance will greatly expand. Moreover, AARP is getting special treatment under health reform. Specifically, AARP's Medigap insurance is:[59]

- Exempt from the prohibition on pre-existing condition exclusions.
- Exempt from a $500,000 cap on executive compensation for insurance industry executives.
- Exempt from the tax on insurance companies.
- Exempt from a requirement imposed on Advantage plans to spend at least 85 percent of their premium dollars on medical claims.

What If I Have a Health Savings Account?

If you are one of the more than 22 million people[60] enrolled in a Health Savings Account (HSA) or a Health Reimbursement Arrangement or if you work for the one of every two employers who now offer one of these consumer-driven health plans, in the future you will have fewer options. The new healthcare law does not outlaw HSA-eligible plans, but it takes away HSA options and future regulations could make these plans impractical and undesirable.

Current Law

Instead of giving all of your healthcare dollars to an insurance company, the current law allows you to choose a plan with a high deductible and more limited benefits and put the premium savings in an account you own and control. Deposits to these accounts may be made with pre-tax dollars, just like employer-paid premiums, and the accounts grow tax-free. Because you get to keep the money you don't spend, self-insuring in this way allows you to directly benefit from being a prudent consumer in the medical marketplace.

Lower Deductibles

The new law reduces the allowed deductible for small-group plans (those with fewer than 100 employees) to $2,000 for singles and $4,000 for families, beginning in 2014. This is roughly one-third the level allowed under current HSA law. This will limit your ability to save on insurance premiums by joining a higher deductible plan.[61]

Larger Penalties

If you take money out of your HSA for a nonmedical purpose, the law has already increased the penalty from 10 percent to 20 percent, and you will have to pay ordinary income taxes as well. As noted above, patients may no longer use their HSA funds to purchase over-the-counter (OTC) drugs. This is especially unfortunate since there is a trend for off-patent drugs to become less expensive OTC drugs.

Additional Risks

The Secretary of Health and Human Services has the authority to review health plan benefits on an annual basis and determine the "essential" benefits that should be included in all health plans. If the secretary determines that all plans must have a benefit that violates the regulations for HSA-eligibility, HSAs could essentially be outlawed by the stroke of a (regulatory) pen.

Other restrictions could make HSA plans impractical. For example, one proposal would require your employer to verify that every single HSA withdrawal is for medical care. This would greatly increase the paperwork cost of administering these accounts.

The Latest Regulatory Risk

As this book goes to press, the Obama administration has announced a regulatory ruling that could effectively eliminate HSA plans from the market for individual insurance. The ruling concerns the minimum medical loss ratio (MLR) requirement that will penalize insurers who fail to spend 80 percent or

85 percent (depending on circumstance) of their premium dollars on healthcare. The problem: The administration wants to count third-party spending on medical care but exclude deposits made to a Health Savings Account before the deductible is met. Such a regulation will make it almost impossible for HSA plans to survive in the new health insurance exchanges.[62]

What If I Have a Flexible Spending Account?

The most significant change is an annual limit on contributions you can make to a Flexible Spending Account. About 35 million people are using FSAs to pay for such things as medical expenses, dental insurance premiums, long-term care, and child care with pre-tax dollars. Funds must be used in the year they are set aside, however. Although most employers limit the amount you can contribute to $5,000, the new law will limit contributions to no more than $2,500 a year—indexed to inflation for future years.

As noted, the new law also changes the definition of a *qualified medical expense,* making over-the-counter medications and products no longer eligible for payment through an FSA. Virtually everything in your medicine cabinet that used to be tax-free (through an FSA) is now taxable. The list includes aspirin, bandages, cough syrup, cold medications, antibiotic ointment, first aid creams, pain relievers, cough drops, antacids, sinus medications, allergy medications, and nasal sprays. If you are one of millions of people with a chronic condition, the increased cost to you could be substantial.

The impact may be even greater if you are one of the millions of people who use these accounts for long-term care for family members with chronic illnesses. For example, families raising special needs children often deposit funds into an FSA to pay for costly education and behavior therapy. This allows them to use pre-tax dollars—at a savings of nearly 50 percent in some cases—to pay for tuition that can top $1,000 per month.

What If I Am Young?

Like all other individuals, you will be required by federal law to purchase health insurance with the specific benefits the federal government says you must have, regardless of whether you want to pay for them and regardless of whether they are useful. For instance, young single males will be required to purchase a plan that has maternity benefits and well-baby coverage.

Benefits of Reform

Young adults up to age 26 (whether married or unmarried) are now able to enroll in their parents' health plans. Currently, this option is limited to children who do not have access to an employer plan. However, beginning in 2014, children will be able to join or stay on their parents' plan even if they have access to an employer plan of their own.

Costs of Reform

If you are like most young people, you are healthier and have lower expected costs than older adults. For example, people in their 20s today typically face premiums that are only one-fifth or one-sixth as high as people in their 60s. The likelihood of ill health, and therefore the cost of health insurance, tends to rise with age, but fortunately so does income. People in their 50s and 60s typically pay higher premiums, but their higher incomes allow them to do so.

Regulations that take effect in 2014 will dramatically change things, however. Insurers will be required to accept all applicants at rates that are not adjusted for health status. Also, premiums can be adjusted for age, but the highest premium can exceed the lowest one by no more than a ratio of three to one. This means that you will face premiums that will be much higher than your expected cost so that older, less healthy adults can pay premiums that will be much lower than their expected costs.

The result: You will have to pay a lot more for your coverage, perhaps even double or triple your current premium. For example, studies based on actual insurance claims data show:[63]

- The premium for a healthy 25 year old in California would more than double—rising from $107 per month to $221.
- The family premium for a 40 year old husband and wife with two children in California would rise by 42 percent—from $536 per month to $763.
- By contrast, a 60 year old, less healthy couple living in California would see a drop in their premiums of about 41 percent—from $1,979 to $1,165.

Exceptions for Young Adults

If you are under the age of thirty, you will have access to health plans that have fewer mandated benefits than the standard plans. These plans will be allowed to have higher deductibles and higher cost-sharing, but your out-of-pocket exposure will be no higher than HSA limits (currently $6,050 for an individual and $12,100 for a family).[64] Presumably, these plans will have lower premiums. They will not qualify for premium subsidies in the exchange, however.

Does Marriage Help or Hurt?

It almost always hurts. The reason: subsidies in the newly created health insurance exchange will treat two singles better than a married couple. Suppose you are earning 200 percent of the federal poverty level (currently $21,660). You will be required to pay a premium equal to 6.3 percent of your income in the exchange—or about $1,365 for a health plan that has an actual cost of, say, $5,000. Thus, you and a cohabitating partner who also earns 200 percent of the federal poverty level could both obtain health coverage for about $2,730. However, if you marry your partner, the two of you will be required to pay 9.5 percent of your income in premiums—or about $4,115. Being married will cost the two of you $1,385 a year.

In some cases, getting married may be worth the financial penalty, however. If you and your partner each earn 100 percent of the federal poverty level (currently $10,830), you would (individually) qualify for Medicaid and would not be allowed to purchase private coverage in the exchange. However, if you are married, your combined income would disqualify you for Medicaid. If you bought insurance in the exchange, you would be required to pay 4 percent of your household income (or $866). The ability to get out of Medicaid (which pays low doctor fees) and into a private plan (which may pay market rates) may be worth the extra premium you have to pay—especially if you value more ready access to care.

What If I Run a Small Business?

Unless you employ mainly high-income people, your best option is probably to avoid providing health insurance altogether. The reason: your employees will be able to obtain insurance that is cheaper (for them) in a new health insurance exchange than you can purchase as an employer. This conclusion is probably valid even if you have to pay a fine for not insuring your employees and even if you forgo the new health insurance tax credit the government will be offering you.

Mandated Health Insurance

If your company employs fewer than fifty-one fulltime workers, you will be exempt from penalties for failing to offer health coverage. The fifty-first worker, however, could be a very expensive hire. If you employ fifty-one or more workers, failure to provide insurance will subject you to a tax penalty of $2,000 for each uninsured employee beyond the first thirty employees. So growing from fifty to fifty-one uninsured workers would subject you to a fine of $42,000 [(51–30) × $2,000] for adding the last worker. This fine, however, will be much smaller than the cost of providing fifty-one employees with the insurance mandated under the Affordable Care Act. Moreover, the fine is much smaller if a firm hires a significant number of part-time workers (those working less than 30 hours per week). In the example above, if twenty of the firm's fifty-one workers were replaced by part-time workers, the firm's penalty would fall from $42,000 to only $2,000.[65] One implication: Many workers who want full-time work may only find part-time work.

A Catch-22

If you are an employer who already provides insurance, you may be able to retain your current health plan by claiming grandfather status. This would make you immune from cost-increasing regulatory burdens, since the mandated benefit package is likely to be more generous and more costly than what you have now.

Any substantial change in your health plan, however, such as switching to a new insurance carrier, will cause you to lose your grandfather status—even though changing insurers is the main way small firms keep premiums down. As a result, you can accept double-digit premium increases for your existing insurance or you can shop around for new coverage, in which case you will lose your grandfather status and have to comply with dozens of costly new mandates.

Under a mid-range estimate, two-thirds of small-business employees will lose their grandfather status by 2013 and will no longer be able to keep the plan they now have. Under the worst-case scenario, as many as 80 percent will lose their grandfather status.[66] By contrast, a self-insured, large company plan or union plan is free to change its third-party administrator as often as it likes and still keep its grandfather status.[67]

Employer Access to an Exchange

If you have fewer than 100 employees, you will be able to purchase coverage in a health insurance exchange rather than buy insurance in the small-group market. However, your employees will not be able to obtain the subsidies that individuals will receive if they are buying their own insurance. Also, just as insurers selling in the exchange will not be allowed to charge premiums based on health status, that same requirement will also govern the small-group market outside the exchange. So at this point, it is unclear whether there will be any financial advantage to using the exchange, if you are paying the premiums.

Uninsured Employees' Access to an Exchange

We do not know at this point what health insurance in a health insurance exchange is going to look like. However, the CBO estimates the average cost of a health plan will be about $5,800 (individual) or $15,200 (family) in 2016.[68] This suggests that the insurance will look a lot like a standard BlueCross plan paying BlueCross fees to providers. Moreover, most people earning less than $70,000 or $80,000 per year will be able to get a subsidy in the exchange that is much more generous than the tax subsidy available for employer-provided coverage.

Take a 40-year-old employee with a family who is earning, say, $30,000. If you provide the government-mandated insurance at work, you will have to spend an amount equal to about half the employee's salary. The only subsidy is the ability to pay premiums with dollars that are not included in the taxable income of the employee. Since this employee makes too little to pay income taxes, you will only be avoiding a 15.3 percent (FICA) payroll tax, and that is worth about $2,800.

If this same employee enters a health insurance exchange, however, he will be charged a premium of only $1,000. The government will pay the remaining premium and reimburse the family for most of its out-of-pocket costs—bringing the total expected annual subsidy to about $11,200.[69]

So, combining your financial interest with your employee's, there is a potential gain of $6,400 if the employee gets health insurance in the exchange rather than at your place of work. That is money that could be used to pay higher wages, provide other benefits, or add to company profits. Note also that the financial gain from sending the employee to the exchange in this case far exceeds a potential $2,000 fine. It also exceeds the value of any small-business health insurance tax credit.

Potential Benefit: A New Small Business Subsidy

The new law includes a health insurance tax credit that may help you purchase health insurance for your employees. However, the credit is available for only six years and only for firms that have twenty-five or fewer employees and pay wages that average less than $50,000. Moreover, most businesses will not meet the strict (and complex) criteria for claiming the credit. In fact, fewer than one-third of small businesses will qualify according to the National Federation of Independent Business, the trade association that represents small business.[70] Also, the credit is not available to sole proprietorships and their families.

Even so, the big surprise is that so few businesses are claiming the credit. The IRS estimates that 4.4 million firms are eligible, and the CBO expected $2 billion in subsidies would be paid out in 2010 alone.[71] Yet at a hearing of the House Ways and Means Committee, the Treasury Department's Inspector General J. Russell George reported that as of mid-October, 2011, only 309,000 businesses had claimed the credit, for a total payout of $416 million.[72]

Why so few? Patricia Thompson of the American Institute of Certified Public Accountants explained that the tax credit violates all of the organization's principles for sound tax policy. Among other flaws, the small-business tax credit is astoundingly complicated and opaque. Ms. Thompson testified:[73]

> In order for an incentive to be effective, taxpayers must know of its existence, know whether it applies to them and how it applies to them. Since most small employers did not know until the end of the year (or after the year ended when their income tax returns were prepared) whether or not they qualified for the credit, there was no incentive for them to provide health insurance coverage.

Limits on Employee Premiums

If you do decide to provide the mandated health insurance benefit to your employees, you may be required to limit the amount of premiums some employees pay to a percentage of their income. For example, health plans are considered unaffordable if workers earning less than 400 percent of the federal poverty level (about $88,200 for a family of four) are required to pay a premium that is more than 9.5 percent of the worker's wage. The premium for an employee earning $30,000, for example, would be deemed unaffordable if it were higher than $2,850. For firms with more than fifty workers, employing a worker whose premium is unaffordable may result in a $3,000 fine.

What If I Am an Early Retiree?

The new law creates subsidies for employer-provided insurance for retirees, but these new subsidies phase out in 2014.[74] Moreover, the subsidies go not to individuals but to employers. Indeed, one of the ironies of the new health law is that the first subsidies are going not to low-income, uninsured families, but to General Motors, General Electric, Procter & Gamble, PepsiCo, Alcoa, Intel, Pfizer, and other large companies. And because higher income employees are more likely to have an employer promise of postretirement care, the subsidies will help those early retirees who least need help.

When these subsidies end in 2014, insurers—selling in a newly created health insurance exchange—will have to accept all applicants regardless of health condition. Since the difference in premiums an insurer charges in the exchange cannot exceed three to one (rather than the more normal cost ratio of six to one), the likely impact will be that young people will be overcharged so that 50 and 60 year olds can be undercharged.

One problem: it appears the mandate may be weakly enforced. If people wait until they get sick to insure, the average premium in the exchange will have to be quite high to cover the costs. As a result, retirees could face higher premiums in the exchange than they would have faced with no reform at all. As noted, millions of seniors also will pay higher premiums for their Medicare (Part D) drug plan because of the cost of closing the donut hole. Expect your premiums to rise in future years.[75]

What If I Am an Immigrant?

If you are a legal resident alien, you will be required to obtain the same government-mandated health coverage that US citizens must obtain. However, if you have been here for less than five years, and if your income falls below 133 percent of the federal poverty level, you will not be allowed to enroll in Medicaid. Instead, you will be able to do something low-income US citizens cannot do: obtain highly subsidized insurance (paying a premium, say, of ten cents on the dollar) in a health insurance exchange. If, as we expect, Medicaid insurance is lower quality insurance, you will have access to better insurance than a US citizen with the same income!

If you are an undocumented immigrant you will not be subject to the individual insurance mandates, and you will not be fined if you fail to purchase health insurance. Nor will you be allowed to enroll in Medicaid or buy insurance in the health insurance exchange. However, hospital emergency rooms will not be able to deny you healthcare if you are in need. What makes this surprising is that the most common argument for an individual mandate is that the uninsured should have to contribute to their own healthcare instead of getting it for free in the emergency room. This is why US citizens will be required to pay hefty fines if they do not obtain insurance. If you are here illegally, however, you're an exception to this rule.

What About Preventive Care?

The new healthcare law promises people on Medicare annual wellness exams, mammograms, prostate cancer screenings, and other preventive services—without any co-payment or deductible. The rest of the population will also have access to a lengthy list of preventive services. Unfortunately, the law that mandated these benefits contained no provision to make sure doctors will be able to deliver the services.

What Services Will I Be Entitled To?

All new health plans (plans that are not grandfathered) must now cover the preventive services recommended by the US Preventive Services Task Force, without cost-sharing. Depending on your age and sex, the following preventive services must be covered by your health insurance:[76]

- Blood pressure, diabetes, and cholesterol screening
- Cancer screenings

- Counseling on weight loss, healthy eating, smoking cessation, alcohol use, and depression.
- Vaccines for measles, polio, meningitis, and the human papillomavirus (HPV).
- Shots for flu and pneumonia prevention.
- Screening, vaccines, and counseling for healthy pregnancies.
- Well-baby and well-child visits up to the age of 21, as well as vision and hearing, developmental assessments, and body mass index (BMI) screenings for obesity.
- Mammograms for women over age 40.
- Pap smears for cervical cancer prevention.
- Colon cancer screening tests for adults over age 50.

Will I Be Able to Get the Preventive Services Promised Me?

The answer is probably not. Providing preventive care takes time, and most primary care physicians already have their hands full. Nationwide, more than one out of every five people is living in an underdoctored area, and the shortage of primary care physicians is expected to grow worse in future years.[77] Furthermore, since preventive screenings are often reimbursed at lower rates than other services, when you call your doctor for a preventive care appointment, you may find there is a long wait.

Is Preventive Medicine Cost-Effective?

Much rhetoric suggests that preventive care pays for itself. If a disease is caught in its early stages, so it is said, treatment costs will be lower. So can wider access to preventive care lower the nation's healthcare costs? In general, no.

For an individual with a health problem, the old adage that an ounce of prevention is worth a pound of cure is true.[78] For the few patients who are diagnosed with a disease, preventive screenings are definitely worth the cost. But the cost of screening thousands of healthy patients to find one patient with a problem usually swamps any savings on patients whose diseases are diagnosed early.

In general, preventive medicine adds to healthcare costs, rather than reducing costs. Mammograms don't pay for themselves. Nor do Pap smears, prostate cancer tests, or general checkups for healthy people.[79] That doesn't mean we should avoid these tests, but we should obtain them judiciously.

There are some exceptions—childhood immunizations and prenatal care for at-risk mothers, for example. But the exceptions are few and far between. Louise Russell, who has studied the economics of preventive care for many years, explained this in a recent article in *Health Affairs*:[80]

> Over the past four decades, hundreds of studies have shown that prevention usually adds to medical spending. [Data] from 599 studies published between 2000 and 2005 [show that] less than 20 percent of the preventive options (and a similar percentage for treatment) fall in the cost-saving category—*80 percent add more to medical costs than they save.*" [Italics added.]

Why Can't We Use Medical Science to Decide What Preventive Care People Should Get?

Who should get a mammogram? At what age? How frequently? What about Pap smears and prostate cancer tests and colonoscopies? Aren't these questions experts can decide? Unfortunately, no. Any reader of daily newspapers knows that we are forever getting conflicting advice from well-meaning people. Part of the problem is that people differ in their attitude toward risk and in their willingness to spend money to reduce risk. A danger in a one-size-fits-all approach fashioned in Washington, DC, is that the experts may not share your values. Their attitude toward risk reduction may be different from yours.

The Danger of Cookbook Medicine

Another danger is that, harried by far more requests for services than they can possibly deliver, doctors will take a routine approach to all their patients and ignore what makes you unique as an individual. What if you feel you are at a heightened risk for breast cancer because your mother or grandmother had breast cancer—but you fall outside the guidelines for early breast cancer screening before age forty? Women at higher risk of breast cancer might want to begin them at age twenty-five, as recommended by Susan G. Komen for the Cure.[81] But will you be allowed to do so? If necessary, will you be allowed to pay for the test yourself? The answers to these questions are not clear.

The Dangers of the Politics of Medicine

Both Congress and the current administration have already shown that they are unwilling to let experts set the guidelines for preventive care. For example, the new law stipulates that seniors are entitled to an annual physical and that males are entitled to an annual prostate cancer test—even though neither is recommended by the Preventive Services Task Force. Also, HHS Secretary Sebelius has chosen to include annual mammograms for women in their 40s, even though the task force recommended against it.

Expect more politics to come. Women's groups have already successfully pushed for free contraceptives under the guise of prevention.[82] Also, while more free services may sound good, remember that the doctor's time is limited, as are the number of healthcare dollars. Granting more marginal care to one person may mean less really serious care for another.

Letting Individuals Make Their Own Choices

There is a better way. Instead of giving all of your healthcare dollars to an impersonal, bureaucratic insurance company, you should be allowed to put some of those dollars in a Health Savings Account that you own and control. That way, you could consult the advice of the Preventive Services Task Force on your own. You could also consider the advice of other experts, including your doctor, and take into consideration personal data about you and your family.

Preventive care is not like an *investment good* that pays a positive rate of return. Instead, it's like a *consumption good*. Preventive care leads to better health. But the enjoyment of that result must be compared with the benefit of other goods and services we could have purchased with the same money.

17

What Most Needs Repealing and Replacing in the New Healthcare Law

THE ORIGINAL LEGISLATION creating ACA was 2,700 pages long. Since then, more than 10,000 pages of regulations have been added.[1] I have identified ten problems so severe that even the White House and Democratic leaders in Congress are going to want to reopen the healthcare reform process and deal with them.

1. An Impossible Mandate

Most Americans will be required to have health insurance beginning on January 1, 2014. The type of insurance you have, where you will get it, and what you will pay will be determined not by you and your employer or by free choice in the marketplace, but by government. Here are the biggest problems the mandate will create.

Crowding Out Other Consumption

Health costs per capita have been rising at twice the rate of per capita income for the past forty years. President Obama did not create the underlying problem. Nor is this a uniquely American problem.[2] The result: healthcare spending will consume more and more of our income with each passing year.

To make matters worse, the normal consumer reactions to rising premiums are going to be disallowed. For example, most people would react to unaffordable premiums by choosing a more limited package of benefits, or opting for catastrophic coverage only or relying more on Health Savings Accounts. But these and other responses are limited or barred altogether under the new law.

The provisions governing preventive care illustrate the problem. Everyone will have to have a plan that covers preventive care (mammograms, Pap smears, colonoscopies, etc.) with no deductibles or co-payments. Since there will be no out-of-pocket payment, no one will have any incentive to comparison shop and try to minimize the cost of these services. Could some preventive care be provided by a nurse at a walk-in clinic more cheaply than at a doctor's office? Undoubtedly. But the new law will prevent you from being in a health plan that gives you economic incentives to economize and reduce those costs.

Crowding Out Wage Increases

Most people will continue to obtain health insurance through an employer. The Congressional Budget Office estimates the average annual cost of a minimum benefit package at $4,500 to $5,000 for individuals and $12,000 to $12,500 for families in 2016.[3] Thus, the minimum cost of labor will be a $7.25 cash minimum wage and a $5.89 health minimum wage (family), for a total of $13.14 an hour or about $27,331 a year.

Imagine you are an employer. You certainly aren't going to pay an employee more than his value to the organization, and competition from other employers will tend to prevent you from paying less. If the government forces you to spend more on health insurance, you will spend less in wages in order to pay for the mandated benefits.

For above-average-wage employees, this is all straightforward. Expect wage stagnation over the foreseeable future, as employers use potential wage increases to pay for expanded (and mandated) health benefits instead. At the low end of the wage scale, however, the effects of this new law are going to be devastating.

Crowding Out Jobs

Ten-dollar-an-hour workers and their employers cannot afford $6-an-hour health insurance. If they bought it, only $4 would be left for cash wages and that would violate the (cash) minimum wage law. This is not a small problem. One-third of uninsured workers earn less than $3 above the minimum wage.[4]

Further, although health economists have known for decades that these are the workers that most need help in obtaining insurance, there are no new subsidies to help employees at Wal-Mart or McDonald's or Denny's or any other restaurant chain buy health insurance. These workers and many others are at risk of losing their jobs.

Do We Really Need a Mandate?

The idea of a health insurance mandate has seemed reasonable to many people on the right as well as the left because of the free-rider problem: those who remain willingly uninsured will have extra money to spend, and if they become sick and need care they cannot pay for, they will look to everyone else to provide that care for free. Are we not rewarding them for being irresponsible and allowing them to be free-riders on the rest of society?

That argument seems persuasive until we ask this question: if we require everyone to have health insurance, what is the appropriate punishment for someone who doesn't? The only practical way to enforce a mandate is with a fine. And if that is all we have in mind by way of enforcement, we do not need a mandate. All we need is a system that fines people who don't purchase insurance.

In fact, the income tax already provides this "fine." Middle-income families who have employer-provided health insurance (as opposed to higher wages) receive a generous tax subsidy. The flip side of that subsidy is a penalty: People who don't have employer-provided insurance pay higher taxes as a result of that fact.

Why is it good not to have a mandate? Because once the government tells us what insurance we must have, every special interest imaginable will lobby Congress to become part of the mandated benefit package. This has already happened at the state level, where insurance plans in various states are required to cover providers ranging from acupuncturists to naturopaths and services ranging from in vitro fertilization to marriage counseling. All told, there are 2,156 mandates at the state level.[5] They increase the price of insurance and have priced as many as one-in-four uninsured people out of the market.[6]

2. A Bizarre System of Subsidies

The Affordable Care Act offers radically different subsidies to people at the same income level, depending on where they obtain their health insurance—at work, through an exchange, or through Medicaid. These subsidies are arbitrary, unfair, and even regressive. Along with the accompanying mandates, they will cause millions of employees to lose their employer plans and maybe their jobs as well.

Subsidies Create Perverse Incentives

Take the maids, waiters, waitresses, busboys, custodians, and groundskeepers at a hotel, making about $15 an hour. The government provides no help for the purchase of employer-provided health insurance. The only subsidy available is the one that has been there all along in the tax code: by purchasing health insurance with pre-tax dollars, employees at this income level will avoid a 15.3 percent (FICA) payroll tax—about $2,800.

Now consider a standard family plan offered in a health insurance exchange. If the $15-an-hour employees are eligible for such a plan, the government will pay anywhere from 90 to 94 percent of the premium depending on the age of the employee and the region of the country. The government subsidy amounts to about $13,617.[7]

Which is better? A $13,617 subsidy or a $2,800 one? If a hotel didn't send its low-wage workers to the exchange and a competitor down the road did so, the hotel would face about 50 percent higher labor costs than the competitor.

But not so fast. There is another wrinkle in this calculation. Although low- and moderate-wage employees get generous subsidies in the health insurance exchange, higher income employees (say about $94,000 and up) get no subsidy at all. If they obtain employer-provided insurance, however, they can take full advantage of the tax law provision. When the hotel buys insurance for a manager, for example, the premiums not only avoid the 15.3 percent payroll tax, they also avoid a 25 percent federal income tax and, say, a 5 or 6 percent state and local income tax. The upshot: through the tax subsidy, government is "paying" for almost half of the cost of the insurance.

Subsidies that Are Regressive and Unfair

Quite apart from the perverse economic incentives the subsidies create, they are completely arbitrary and unfair. As Figure 17.1 shows, a $31,200-a-year family (about 133 percent of poverty) getting health insurance at work gets less than

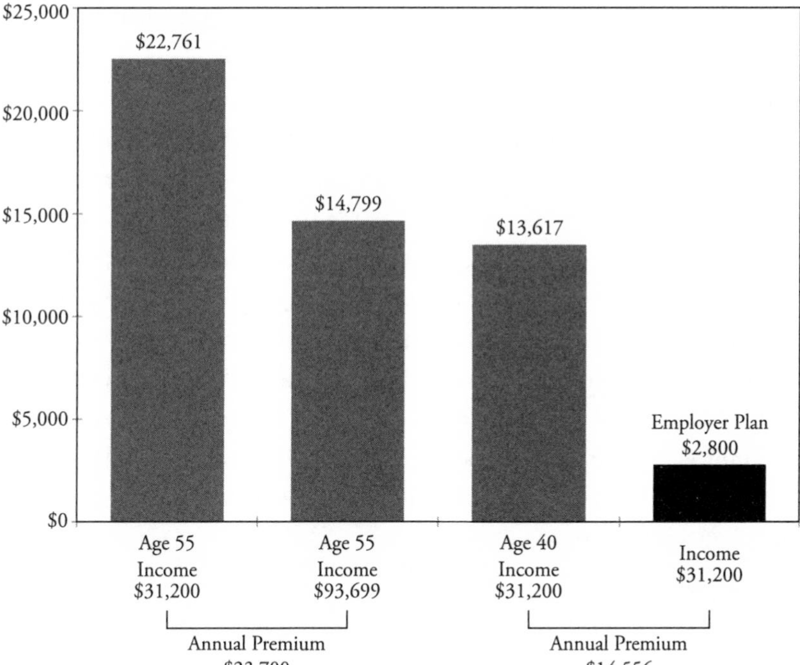

Figure 17.1. Health Insurance Subsidies for a Family of Four (high-cost region)
Sources: Author calculations, Stephen Entin and Kaiser Family Foundation Subsidy Calculator.

one-fourth as much help from the government, compared to a family making nearly three times that much income and getting insurance in the exchange.

Subsidies that Create High Marginal Tax Rates

Starting in 2014, subsidies in the health insurance exchanges will be available to families with incomes between 133 percent and 400 percent of the federal poverty line. The range is from $31,389 to $93,699 for a family of four. (People below 133 percent of poverty will be forced to turn to Medicaid.) An analysis by Daniel Kessler predicts that health coverage will cost $23,700 for a family of four headed by a 55 year old, living in a high-cost region.[8] The subsidy for this plan starts at $22,740 at the low end and falls to zero as income rises.

Figures 17.2 and 17.3 show the average marginal tax rates that individuals and families can expect to pay under the new law, on the average. Note that the highest marginal tax rates fall on moderate-income earners. An individual earning between $20,000 and $30,000, say, will face a marginal tax rate substantially higher than the rate paid by Bill Gates or Warren Buffett.

What is the highest marginal tax rate a family could face? Although premiums for health insurance sold in the exchange are capped at 9.5 percent of income for the families earning between 350 and 400 percent of poverty, there are no subsidies for families earning more than 400 percent of poverty. That means premiums would be capped at $8,901—resulting in a subsidy of $14,799 ($23,700 – $8,901) for a family earning $93,699 (400 percent of poverty). But if the family earns $1 more ($93,700), they no longer qualify for a subsidy. Thus $1 in additional income results in a subsidy loss of $14,700, for an *implicit tax rate of 1.47 million percent.*

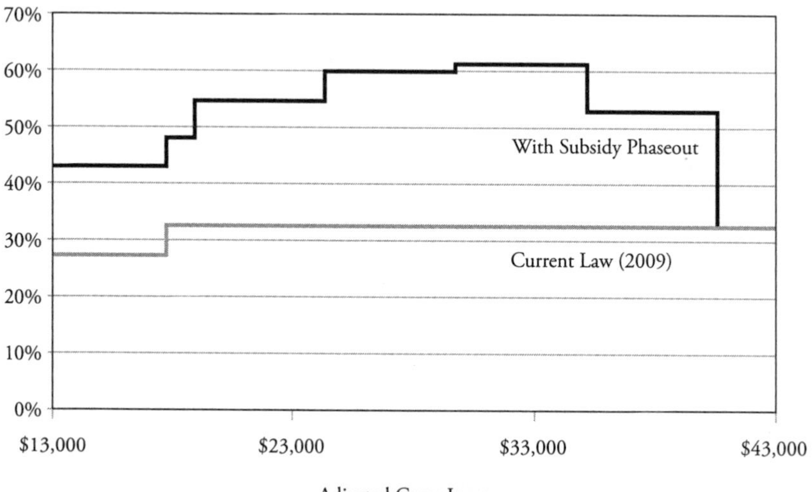

Figure 17.2. Effective Marginal Tax Rates with the Phaseout of the Health Exchange Subsidies (Single Individual)

Source: Michael Schuyler, "Health Exchange Subsidies Would Impose High Marginal Taxes," National Center for Policy Analysis, Brief Analysis No. 697, March 3, 2010.

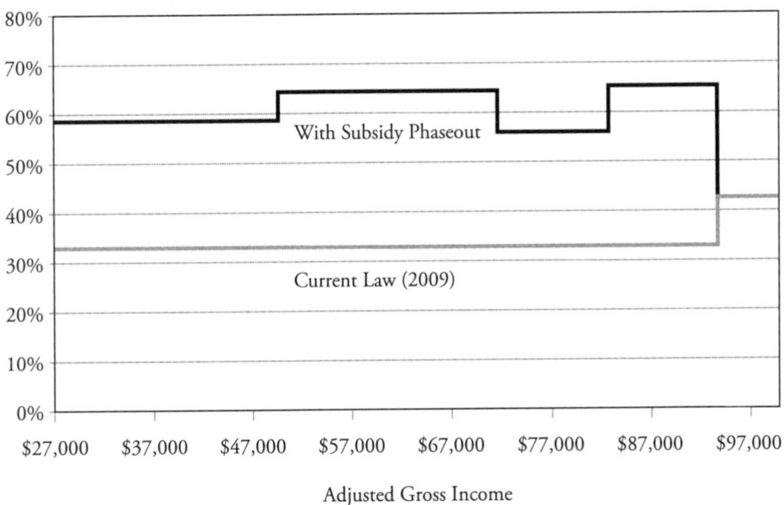

Figure 17.3. Effective Marginal Tax Rates with the Phaseout of the Health Exchange Subsidies (Couple with Two Children)

Source: Michael Schuyler, "Health Exchange Subsidies Would Impose High Marginal Taxes," National Center for Policy Analysis, Brief Analysis No. 697, March 3, 2010.

A Better Way to Encourage Private Insurance

To achieve the ideal, the federal government should offer people the same tax relief for the purchase of health insurance, regardless of where it is obtained—at work, in the marketplace, in a health insurance exchange, through a cooperative, and so on. In addition, we should end the regressive practice of giving the largest subsidies to those taxpayers who need help the least. A reasonable system would be one in which every taxpayer receives the same subsidy, regardless of income. If it is socially desirable to encourage people to insure and if the cost of insurance is largely independent of income, the financial help coming from government should also be independent of income.

Finally, we should end the wasteful practice of allowing people unlimited opportunity to lower their tax burden by buying more expensive insurance. Instead of generously subsidizing the last dollar of premium people pay, we should subsidize the first dollars more heavily and let them pay the last dollars out of their own pockets. A straightforward way of doing this is with a lump sum tax credit. A family would get, say, $8,000 to apply dollar for dollar to the first $8,000 of health insurance premiums. Since many employer plans cost almost twice that amount for family coverage, the tax credit would not cover the entire amount people are likely to spend on health insurance. Nor should it.

Families would be encouraged to think carefully about what value they get from the second $8,000 they and their employers have been spending. If they can find ways to economize, each dollar not spent on health insurance would be a dollar available for some other purpose.

3. Perverse Incentives for Insurers

Under the current system virtually all employers and group insurers have perverse incentives to attract the healthy and avoid the sick. Once people have enrolled, the incentives are to overprovide to the healthy (to encourage them to stay) and underprovide to the sick (to encourage them to leave).

Managed Competition in ACA Exchanges

The problem with managed competition under ACA is that the pressures to act on the incentives will be much more intense. In the health insurance exchanges, health plans will be forced to charge the same premium, regardless of health status, and potential enrollees will be able to easily compare premiums. In this way, the insurers will be forced to aggressively compete on price. To the degree that a plan succeeds in attracting an above average share of healthy enrollees or a below-average share of sick enrollees, its average cost will be lower than that of competing plans. That means it will be able to charge a lower premium than other plans and enjoy a competitive advantage in the health insurance exchange. There are provisions to offset some of the expected perversity with so-called "risk adjustments." Yet no system of risk adjustment works well. Currently, the Medicare Advantage program has the most sophisticated risk adjustment mechanism—employing as many as 60 or 70 variables. However, studies show that the system predicts individual health costs very poorly[9] and the health plans are still able to game the system and attract an above-average healthy enrollment.[10]

A Better Alternative: Creating a Market for the Care of the Sick

Instead of requiring insurers to ignore the fact that some people are sicker and more costly to insure than others, we should adopt a system that compensates them for the higher expected costs—ideally, making a high-cost enrollee just as attractive to an insurer as a low-cost enrollee. At a minimum, this means that when individuals switch health plans, they always move at market prices, not artificial prices.

4. Perverse Incentives for Individuals

A poorly reported development in Massachusetts is the growing number of people who are gaming the system.[11] People remain uninsured while they are healthy and get insurance after they get sick. Then, after they receive care and their medical bills are paid, they drop their coverage again. In the industry, they are called "jumpers and dumpers." They jump in after they get sick and dump the plan after they get well. This behavior is more likely the lower the penalty for being uninsured and the more weakly the individual mandate is enforced.

Under ACA, the fines for being uninsured are low. When fully phased in, the fine is $695 for individuals and $2,085 for families. But these fines do not apply to people who do not file tax returns—and that is more than 20 million households. To make matters worse, the IRS is hinting that it has no plans to enforce these fines.[12]

Individuals gaming the system could be the death knell for private insurance—leading to what many in Congress wanted all along: a single-payer, public plan.

5. Impossible Expectations

Suppose that Congress passed a law requiring all health plans to pay for an hour of free conversation every year between patients and doctors. The logical question would be: where are the doctors going to find all the additional hours to provide this service? The same question is relevant for the Affordable Care Act. It promises almost everyone in the country access to annual physicals, mammograms, Pap smears, prostate cancer (PSA) tests, colonoscopies and other services most are not now getting—with no deductible and no co-payment.[13] Who is going to deliver these services?

The Demand for Free Preventive Care

There's an even more important question: when millions of Americans line up for additional preventive care, how will this affect cost, quality and access to care? In a 2003 study researchers at Duke University Medical Center estimated that it would require 1,773 hours a year of the average doctor's time—or 7.4 hours every working day—for the average doctor to counsel and facilitate patients for every procedure recommended by the US Preventive Services Task Force.[14] And remember, every so often a screening test turns up something that requires more testing and more doctor time. The current supply of medical personnel cannot come anywhere close to providing what has been promised.

In addition, screening tests and similar services add to healthcare costs, rather than reduce them,[15] and sick patients may be crowded out in the process. Patients in higher-paying plans seeking preventive services could displace the more urgent needs of sick patients in lower-paying plans. The most vulnerable patients will be the elderly and the disabled on Medicare, poor families on Medicaid, and newly insured enrollees in subsidized private plans sold in the health insurance exchanges.[16]

Impact of Concierge Doctors

A major increase in demand and no change in supply will cause increased waiting for care almost everywhere, and one place patients will turn is to concierge doctors. In return for an annual fee, patients receive increased access and additional services.[17] Whereas a doctor in a regular practice typically has about 2,500 patients, however, a concierge practice usually has only about 500 patients. The more doctors that opt out of conventional care for concierge care, the greater the rationing problem becomes for everyone left behind. This could result in a two-tiered system in which those with more financial resources have concierge care, and everyone else is subjected to rationing by waiting.

The Administration's Options

For its part, the Obama administration is caught on the horns of a dilemma. While it wants to be seen as the champion of preventive care, a vast increase in this kind of coverage will increase healthcare costs and crowd out access to care for those who have more serious medical needs. Even before healthcare reform, the Association of American Medical Colleges was predicting a 21,000 primary care physician shortfall by 2015, while the Health Resources and Services Administration at HHS estimated a shortage of between 55,000 and 150,000 physicians by 2020.[18]

The Obama administration knows the problem and is quite worried about it. Is there anything it can do to ameliorate the situation?

Apparently, Health and Human Services Secretary Kathleen Sebelius plans to use $250 million targeted for "prevention and public health" in the Patient Protection and Affordable Care Act for physician training instead.[19] The funds would train 500 physicians, 600 physician assistants, and 600 nurse practitioners. Also, she plans to raid pots of "stimulus" money created under the American Recovery and Reinvestment Act to subsidize the training of doctors and nurses. All told, the administration now claims it will train 16,000 primary care providers by 2015.[20]

However, this initiative will not create any new medical residency slots, which are required before a medical graduate can practice medicine. Thus, it is unlikely that any additional physicians will be trained. Moreover, virtually all of the medical students and nursing students who will be subsidized are already enrolled in medical training programs.

A Better Alternative: Liberate the Supply Side of the Market

The most obvious way to avoid a huge imbalance between the supply and the demand for medical care (especially primary care) is to abolish the requirement that health plans provide a long list of preventive services with no co-pay or deductible. In addition, nurses, physicians' assistants, and other paramedical personnel should have greater freedom to offer their services to the marketplace.

In Oregon, nurse practitioners with the proper credentials and licensure may open their practices anywhere they choose and operate in the same capacity as a primary care physician without oversight from any other medical professionals.[21] They can draw blood, prescribe medications, and admit patients to the hospital. In Texas, however, which has some of the most stringent regulations in the country, a nurse practitioner can't do much of anything without being supervised by a doctor who must:[22]

- Not oversee more than four nurses at one time.
- Not oversee nurses located outside of a 75-mile radius.
- Conduct a random review of 10 percent of the nurses' patient charts every 10 days.
- Be on the premises 20 percent of the time.

Walk-in clinics manned by nurses in pharmacies and shopping malls seem to have overcome these legal barriers. But in poorer areas—especially in poor, rural areas—the obstacles may be insurmountable. In 2009, about 30 percent of Texas counties, most of them rural, had poverty rates of 20 percent or more.[23] Yet the farther a nurse is located from a doctor's office, the less likely the doctor will be to travel to supervise the practice. In medically underserved areas, a doctor must visit a nurse practitioner at least once every tenth business day. Because of the shortage of practitioners, people living in poverty-stricken counties in Texas must drive long distances in order to get simple prescriptions and uncomplicated diagnoses.

California provides another example of the harmful effects of medical practice statutes: after more than 6,600 people overwhelmed volunteers at a free mobile health clinic in Los Angeles in 2010, California legislators passed a law making it easier for out-of-state medical personnel to assist with future events.[24] But because the state failed to adopt needed regulations, only medical personnel licensed in California could treat patients. Think about that: doctors from Nevada, Arizona, and Oregon can't cross state lines to deliver free care to people who need it.

6. A Tattered Safety Net

One of the most oft-repeated arguments for health reform is to reduce costly and delayed trips to the emergency room by uninsured patients. But will that happen? The heaviest users of the ER (in proportion to their numbers) are Medicaid patients (perhaps because many doctors won't accept them), and more than half of the people who gain insurance under the new health reform bill will enroll in Medicaid.

What to Expect Under ACA

While the increased demand for services may turn some people to concierge doctors, many more are likely to turn to the emergency room when they cannot get their needs met at doctors' offices:[25] if, say, only one-third of those newly insured turn to the emergency room because of inadequate primary care supply, that would equal *between 39 million and 41 million additional emergency room visits every year.*

A Better Approach

To protect the institutions that deliver care to our most vulnerable populations, we need a dedicated flow of funds that rises and falls with the objective need. One source of funds is the money represented by unclaimed tax credits. These funds could be redirected to the safety net institutions in the areas where the uninsured live to provide a source of funds in case they cannot pay their own medical bills.

7. Impossible Benefit Cuts for the Elderly and the Disabled

Senior citizens are major losers in health reform. More than half the cost of the reform will be paid for by $523 billion of cuts in Medicare spending over the next ten years.[26] Although there are some new benefits for seniors (mainly new drug coverage), the costs exceed the benefits by a factor of more than ten to one.

Cuts in Medicare Fees to Providers and in Advantage Plans

Medicare actuaries predict that:[27]

- By 2020, Medicare nationwide will pay doctors and hospitals less than what Medicaid pays.[28]
- By 2019, one in seven facilities will become unprofitable and will probably be forced to leave the Medicare program.
- That number will grow to 25 percent of all facilities by 2030 and to 40 percent by 2050.

Moreover, in the not-too-distant future, Medicare patients could find themselves in the same position as Medicaid enrollees—who often are forced to get all their care at community health centers and safety net hospitals.[29] Ultimately, if Medicare spending grows at a lower rate than the healthcare system as a whole, the elderly and the disabled will end up in a completely different healthcare system. They will not be able to see the same doctors, enter the same hospitals, or get the same quality of care other Americans have access to.

In defense of its plan, the Obama administration claims that it will target Medicare cuts to eliminate waste—to encourage low-cost, high-quality care and discourage high-cost, low-quality practices. Yet, the cuts in Medicare Advantage subsidies, for example, appear to be based on special interest politics alone, not on any lofty goals.[30] Moreover, the plans that are being defunded are ostensibly doing everything President Obama says he wants to accomplish with health reform:[31]

- They provide subsidized coverage to low- and moderate-income people who could otherwise not afford it.
- They control costs better than conventional insurance by eliminating unnecessary care.
- They provide higher quality care.
- They have no pre-existing condition limitations, and some plans actually specialize in attracting and caring for patients with multiple illnesses.
- They provide an annual choice of plans.
- They even compete against a public plan (traditional Medicare).

A Better Solution: Reform Medicare the Right Way

Many of the cuts to Medicare will have to be restored. However, Medicare cost increases can be slowed by empowering patients and doctors to find efficiencies and eliminate waste.

On the demand side, seniors should be able to have Health Savings Accounts. In this way, those who avoid unnecessary or wasteful spending would be able to use those same dollars for other consumption spending. Patients, in other words, would have a financial self-interest in keeping costs down.

On the supply side, doctors, hospital administrators, and other providers should be able to approach Medicare and request to be paid in more efficient ways. The ground rules are: the change cannot increase Medicare's costs, and the quality of care for the patients cannot go down. With this opportunity in place, providers would find it in their self-interest to find ways to eliminate inefficiencies and waste.

8. Impossible Burden for the States

The Affordable Care Act is expected to add up to 16 million more Medicaid enrollees and will significantly expand eligibility for families with incomes up to 133 percent of the federal poverty level. Initially, the federal government will pay 100 percent of the cost of the newly eligible, newly enrolled populations and 95 percent of costs through 2019. However, hidden costs will strain state budgets, and states will still find their share unaffordable.

The Cost of Enrolling the Already Eligible

An estimated 10 million to 13 million uninsured people are already eligible for Medicaid—but not enrolled. When the individual mandate to obtain health coverage takes effect in 2014, many states will find the cost of their Medicaid programs higher as a result.

For example, a decade after the new law's implementation, Texas Medicaid rolls are predicted by the Texas Department of Health and Human Services to rise by 2.4 million people. Of these, only 1.5 million enrollees will be newly eligible, so a significant share of the cost for the remaining 9 million will have to be borne by the state.[32]

Low Medicaid Provider Payments

On the average, reimbursements for Medicaid providers are only about 59 percent of what a private insurer would pay for the same service, but it varies from state-to-state. For example:[33]

- New York pays primary care physicians only about 29 percent of what private insurers pay for primary care.
- The comparable figure in New Jersey is 33 percent.
- California pays primary care providers 38 percent of what private insurers pay.
- Texas reimburses primary care physicians for about 55 percent of what private insurers pay.

Low provider reimbursement rates make it more difficult for Medicaid enrollees to find physicians willing to treat them. Initially, the federal government will bear the cost of raising Medicaid provider fees to Medicare levels — but only for two years, 2014 and 2015. Then the rates will fall back to their previous levels, or the states will bear much of the cost of keeping Medicaid provider fees at a level necessary to ensure enough physicians are willing to participate in the program.

Lower Payment to Safety Net Hospitals

Disproportionate share hospital (DSH) payments are used to compensate hospitals that treat a disproportionate share of indigent and uninsured patients. The federal government distributes about $12 billion annually to offset part of the cost.

The ACA reduces DSH payments by about one-quarter, on average, through 2019. Beginning in 2018, annual reductions are about $5 billion per year. The federal government will initially deduct about three-quarters of hospitals' historic allotment and then give back a portion of the funding reduction using complex formulas. The rationale is that as more patients have coverage, hospitals will have fewer uninsured patients. However, 23 million people will remain uninsured—

some of whom may seek uncompensated care. States may have to bear some of the additional costs if their hospitals are to stay solvent.

Crowd Out of Private Insurance

Many of the newly insured under Medicaid will likely be those who previously had private coverage. Research dating back to the 1990s consistently confirms that when Medicaid eligibility is expanded, 50 percent to 75 percent of the newly enrolled are those who have dropped private coverage.[34]

A Better Solution: Give the States Control Over Medicaid

A good argument can be made for abolishing Medicaid. Given the freedom to spend the same money in other ways, state governments should be able to deliver more care and better care. Even if they decide to retain the basic structure of Medicaid, the states can implement a slew of reforms that will lower costs, improve quality and increase access to care.

The most straightforward solution is to give the states their share of Medicaid dollars with no strings attached except the requirement to spend the money on indigent care. The fairest allocation system is to let each state's block grant reflect the proportion of the nationwide poverty population living in the state.

9. Impossible Insurance Company Regulations

Regulating the Medical Loss Ratio

A medical loss ratio is the percentage of health insurance premiums that is spent on medical care. The popular term for the remainder is "administrative costs." The new law requires plans to spend at least 85 percent of their premium income on medical care and no more than 20 percent on administration.[35]

Here's one immediate problem: no one knows how to define "administration." Just as there is no line item in the federal budget called "waste fraud and abuse," there is also no line item in any organization's budget called "administrative costs." Most of us think we vaguely know what it is. But pinning it down is sort of like trying to nail Jell-O to the wall.

Think about a doctor's office and ask yourself what goes on there that you would be inclined to call "administration" or "overhead" and what you would call "medical care." Arguably, the physical facility, the equipment, and the utilities are all overhead. The personnel who admit you and discharge you are engaged in administration, are they not? Ditto for the taking of your medical history and your vitals—and even ascertaining the nature of the complaint that brought you there. In fact, you could make a case that unless someone is actually drawing blood, giving you a shot or ordering a prescription, *it's all overhead.*

Looking at it this way, you could argue that about 95 percent of everything that goes on in a doctor's office is administration and overhead. Conversely, a clever accountant might also be able to argue the reverse—that only 5 percent is really overhead.

Now, let's think about insurance companies for a moment. The MLR is a constraint that potentially limits sales efforts, profit, efforts to ferret out fraud, and any other nonmedical expense—insurers will no doubt see it as an *undesirable* constraint. Sales commissions to insurance brokers who service health policies are also considered overhead. So is the activity of answering the enrollees' questions about the plan.

Five Perverse Incentives

Of all the perverse incentives this kind of regulation creates, I want to focus on five that I think will be especially pernicious.

First, just about any payment an insurer makes to a doctor or hospital is going to count as medical care, no matter how large the administrative costs are for the provider. So both entities have an incentive to find ways of shifting administrative costs from the insurer to the providers. The most obvious way of doing that is for the insurer to contract with an HMO, give the HMO a fixed fee per enrollee, and let the HMO manage all the care, no questions asked.

Second, almost anything the insurer does that conforms to the Obama administration's view of "improving quality"—managed care, coordinated care, integrated care, electronic medical records—will count as "medical care." But efforts to detect and prevent fraud will not count. Doctor credentialing won't count either. One way to think about this is to realize that everything insurers are doing today to hassle *good* doctors will be encouraged and much of what they do to get rid of *bad* doctors will be discouraged.

Third, the days of the insurance broker are probably numbered. Since broker commissions won't count as "medical care" and since the MLR is averaging about 70 percent, rather than 80 percent, in the individual market, insurers will cut back on commissions, and brokers may leave the market completely. Why should you care? Because in today's bureaucratic health insurance system, brokers (along with employers) act as advisers and protectors. They answer questions, correct mistakes, eliminate confusion, and offer other customer services. Once they're gone, you will be left on your own to navigate the complexities of the system.

Fourth, the minimum MLR restricts what insurers can spend to compete with each other in a way that favors larger firms and discriminates against smaller ones. Health insurers across the country are already leaving the small-group and individual health insurance markets, forcing people to find other sources of coverage. In the process, we are left with markets that are more concentrated, less competitive and offering consumers less choice. Here are a few examples, courtesy of the Galen Institute:[36]

- The American Enterprise Group announced in October 2011 that it would drop non-group coverage for 35,000 people in more than 20 states.
- In Indiana, nearly 10 percent of the state's health insurance carriers have withdrawn from the market because they are unable to comply with the federal medical loss ratio requirement.
- Cigna has announced that it is no longer offering health insurance coverage to small businesses in 16 states and the District of Columbia.
- In Colorado, Aetna will stop selling new health insurance to small groups in the state and is moving existing clients off its plans this year, affecting 1,200 companies and 5,200 employees and their dependents.
- In New Mexico, four insurers—National Health Insurance, Aetna, John Alden, and Principle—are no longer offering insurance to individuals or to small businesses.

These announcements are indicative of an accelerating trend that the American Medical Association says leaves four out of five metropolitan areas in the United States without a competitive health insurance market.[37]

Finally, insurers will be constrained in their ability to realize profits on their insurance business, but there will be no constraint on their profits from invested reserves. This means that in the business of insurance, the insurer will be like a regulated utility. There will be no incentive to take risks on developing new products because the insurer will not be able to reap the rewards of successful innovation. On the other hand, the insurer can realize the full return from risky investments outside the business of insurance.

A Better Solution: Deregulation

At a minimum, getting control of healthcare costs requires a vibrant competitive health insurance marketplace. The most important innovations in health insurance are not coming from the largest companies. They are being produced by smaller, more innovative companies aggressively competing to find a market niche. Imposing regulatory requirements that leave only one or two insurers standing will be self-defeating in the long run.

10. Discrimination Against Consumer-Directed Care

Recall that Health Savings Accounts are the fastest growing product in the health insurance marketplace. Currently, about 25 million families are managing some of their own healthcare dollars as a result. Virtually every serious study has found that these plans lower costs without jeopardizing the quality of care people receive. In fact, most employers have decided that giving financial incentives to employees is the most reliable way to rein in spending.

Given that one of the main goals of health reform was to lower the rate of growth of healthcare spending, it would be truly ironic if the new law makes the most reliable way of achieving the goal unavailable to millions of people. But it appears that is about to happen.

Here's the reason. HSA plans achieve their lower premiums by having patients take more control over healthcare dollars. People pay less to the third-party payer because they agree to take responsibility for more of the expenses. Yet under the new MLR rules, the out-of-pocket spending from an HSA is not counted in the MLR calculation—at least for individually owned insurance.[38] Specifically, if an insurer pays for a healthcare service for their insured, that counts as a medical expense in calculating the medical loss ratio. But if an individual pays for a healthcare service to meet her deductible, that expense does not count as a medical expense for purposes of MLR calculation.

Health policy analyst and insurance veteran, Greg Scandlen, gives this illustration:[39]

> Suppose I buy an insurance policy with no deductible that costs $5,000. I have $4,000 in medical expenses. That is 80 percent of my premium, so the health plan is in compliance with the new MLR rule.
>
> However, if I buy a policy with $1,000 deductible for $4,000 in premium and still have $4,000 in medical expenses, I pay the first $1,000 directly to meet my deductible. The health plan pays the remaining $3,000. That is only 75 percent of my $4,000 premium, so the plan is not in compliance.
>
> Both cases have the exact same total cost of coverage. They have the exact same medical expense. But one design complies and the other does not.

Repeal of the new MLR regulations would go a long way toward ensuring that HSA plans remain in the market and continue to thrive. However, more should be done. There is enormous potential to use Health Savings Accounts to meet the needs of the chronically ill. To realize that potential, we need not only to repeal self-defeating regulations produced under ACA, we also need to liberalize the restrictions in the pre-Obama tax code that keep these accounts from reaching their potential.

18

Conclusion

Principles for a New Healthcare Order

I BEGAN THIS book with a promise. I offered to treat you to a unique view of healthcare—one quite different from what you are likely to encounter anywhere else in the health policy world. I hope I have not disappointed. One fear that I had was that the views I am presenting are too radically different from the norm. Readers need to be able to segue from wherever they are to a new place. The greater the leap that is required, the greater the mind's natural resistance.

But if you have made it this far, I have a few more radical ideas for you to consider.

Healthcare, we have seen, is a complex system, undoubtedly the most complex of all social systems. None of us can ever fully grasp or understand a complex system. It is futile to even try. We should understand, however, that perverse incentives usually lead to perverse outcomes. Therefore, it is almost always a bad idea to create them. Where we discover them, it is almost always wise to eliminate them. Perturbations of complex systems always produce unintended and unexpected consequences, even when all we are doing is eliminating perversion. Nonetheless, the wise course of action is usually to admit our ignorance and avoid giving people incentives to engage in antisocial behavior.

The focus of this book has been almost entirely on identifying the perverse incentives created by government policies and considering ways to remove them with a minimum of social disruption. In Chapter 13, we presented an overview of what the policy environment would look like if we eliminated distortions from some of the most important decisions people are forced to make. In each case, we envisioned replacing biased policies with unbiased ones—leaving people free to make their own choices on a level playing field.

I now want to consider three fundamental questions about healthcare and answer them by means of three principles. Further, I want to consider these questions without reference to health insurance. The reason: Our answers to these questions will help guide us to what we want health insurance to allow us to do.

Here are the questions:

- When patients receive a healthcare service, how much should they pay for it?
- When doctors and other providers deliver a healthcare service, how much payment should they receive?
- How should these amounts be determined?

To guide your thinking about these questions, I want to make two suggestions. First, the philosopher John Rawls observed that when we think about institutions and public policies, it's hard not to personalize the issues.[1] (Would a change be good for me? Or bad for me?) To overcome that temptation, Rawls proposed imagining standing behind a "veil of ignorance" where we are forced to make decisions "position blind." That is, imagine that you are about to be born into society, but you don't know who you will be once you get there. You could be born rich or poor, smart or not very smart, talented or not very talented. Put differently think about the 300 million people living in the United States today. Behind the veil of ignorance, you know in advance that you will become one of those, but you don't know which one. You have an equal chance of becoming any of them.

The second aid to thinking is to distinguish between marginal and inframarginal, or all-or-nothing, decisions. If I ask you what it is worth to you to make one more trip to the doctor or to take one more pill, I am asking you to give me a marginal evaluation. On the other hand, if I ask you how much it is worth to be able to see a doctor at all, I am asking for an all-or-nothing evaluation.

Most of the decisions we make in healthcare are (1) elective and (2) made at the margin. Those decisions and the value we place on them are the only ones I want to consider here. I mention this because there is tendency in healthcare to focus on the all-or-nothing (your-money-or-your-life) circumstances. Suppose you were wheeled into an emergency room on a gurney, facing a life-or-death emergency, and I ask you, "How much is it worth to you to have a doctor save your life?" Your answer might well be, "My entire net worth." Neither my question nor your answer would be very interesting or practical, however.

We can turn that question into one that *is* interesting and practical, though. Suppose I asked you, "How much would it be worth to you to pay a slightly higher fee to emergency room doctors in order to attract one more doctor to the staff and increase the probability of your life being saved in a future emergency by some small probability?" Not only is this an interesting question, economists can actually come up with an answer to it—not necessarily for you personally, but for people generally. They can do that by looking at tradeoffs people make between small risks and amounts of money people are willing to spend to avoid them in everyday life.

With those caveats in mind, I want to answer the three questions by proposing three principles that should govern the purchase of healthcare.

- Patients should pay a price for care equal to its marginal social cost.
- Providers should receive a price equal to the marginal social value their care creates.
- Wherever possible, these prices should be determined in competitive markets.

Were this any other market, most economists I know would find these principles unobjectionable. The reasons are straightforward. If patients are charged less than the cost of their care, they will have a perverse incentive to overconsume. If they have to pay more, they will have an incentive to underconsume. On the provider side, the same reasoning applies. If doctors receive a fee that is less than the social value of a service, they will underprovide that service. If their fee is higher than the social value of the service, they will overprovide. As for the third principle, most of the time competitive markets are essential to make the first two principles happen.

This is Economics 101. It is rational. It is sensible. It is unobjectionable. And yet every country in the world has done almost everything imaginable to prevent these three principles from being implemented.

The failure to follow these principles is the main reason why there are so many unmet healthcare needs. Although an estimated 71 million Americans have high levels of bad cholesterol, only about half of them are being treated for the problem.[2] Of those who are being treated, about one-third do not have the problem under control. If National Heart, Lung, and Blood Institute (NHLBI) guidelines were followed for drug treatment of hypertension, the number of people on angiotensin-converting enzyme (ACE) inhibitors would double. If the NHLBI guidelines were followed for the treatment of asthma, the use of asthma medication (inhaled corticosteroids) would rise from two- to tenfold.[3]

Consider for a moment how our healthcare system might be different. In a normal market, all these unmet needs would be viewed as an opportunity for the providers of care. Unsolved problems and unmet needs are the fertile soil from which entrepreneurial ventures inevitably grow.

So why don't we see thousands of doctors, nurses, and other paramedical personnel actively searching for better answers day in and day out? Why don't we see newspaper and television advertisements touting new therapies and new techniques for this huge potential group of customers? If we implemented the three principles governing the purchase of healthcare, we would see that happening.

Let's now turn to the subject of health insurance. From our answers to the previous questions, we know we want insurance to do two things: (1) allow us to purchase care when we need it and (2) do so in a way that does not distort the three principles that should govern the purchase of healthcare.

To make care more accessible, this book has suggested:

- Empowering patients with Health Savings Accounts, Health Stamps, individually managed chronic care accounts, and other mechanisms allowing them to become unrestricted consumers in the medical marketplace.
- Allowing patients in such public insurance plans as Medicaid and Medicare to use their insurance to gain easy access to walk-in clinics and other convenient, low-cost sources of care.
- Encouraging providers to offer telephone and email consultations and other more convenient methods of care.
- Encouraging providers in other ways to compete for patients based on price, quality, and convenience.
- Loosening medical practice statutes to allow a broader array of providers into the market for direct care.

These ideas aren't all that novel. They would seem to be natural solutions if the primary interest were access to healthcare.

With respect to health insurance, we have argued that insurance should be purchased in a competitive market, and everyone should receive the same amount of help from government, regardless of where the insurance is obtained. Failure to encourage all insurance uniformly gives people perverse incentives. It's also arbitrary and unfair. Beyond that, there are three fundamental questions to be asked:

- Who should own the insurance?
- What happens when people change their insurance?
- What should be the role of self-insurance?

The answers form three additional principles:

- Insurance should be individually owned and should travel with people from job to job and in and out of the labor market.
- When people change insurance plans, they should always move at real prices, not artificial prices.
- People should be able to freely move between individual self-insurance and third-party insurance based on individual preference and market opportunities; and almost all marginal decisions should be made by patients spending their own money.

Portability, we have seen, is about the only rational solution to the problems of pre-existing conditions. Without it, employers and employees face all manner of perverse incentives in the labor market.

In an ideal world, health insurance is a secondary institution. Its only real purpose is to facilitate the market for medical care, rather than be a substitute for it. Failure to understand this one fact is the single most important reason for the crisis of healthcare policy that we see in this country and throughout the developed world.

Notes

Preface

1. John C. Goodman and Gerald L. Musgrave, *Patient Power: Solving America's Healthcare Crisis* (Washington, DC: Cato Institute, 1992).
2. Roger Feldman, ed. *American Health Care: Government, Market Processes, and the Public Interest* (New Brunswick, NJ: Transaction Publishers for the Independent Institute, 2000).
3. Chapin White, "A Comparison of Two Approaches to Increasing Access to Care: Expanding Coverage versus Increasing Physician Fees," *Health Services Research*, 2012, http://www.hschange.org/CONTENT/1273/1273.pdf.
4. Mark V. Pauly and John C. Goodman, "Tax credits for health insurance and medical savings accounts," *Health Affairs* 14, no.1 (1995):125-139.
5. J.D. Kleinke, "Access versus Excess: Value-Based Cost Sharing For Prescription Drugs," *Health Affairs* 23, no. 1, January 2004, 34-47, http://content.healthaffairs.org/content/23/1/34.full#fn-group-1
6. Regina E. Herzlinger, *Consumer-Driven Healthcare: Implications for Providers, Payers and Policy Makers* (New York: Basic Books, 1999).
7. John C. Goodman, Gerald L. Musgrave, and Devon M. Herrick, *Lives at Risk* (New York: Rowman & Littlefield Publishers), 2004.
8. John C. Goodman, Michael Bond, Devon Herrick, Gerald Musgrave, Pamela Villarreal and Joe Barnett, "Handbook on State Health Care Reform," National Center for Policy Analysis, 2007, http://www.ncpa.org/email/State_HC_Reform_6-8-07.pdf.
9. John C. Goodman, Linda Gorman, Devon Herrick and Robert Sade, "Health Care Reform: Do Other Countries Have the Answers?" National Center for Policy Analysis, Brief Analysis, 2009, http://www.ncpa.org/pdfs/sp_Do_Other_Countries_Have_the_Answers.pdf.

Chapter 1: Introduction

1. Uwe E. Reinhardt, "The Supreme Court and Healthcare," *New York Times, Economix* (blog), November 25, 2011, http://economix.blogs.nytimes.com/2011/11/25/the-supreme-court-and-health-care-2/.

2. Amy Finkelstein, "The Aggregate Effects of Health Insurance: Evidence from the Introduction of Medicare," *Quarterly Journal of Economics* 122 (2007): 1–38, http://www.dartmouth.edu/~jskinner/documents/FinkelsteinATheAggregate_000.pdf.
3. "The Medicare/Social Security Trustees Spring Report: A Bleak Future," National Center for Policy Analysis, 2009, http://www.ncpa.org/pdfs/A_Bleak_Future.pdf.
4. Andrew J. Rettenmaier and Zijun Wang, "Medicare Prescription Drug Benefit: What Difference Would It Make?" National Center for Policy Analysis, Brief Analysis, No. 463, Monday, November 17, 2003, http://www.ncpa.org/pdfs/ba463.pdf.
5. J. Michael McWilliams, Alan M. Zaslavsky, and Haiden A. Huskamp, "Implementation of Medicare Part D and Nondrug Medical Spending for Elderly Adults With Limited Prior Drug Coverage," *Journal of the American Medical Association* 306 (2011): 402–409.
6. Atul Gawande, "The Hot Spotters," *New Yorker*, January 24, 2011, http://www.newyorker.com/reporting/2011/01/24/110124fa_fact_gawande.

Chapter 2

1. Friedrich Hayek, *The Fatal Conceit: The Errors of Socialism* (Chicago: University of Chicago, 1988).
2. Hospital costs are derived using a complex formula and filed with Medicare as a report that hospitals refer to as a Medicare Cost Report. These reports are periodically audited to ensure accuracy and the absence of fraud.
3. John C. Goodman and Gerald L. Musgrave, *Patient Power: Solving America's Healthcare Crisis* (Washington, DC: Cato Institute, 1992), 7.
4. Devon Herrick, "Medical Tourism: Have Insurance Card, Will Travel," National Center for Policy Analysis, Brief Analysis, No. 724, September 22, 2010, http://www.ncpa.org/pdfs/ba724.pdf.
5. MediBid.com website, correspondence, and discussions with Ralph Weber, president and CEO of MediBid.
6. Kelly Kennedy, "Healthcare costs vary widely, study shows," *USA Today*, June 30, 2011, http://www.usatoday.com/money/industries/health/2011-06-30-health-costs-wide-differences-locally_n.htm.
7. John D. Shatto and M. Kent Clemens, "Projected Medicare Expenditures under an Illustrative Scenario with Alternative Payment Updates to Medicare Providers," Centers for Medicare & Medicaid Services, US Department Of Health & Human Services, August 5, 2010, https://www.cms.gov/ReportsTrustFunds/downloads/2010TRAlternativeScenario.pdf#page=7.
8. Michael Ettlinger, Michael Linden, and Seth Hanlon, "Budgeting for Growth and Prosperity: A Long-Term Plan to Balance the Budget, Grow the Economy and Strengthen the Middle Class," in *The Solutions Initiative*, Peter G. Peterson Foundation, Washington, DC, May 2011, 40–47, http://www.pgpf.org/Issues/Fiscal-Outlook/2011/01/20/~/media/4595173EB72C47EF9E8E85DE680A22B0.ashx.
9. John C. Goodman, "Emergency Room Visits Likely to Increase under ObamaCare," National Center for Policy Analysis, Brief Analysis No. 709, June 18, 2010, http://www.ncpa.org/pdfs/ba709.pdf.

10. Jonathan Gruber, "The Impacts of the Affordable Care Act: How Reasonable Are the Projections?" National Bureau of Economic Research, NBER Working Paper 17168, June 2011, http://www.nber.org/papers/w17168.pdf.
11. "Hospital Waiting Times/List Statistics," Department of Health, United Kingdom, 2nd Quarter, 2008/2009, http://www.performance.doh.gov.uk/waitingtimes/index.htm.
12. Jim Landers, "Trust your doctor to save?" *Dallas Morning News*, January 9, 2012, http://www.dallasnews.com/business/columnists/jim-landers/20120109-trust-your-doctor-to-save.ece.
13. Karen Davis, Cathy Schoen, and Kristof Stremikis, "Mirror, Mirror on the Wall: How the Performance of the U.S. Healthcare System Compares Internationally, 2010 Update," Commonwealth Fund, June 2010, http://www.commonwealthfund.org/~/media/Files/Publications/Fund%20Report/2010/Jun/1400_Davis_Mirror_Mirror_on_the_wall_2010.pdf.
14. "How to Start a Cell Phone Repair Business," eHow.com, http://www.ehow.com/how_5635463_start-cell-phone-repair-business.html.
15. Daniel Vitiello, "Business Idea: iPhone Repair Business," PowerHomeBiz.com, December 4, 2010, http://www.powerhomebiz.com/News/122010/iphone-repair-business.htm.
16. Website for Onsite Cellular Repair: http://onsitecellularrepair.com/index.php.
17. Timothy M. Dall, Yiduo Zhang, Yaozhu J. Chen, William W. Quick, Wenya G. Yang, and Jeanene Fogli, "The Economic Burden of Diabetes," *Health Affairs*, Vol. 29, No. 2, February 2010, pp. 297–303.
18. John C. Goodman, "Markets and Medicare," *Wall Street Journal*, February 23, 2008, http://online.wsj.com/article/SB120373015283387491.html; John C. Goodman, "A Framework for Medicare Reform," National Center for Policy Analysis, Policy Report No. 315, September 2008, http://www.ncpa.org/pdfs/st315.pdf; John C. Goodman, "Reforming Medicare the Right Way," *John Goodman's Health Policy Blog*, June 13, 2011, http://healthblog.ncpa.org/the-only-way/.
19. Kenneth J. Arrow, "Uncertainty and the Welfare Economics of Medical Care," *The American Economic Review*, December 1963, http://www.who.int/bulletin/volumes/82/2/PHCBP.pdf.
20. Ha T. Tu and Jessica H. May, "Self-Pay Markets In Healthcare: Consumer Nirvana Or Caveat Emptor?" *Health Affairs* 26 (2007): w217–w226, doi: 10.1377.
21. Roger Koppl, Editor; Wendell Cox, Jennifer Dirmeyer, Devon M. Herrick, Kai Jaeger, Edward P. Stringham, Shirley Svorny, Diana W. Thomas and Michael D. Thomas, "Enterprise Programs: Freeing Entrepreneurs to Provide Essential Services to the Poor," National Center for Policy Analysis, Special Publication, August 2011.
22. John C. Goodman, "Why the Poor Need the Marketplace," *John Goodman's Health Policy Blog*, August 24, 2011, http://healthblog.ncpa.org/poor-need-the-marketplace/.
23. Devon M. Herrick and Pamela Villarreal, "Healthcare for Hurricane Victims," National Center for Policy Analysis, Brief Analysis No. 532, October 6, 2005.
24. Megan McArdle, "Why Pilot Projects Fail," *The Atlantic*, December 21, 2011, http://www.theatlantic.com/business/archive/2011/12/why-pilot-projects-fail/250364/; and Megan McArdle, "The Value of Healthcare Experiments," *The Atlantic*, December 24, 2011, http://www.theatlantic.com/business/archive/2011/01/the-value-of-health

-care-experiments/70106/; and John C. Goodman, "Pilot Programs," *John Goodman's Health Policy Blog*, September 8, 2010, http://healthblog.ncpa.org/pilot-programs/.

25. Douglas W. Elmendorf, "Letter to the Honorable Nancy Pelosi," Congressional Budget Office, March 18, 2010, Table 3, p. 4, http://www.cbo.gov/ftpdocs/113xx/doc11355/hr4872.pdf; and "Budget Options, Volume I: Healthcare," Congressional Budget Office, December 2008, http://www.cbo.gov/ftpdocs/99xx/doc9925/12-18-Health Options.pdf.
26. David M. Cutler, *You Money or Your Life: Strong Medicine for America's Healthcare System* (Oxford: Oxford University Press, 2004).
27. The elderly took advantage of innovations in medical science, but the existence of Medicare did not seem to affect mortality. Amy Finkelstein and Robin McKnight, "What Did Medicare Do? The Initial Impact of Medicare on Mortality and Out of Pocket Medical Spending," *Journal of Public Economics* 92 (2008): 1644–1669. Also see Amy Finkelstein, "The Aggregate Effects of Health Insurance: Evidence from the Introduction of Medicare," *Quarterly Journal of Economics* 122, 3 (2007): 1–37.
28. Joseph P. Newhouse, *Free for All?: Lessons from the Rand Health Insurance Experiment* (Cambridge: Harvard University Press, 1993).
29. Jack Hadley and John Holahan, "Covering the Uninsured: How Much Would It Cost?" *Health Affairs* 22 (2003). doi: 10.1377/hlthaff.w3.250.
30. From time to time readers may come across the claim that thousands of people die every year because they are uninsured. As we show in Chapter 7, careful analysis by former Congressional Budget Office director, June O'Neill, health economist Linda Gorman and other scholars find these claims to be completely unsubstantiated.
31. Robin Hanson, "Cut Medicine in Half," Cato Institute, *Cato Unbound*, September 10th, 2007, http://hanson.gmu.edu/CutMed.htm.
32. Steven B. Cohen and William Yu, "The Concentration and Persistence in the Level of Health Expenditures over Time: Estimates for the US Population, 2008–2009," Agency for Healthcare Research & Quality, Statistical Brief No. 354, January 2012, http://meps.ahrq.gov/mepsweb/data_files/publications/st354/stat354.pdf.
33. Lois Snyder, editor, "American College of Physicians Ethics Manual, Sixth Edition," *Annals of Internal Medicine* (2012): 73–104.
34. Rob Stein, "Physicians Group: Weigh Costs in Treating Patients," National Public Radio, All Things Considered, January 2, 2012. http://www.npr.org/2012/01/02/144591018/physicians-group-weigh-costs-in-treating-patients.
35. Aaron Caroll, "Is it unethical for physicians not to consider costs?" *The Incidental Economist* (blog), January 4, 2012, http://theincidentaleconomist.com/wordpress/is-it-unethical-for-physicians-not-to-consider-costs/.
36. Ezekiel J. Emanuel, "It Costs More, but Is It Worth More?" *New York Times Opinionator* (blog), January 2, 2012, http://opinionator.blogs.nytimes.com/2012/01/02/it-costs-more-but-is-it-worth-more/.

Chapter 3

1. See http://en.wikipedia.org/wiki/Pareto_optimality.
2. See Kenneth J. Arrow, *Social Choice and Individual Values, 2nd edition* (New York: John Wiley and Sons, 1963).
3. Helene Cooper and Laurie Goodstein, "Rule Shift on Birth Control Is Concession to Obama Allies," *New York Times,* February 10, 2012, http://www.nytimes.com/2012/02/11/health/policy/obama-to-offer-accommodation-on-birth-control-rule-officials-say.html.
4. Gina Kolata, "Mammogram Debate Moving From Test's Merits to Its Cost," *New York Times*, December 27, 1993.
5. David Henderson, "How to Cut the Cost of Contraceptives by Regulating Less," *EconLog* (blog), February 13, 2012, http://econlog.econlib.org/archives/2012/02/how_to_increase_1.html.
6. Cheryl P. Weinstock, "Lawyers Debate the Insurability of Bone-Marrow Transplants," *New York Times*, March 20, 1994, http://www.nytimes.com/1994/03/20/nyregion/lawyers-debate-the-insurability-of-bone-marrow-transplants.html.
7. Alex Sundby, "Organ Transplants Denied in Arizona after Medicaid Agency's Budget Cut," CBS News *HealthPop* (blog), November 17, 2010, http://www.cbsnews.com/8301-504763_162-20023102-10391704.html.
8. Karol Sikora, "Cancer survival in Britain," *BMJ* 319 (1999): 461, doi: 10.1136/bmj.319.7208.461.
9. John C. Goodman, "It's Still Not What I'm Looking For," *John Goodman's Health Policy Blog*, February 20, 2009, http://healthblog.ncpa.org/its-still-not-what-im-looking-for/.
10. Atul Gawande, "The Velluvial Matrix," *New Yorker* (blog), June 16, 2010, http://www.newyorker.com/online/blogs/newsdesk/2010/06/gawande-stanford-speech.html.
11. Karen Davis, "How Will the Healthcare System Change Under Health Reform?" *The Commonwealth Fund Blog* (blog), June 29, 2010, http://www.commonwealthfund.org/Blog/How-Will-the-Health-Care-System-Change.aspx.
12. Atul Gawande, Donald Berwick, Elliott Fisher, and Mark B. McClellan, "10 Steps to Better Healthcare," *New York Times*, August 12, 2009, http://www.nytimes.com/2009/08/13/opinion/13gawande.html. See also John C. Goodman, "The Demand-Side Approach to Changing What Doctors Do," *John Goodman's Health Policy Blog*, November 16, 2009, http://healthblog.ncpa.org/the-demand-side-approach-to-changing-what-doctors-do/.
13. Mark Kelley, "Productivity Still Drives Compensation in High Performing Group Practices," *Health Affairs Blog*, December 20, 2010, http://healthaffairs.org/blog/2010/12/20/productivity-still-drives-compensation-in-high-performing-group-practices/.
14. Robin Hanson, "Showing that You Care: The Evolution of Health Altruism," Department of Economics, George Mason University, August 2007 (first version May 1999), http://hanson.gmu.edu/showcare.pdf.
15. For an economic explanation of profit, see "Profit (Economic)," Wikipedia.com, June 2011, http://en.wikipedia.org/wiki/Profit_(economics).
16. Joe Nocera, "Dr. Berwick's Pink Slip," *New York Times*, December 5, 2011, http://www.nytimes.com/2011/12/06/opinion/nocera-dr-berwicks-pink-slip.html?_r=1.

17. Robert Pear, "Health Official Takes Parting Shot at 'Waste'," *New York Times*, December 3, 2011, http://www.nytimes.com/2011/12/04/health/policy/parting-shot-at-waste-by-key-obama-health-official.html.
18. Robert Kocher, Ezekiel J. Emanuel, and Nancy-Ann M. DeParle, "The Affordable Care Act and the Future of Clinical Medicine: The Opportunities and Challenges," *Annals of Internal Medicine* E-274 published ahead of print (2010). http://www.annals.org/content/early/2010/08/23/0003-4819-153-8-201010190-00274.1.full.
19. "2009 Survey of Physician Appointment Wait Times," Merritt Hawkins & Associates, 2009, http://www.merritthawkins.com/pdf/mha2009waittimesurvey.pdf.

PART II

Chapter 4

1. Adam Smith, *The Wealth of Nations, 5th edition* (London: Methuen & Co., Ltd., 1904).
2. More than half of people in one survey reported using the Internet to gather health information. Sixty percent of those felt the information they gathered was the "same as" or "better than" the information they receive from their doctor. See Joseph A. Diaz, Rebecca A. Griffith, James J. Ng, Steven E. Reinert, Peter D. Friedmann, and Anne W. Moulton, "Patients' Use of the Internet for Medical Information," *Journal of General Internal Medicine* 17, No. 3 (2002): 180–185.
3. Donald M. Berwick, "Medicare Program; Hospital Inpatient Value-Based Purchasing Program," Final Rule 42 CFR Parts 422 and 480, Centers for Medicare & Medicaid Services, Department of Health and Human Services, May 6, 2011.
4. "2011 Physician Quality Reporting System (Physician Quality Reporting) Measures List," Centers for Medicare & Medicaid Services, Department of Health and Human Services, March 31, 2011, https://www.cms.gov/PQRS/Downloads/2011_PhysQualRptg_MeasuresList_033111.pdf.
5. Lauren H. Nicholas, Nicholas H. Osborne, John D. Birkmeyer, and Justin B. Dimick, "Hospital Process Compliance and Surgical Outcomes in Medicare Beneficiaries," *Archives of Surgery* 145(10) (2010): 999–1004.
6. Brian Serumaga et al., "Effect of Pay for Performance on the Management and Outcomes of Hypertension in the United Kingdom: Interrupted Time Series Study," *BMJ* 342 (2011): 108. doi: 10.1136/bmj.d108.
7. "Screening for Breast Cancer," US Preventive Services Task Force, US Department of Health & Human Services, November 2009, http://www.uspreventiveservicestaskforce.org/uspstf/uspsbrca.htm; see also Gina Kolata, "Mammograms' Value in Cancer Fight at Issue," *New York Times*, September 22, 2010; Gina Kolata, "Study Sets Off Debate Over Mammograms' Value," *New York Times*, December 9, 2001; and Gina Kolata, "Dispute Builds Over Value of Mammography," *New York Times*, February 01, 2002.
8. Thomas R. Burton, "Study Cites Cardiology Conflicts," *Wall Street Journal*, March 28, 2011, http://online.wsj.com/article/SB10001424052748703739204576228850121858250.html.

9. Ronen Avraham, "A Market Solution for Malpractice," *New York Times*, March 28, 2011, http://www.nytimes.com/2011/03/29/opinion/29Avraham.html.
10. Diedtra Henderson, "Article Questions Eli Lilly Marketing Push," *Boston Globe*, October 19, 2006, http://www.boston.com/business/globe/articles/2006/10/19/article_questions_eli_lilly_marketing_push/.
11. Don Taylor, "More on Generalizability," *The Incidental Economist* (blog), March 29, 2011, http://theincidentaleconomist.com/wordpress/more-on-generalizability/.
12. Don Taylor, "COPD and Generalizability," *The Incidental Economist* (blog), March 28, 2011, http://theincidentaleconomist.com/wordpress/copd-and-selection-bias/.
13. Steven Goldberg, "Deciding What Works Responses," *The Healthcare Blog*, March 28, 2011, http://thehealthcareblog.com/blog/2011/03/28/deciding-what-works/.
14. Anirban Basu, "Economics of Individualization in Comparative Effectiveness Research and a Basis for a Patient-Centered Healthcare," National Bureau of Economic Research, NBER Working Paper 16900, March 2011, http://www.nber.org/papers/w16900.
15. Reed Abelson, "In Bid for Better Care, Surgery with a Warranty," *New York Times*, May 17, 2007.
16. L. J. Goes, "A Day in the Life of an Autism Mom," *Age of Autism*, August 28, 2011, http://www.ageofautism.com/2011/08/a-day-in-the-life-of-an-autism-mom-1.html.
17. Ha T. Tu and Ralph C. Mayrell, "Employer Wellness Initiatives Grow, but Effectiveness Varies Widely," Center for Studying Health System Change, NIHCR Research Brief No. 1, July 2010.
18. "Trim Staff, Fat Profits?" *Economist*, July 30, 2011, http://www.economist.com/node/21524905.
19. Julie Appleby, "Specialty Drugs Offer Hope, But Can Carry Big Price Tags," *USA Today*, August 22, 2011, http://www.usatoday.com/money/industries/health/drugs/story/2011/08/Specialty-drugs-offer-hope-but-can-carry-big-price-tags/50090368/1.
20. For a discussion of rationing under managed care, see Emily Friedman, "Managed Care Rationing and Quality: A Tangled Relationship," *Health Affairs* 16 (3) (1997):174–182.
21. Mark W. Stanton, "The High Concentration of US Healthcare Expenditures," Agency for Healthcare Research and Quality, *Research in Action* 19 (2006), http://www.ahrq.gov/research/ria19/expendria.pdf.
22. John C. Goodman, Gerald L. Musgrave, and Devon M. Herrick, *Lives at Risk: Single-Payer National Health Insurance Around the World* (Lanham, MD: Rowman & Littlefield Publishers, 2004), 62.
23. Canadian Agency for Drugs and Technology in Health, "Publicly Funded PET Scanners and Cyclotrons in Canada," undated, http://www.cadth.ca/media/healthupdate/Issue8/pet.pdf; and Society for Nuclear Medicine, "Referring Physicians: Positron Emission Tomography (PET) Scan," Center for Molecular Imagining Innovation and Translation, undated. http://www.molecularimagingcenter.org/index.cfm?PageID=7608.
24. For an explanation of Medicare cost-sharing see "Summary of Medicare Benefits and Cost-Sharing for 2012," California Health Advocates, November 15, 2011, http://www.cahealthadvocates.org/basics/benefits-summary.html.

25. William J. Scanlon, "Medigap: Current Policies Contain Coverage Gaps, Undermine Cost Control Incentives," Testimony before the Subcommittee on Health, Committee on Ways and Means, House of Representatives, March 14, 2002, http://www.gao.gov/new.items/d02533t.pdf; also see Noam N. Levey, "Once Politically Taboo, Proposals to Shift More Medicare Costs to Elderly Are Gaining Traction," *Los Angeles Times*, July 15, 2011.
26. "2012 Medicare Part D Outlook," Q1Medicare.com, undated, http://www.q1medicare.com/PartD-The-2012-Medicare-Part-D-Outlook.php.

Chapter 5

1. Uwe E. Reinhardt, Peter S. Hussey, and Gerard F. Anderson, "US Healthcare Spending in an International Context," *Health Affairs* 23 (2004): 10–25, doi: 10.1377/hlthaff.23.3.10.
2. G. William Hoagland, "Public Policy Meets Private Sector: A Crossroads for the Healthcare Industry," Payors, Plans & Managed Care Law Institute, December 6, 2011, p. 6, http://www.healthlawyers.org/Events/Programs/Materials/Documents/PPMC11/papers/hoagland_slides.pdf.
3. Note, however, that this unfunded liability was officially cut in half by the passage of the Affordable Care Act, which requires enormous cuts in future Medicare spending. Whether these spending cuts will actually take place, however, is highly questionable. See the discussion in Chapter 13.
4. Laurence Kotlikoff, "US Is Bankrupt and We Don't Even Know It," *Bloomberg Opinion*, August 10, 2010, http://www.bloomberg.com/news/2010-08-11/u-s-is-bankrupt-and-we-don-t-even-know-commentary-by-laurence-kotlikoff.html.
5. On average, patients pay only 12 percent of medical care out of pocket. "National Health Expenditures by Type of Service and Source of Funds: Calendar Years 1960 to 2009," Centers for Medicare and Medicaid Services, US Department of Health and Human Services, January 4, 2011, https://www.cms.gov/NationalHealthExpendData/downloads/nhe2009.zip.
6. Mike Offit, "The Big Physical: Where to Go, What to Get," Departures.com, Jan/Feb-2008, http://www.departures.com/articles/the-big-physical-where-to-go-what-to-get.
7. Simon Rottenberg, "Unintended Consequences: The Probable Effects of Mandated Medical Insurance," *Regulation,* Cato Institute, undated, http://www.cato.org/pubs/regulation/regv13n1/reg13n1-rottenberg.html.
8. For example, see "ASHG Statement on Direct-to-Consumer Genetic Testing in the United States," *The American Journal of Human Genetics* 81 (2007): 635–637.
9. Krista Conger, "Study first to analyze individual's genome for risk of dozens of diseases, potential responses to treatment," *Inside Stanford Medicine,* Stanford School of Medicine, April 29, 2010, http://med.stanford.edu/ism/2010/april/genome.html.
10. Ron Winslow and Shirley S. Wang, "Soon, $1,000 will Map Your Genes," *Wall Street Journal*, January 10, 2012.
11. Megan McArdle, "Why Pilot Projects Fail," *The Atlantic*, December 21, 2011, http://www.theatlantic.com/business/archive/2011/12/why-pilot-projects-fail/250364/; Megan McArdle, "The Value of Healthcare Experiments," *The Atlantic*, December 24, 2011, http://www.theatlantic.com/business/archive/2011/01/the-value-of-health

-care-experiments/70106/; John C. Goodman, "Pilot Programs," *John Goodman's Health Policy Blog*, September 8, 2010, http://healthblog.ncpa.org/pilot-programs/.

12. Douglas W. Elmendorf, "Letter to the Honorable Nancy Pelosi," Congressional Budget Office, March 18, 2010, Table 3, p. 4, http://www.cbo.gov/ftpdocs/113xx/doc11355/hr4872.pdf; "Budget Options, Volume I: Healthcare," Congressional Budget Office, December 2008, http://www.cbo.gov/ftpdocs/99xx/doc9925/12-18-HealthOptions.pdf; Lyle Nelson, "Lessons from Medicare's Demonstration Projects on Disease Management, Care Coordination, and Value-Based Payment," Congressional Budget Office, January 18, 2012.
13. American Medical Group Association, "Medicare Shared Savings Program: Accountable Care Organizations," American Medical Group Association, Letter, May 11, 2011, http://www.amga.org/Advocacy/MGAC/Letters/05112011.pdf.
14. Andrew M. Ryan, Brahmajee K. Nallamothu, and Justin B. Dimick, "Medicare's Public Reporting Initiative On Hospital Quality Had Modest Or No Impact On Mortality From Three Key Conditions," *Health Affairs* 31 (2012): 585–592.
15. David Dranove, "Quality Disclosure and Certification: Theory and Practice," *Journal of Economic Literature*, 48 (2010): 935–963, doi: 10.1257/jel.48.4.935.
16. Brian Serumaga et al., "Effect of Pay for Performance on the Management and Outcomes of Hypertension in the United Kingdom: Interrupted Time Series Study," *British Journal of Medicine* (2011), doi: 10.1136/bmj.d108.
17. Amy Goldstein, "Experiment to Lower Medicare Costs Did Not Save Much Money," *Washington Post*, June 1, 2011.
18. Ashley D. Black et al., "The Impact of eHealth on the Quality and Safety of Healthcare: A Systematic Overview," *PloS Medicine* (2011), http://www.plosmedicine.org/article/info%3Adoi%2F10.1371%2Fjournal.pmed.1000387.
19. Danny McCormick, David H. Bor, Stephanie Woolhandler, and David U. Himmelstein, "Giving Office-Based Physicians Electronic Access To Patients' Prior Imaging and Lab Results Did Not Deter Ordering Of Tests," *Health Affairs* 31 (2012): 499–495.
20. Lyle Nelson, "Care Coordination, and Value-Based Payment," Issue Brief, Health and Human Resources, Congressional Budget Office, January 2012, http://www.cbo.gov/ftpdocs/126xx/doc12663/01-18-12-MedicareDemoBrief.pdf.
21. "Lessons from Medicare's Demonstration Projects on Disease Management, Care Coordination, and Value-Based Payment," *Congressional Budget Office Director's Blog*, January 18, 2012, http://cboblog.cbo.gov/?p=3158.
22. Megan McArdle, "Why Pilot Projects Fail," *The Atlantic*, December 21, 2011, http://www.theatlantic.com/business/archive/2011/12/why-pilot-projects-fail/250364/.
23. Megan McArdle, "The Value of Healthcare Experiments," *The Atlantic*, January 24, 2011, http://www.theatlantic.com/business/archive/2011/01/the-value-of-health-care-experiments/70106/.
24. Banner Health, "40 Years Ago, Surgicenter Created New Model of Patient Care," BannerHealth.com, February 12, 2010, http://www.bannerhealth.com/About+Us/News+Center/Press+Releases/Press+Archive/2010/40+years+ago+Surgicenter+created+new+model+of+patient+care.htm.
25. Roni Caryn Rabin, "Drug Scarcity's Dire Cost, and Some Ways to Cope," *New York Times*, December 12, 2011, http://www.nytimes.com/2011/12/13/health/policy/the-personal-price-paid-for-shortages-of-doxil-and-other-drugs.html.

26. "Survey Reveals 90 Percent of Anesthesiologists Experiencing Drug Shortages of Anesthetics," Press Release, American Society of Anesthesiologists, May 9, 2011, http://www.asahq.org/For-the-Public-and-Media/Press-Room/ASA-News/Survey-Reveals-90-Percent-of-Anesthesiologists-Experiencing-Drug-Shortages-of-Anesthetics.aspx.
27. Ezekiel Emanuel, "Shortchanging Cancer Patients," *New York Times*, August 6, 2011, http://www.nytimes.com/2011/08/07/opinion/sunday/ezekiel-emanuel-cancer-patients.html.
28. Emanuel, "Shortchanging Cancer Patients."
29. Scott Gottlieb, "Drug Shortages: Why They Happen and What They Mean" (Statement before the Senate Finance Committee, United States Senate), December 7, 2011.
30. Peter Loftus, "Attention Disorder Drug Shortage Prompts Finger-Pointing," *Wall Street Journal*, May 5, 2011, http://online.wsj.com/article/SB10001424052748703992704576305482186274332.html.
31. Gottlieb, "Drug Shortages."
32. Gottlieb, "Drug Shortages."
33. "Healthcare Reform: 340B Drug Pricing Program," E-ALERT, Covington Burling LLP, April 2010.
34. Stephen Barlas, "Healthcare Reform Bill Expands Access to Section 340B Discounted Drugs for Hospitals," *P&T* 35, No. 11 (2010), http://www.ptcommunity. com/ptjournal/fulltext/35/11/PTJ3511632.pdf.
35. "Drug Pricing: Manufacturer Discounts in the 340B Program Offer Benefits, but Federal Oversight Needs Improvement," Government Accountability Office, GAO-11-836, September 2011, http://gao.gov/products/GAO-11-836.
36. Physicians for a National Health Program, http://www.pnhp.org/.
37. "Conyers Reintroduces 'Expanded & Improved Medicare For All' Bill (HR 676)," *Healthcare-NOW!* Update, February 14, 2011, http://www.healthcare-now.org/conyers-reintroduces-expanded-improved-medicare-for-all-bill-hr-676/.
38. Paul Krugman, "Medicare Saves Money," *New York Times*, June 12, 2011, http://www.nytimes.com/2011/06/13/opinion/13krugman.html.
39. Aaron Carroll, "In defense of Canada," *The Incidental Economist* (blog), June 5, 2011, http://theincidentaleconomist.com/wordpress/in-defense-of-canada/.
40. Paul Krugman, "Messing with Medicare," *New York Times*, July 24, 2011, http://www.nytimes.com/2011/07/25/opinion/25krugman.html.
41. Robert Reich, "Why Medicare Is the Solution—Not the Problem," *The Healthcare Blog*, July 22, 2011, http://thehealthcareblog.com/blog/2011/07/22/why-medicare-is-the-solution-%E2%80%94-not-the-probl/.
42. Merrill Matthews, "Medicare's Hidden Administrative Costs: A Comparison of Medicare and the Private Sector," (Based in part on a technical paper by Mark Litow of Milliman, Inc.), Council for Affordable Health Insurance, January 10, 2006, http://www.cahi.org/cahi_contents/resources/pdf/CAHI_Medicare_Admin_Final_Publication.pdf.
43. Benjamin Zycher, "Comparing Public and Private Health Insurance: Would a Single-Payer System Save Enough to Cover the Uninsured?" Manhattan Institute for Policy Research, Medical Progress Report No. 5, October 2007, http://www.manhattan-institute.org/html/mpr_05.htm.

44. Robert A. Book, "Medicare Administrative Costs Are Higher, Not Lower, Than for Private Insurance," Heritage Foundation, Web Memo No. 2505, June 25, 2009, http://www.heritage.org/research/reports/2009/06/medicare-administrative-costs-are-higher-not-lower-than-for-private-insurance.
45. Merrill Matthews and Mark Litow, "Why Medicare Patients See the Doctor Too Much," *Wall Street Journal*, July 11, 2011, http://online.wsj.com/article/SB10001424052702304760604576428300875828790.html.
46. New York State Office for the Aging, Health Benefits Fraud Index (estimate provided by the US General Accounting Office), http://www.aging.ny.gov/healthbenefits/FraudIndex.cfm.
47. John D. Shatto and M. Kent Clemens, "Projected Medicare Expenditures under an Illustrative Scenario with Alternative Payment Updates to Medicare Providers" (Memorandum delivered on August 5, 2010), Department of Health & Human Services, Centers for Medicare & Medicaid Services, Office of the Actuary, http://www.cms.gov/ReportsTrustFunds/downloads/2010TRAlternativeScenario.pdf.
48. John C. Goodman and Thomas R. Saving, "Is Medicare More Efficient Than Private Insurance?" *Health Affairs Blog*, August 19, 2011, http://healthaffairs.org/blog/2011/08/09/is-medicare-more-efficient-than-private-insurance/.
49. Michael Ettlinger, Michael Linden, and Seth Hanlon, "Budgeting for Growth and Prosperity: A Long-Term Plan to Balance the Budget, Grow the Economy and Strengthen the Middle Class," in *The Solutions Initiative*, Center for American Progress, 40–47.
50. "Why Is Health Spending in the United States So High?" OECD (2011), *Health at a Glance 2011: OECD Indicators*, OECD Publishing, doi: 10.1787/health_glance-2011-en.
51. Ezekiel J. Emanuel, "Spending More Doesn't Make Us Healthier," *New York Times Opinionator* (blog), October 27, 2011, http://opinionator.blogs.nytimes.com/2011/10/27/spending-more-doesnt-make-us-healthier/.
52. Henry J. Aaron and Paul B. Ginsburg, "Is Health Spending Excessive? If So, What Can We Do About It?" *Health Affairs* 28 (2009): 1260–1275, doi: 10.1377/hlthaff.28.5.1260.
53. Sarah Kliff, "What Does All Our Healthcare Spending Buy Us? Not Much," *Washington Post, Ezra Klein's Wonkblog*, November 15, 2011, http://www.washingtonpost.com/blogs/ezra-klein/post/what-does-all-our-health-care-spending-buy-us-not-much/2011/11/15/gIQAcm5hPN_blog.html.
54. Austin Frakt, "In Healthcare, the US Is on a Different Planet," *The Incidental Economist* (blog), November 15, 2011, http://theincidentaleconomist.com/wordpress/in-health-care-the-us-is-on-a-different-planet/.
55. Karen Davis, Cathy Schoen, and Kristof Stremikis, "Mirror, Mirror on the Wall: How the Performance of the US Healthcare System Compares Internationally, 2010 Update," The Commonwealth Fund, June 2010, http://www.commonwealthfund.org/~/media/Files/Publications/Fund%20Report/2010/Jun/1400_Davis_Mirror_Mirror_on_the_wall_2010.pdf.
56. Paul Krugman, "Vouchers for Veterans," *New York Times, Conscience of a Liberal* (blog), November 13, 2011, http://www.nytimes.com/2011/11/14/opinion/krugman-vouchers-for-veterans-and-other-bad-ideas.html.

57. Charles Forelle, "Health System Reflects Greece's Ills," *Wall Street Journal*, November 12, 2011, http://online.wsj.com/article/SB10001424052970203658804576638812089566384.html?mod=googlenews_wsj.
58. John C. Goodman et al., "Healthcare Reform: Do Other Countries Have the Answers?" National Center for Policy Analysis, Special Publication, March 10, 2009, http://www.ncpa.org/pdfs/sp_Do_Other_Countries_Have_the_Answers.pdf.
59. "Why Is Health Spending in the United States So High?" OECD (2011), *Health at a Glance 2011: OECD Indicators*, OECD Publishing, doi: 10.1787/health_glance-2011-en.
60. Mark Pauly, "US Healthcare Costs: The Untold True Story," *Health Affairs* 12 (1993): 152-159, doi: 10.1377.
61. Robert L. Ohsfeldt and John E. Schneider, "The Business of Health: How Does the US Healthcare System Compare to Systems in Other Countries?" (Health Policy Discussion, American Enterprise Institute) October 2006. Note: This result has been disputed by the OECD, which claimed Ohsfeldt and Schneider relied too heavily on the high US gross domestic product in their estimates of life years lost due to violence and car accidents. See Matthew Dalton, "Violence, Traffic Accidents and US Life Expectancy," *Wall Street Journal Health Blog*, August 25, 2009, http://blogs.wsj.com/health/2009/08/25/violence-traffic-accidents-and-us-life-expectancy/.
62. The relationship of life expectancy to health expenditure is a loose one. For example, Sweden and Denmark spend similar amounts per capita on healthcare, yet life expectancy is nearly four years longer in Sweden than Denmark. See "Healthcare Systems: Getting More Value for Money," Organisation for Co-operation and Development, OECD Economics Department Policy Notes No. 2. (2010), http://www.oecd.org/dataoecd/21/36/46508904.pdf; and "Life Expectancy vs Healthcare Spending in 2007 for OECD Countries," Organisation for Co-operation and Development, OECD Health Data 2010, http://en.wikipedia.org/wiki/Health_care_system#Cross-country_comparisons.
63. "Broken Promises: Reservations Lack Basic Care," Associated Press, June 14, 2009, http://www.msnbc.msn.com/id/31210909/ns/health-health_care/#.TxBITvl2BBk.
64. David R. Henderson, "Mini-Med Plans," National Center for Policy Analysis, Brief Analysis No. 727, October 21, 2010, http://www.ncpa.org/pub/ba727.
65. Karen Stocker, Howard Waitzkin, and Celia Iriart, "The Exportation of Managed Care to Latin America," *New England Journal of Medicine* 340 (1999): 1131–1136.
66. Abby Goodnough and Kevin Sack, "Massachusetts Tries to Rein in Its Health Costs," *New York Times*, October 17, 2011.

Chapter 6

1. Steven M. Aschet et al., "Who Is at Greatest Risk for Receiving Poor-Quality Healthcare?" *New England Journal of Medicine* 354 (2006): 1147–1156.
2. David McKalip, "Do Patients Receive About Half of Recommended Healthcare?" *John Goodman's Health Policy Blog*, June 8, 2009, http://healthblog.ncpa.org/do-patients-receive-about-half-of-recommended-health-care/.
3. Author calculations based on Troyen A. Brennan et al., "Incidence of Adverse Events and Negligence in Hospitalized Patients: Results of the Harvard Medical Practice Study I," *New England Journal of Medicine* 324, No. 6 (1991): 370–376 and Eric J.

Thomas et al., "Incidence and Types of Adverse Events and Negligent Care in Utah and Colorado," *Medical Care* 38, No. 3 (2000): 261–271.

4. Author calculations based on Jon Shreve et al., "The Economic Measurement of Medical Errors," Society of Actuaries, Health Section, June 2010, http://www.soa.org/files/pdf/research-econ-measurement.pdf.
5. John C. Goodman, Pamela Villarreal, and Biff Jones, "The Social Cost of Adverse Medical Events, and What We Can Do About It," *Health Affairs* 30 (2011): 590–595.
6. David C. Classen et al., "'Global Trigger Tool' Shows That Adverse Events in Hospitals May Be Ten Times Greater Than Previously Measured," *Health Affairs* 30 (2011): 581–589.
7. John Dale Dunn, "Patient Safety Research: Creating Crisis," American Council for Science and Health, January 10, 2005, http://www.acsh.org/factsfears/newsID.487/news_detail.asp.
8. "The Benefits and Costs of the Clean Air Act, 1970 to 1990," US Environmental Protection Agency, October 1997, http://www.epa.gov/air/sect812/1970-1990chptr1_7.pdf.
9. Linda Gorman, "The History of Health Care Costs and Health Insurance," Wisconsin Policy Research Institute, Vol. 19, No. 10. October 2006, p. 21. Available at: http://www.wpri.org/Reports/Volume19/Vol19no10.pdf. Also see Baker et al., "The Canadian Adverse Events Study: The Incidence of Adverse Events Among Hospital Patients in Canada," *Canadian Medical Association Journal* 170, No. 11 (2004): 1678–1686.
10. Detroit Medical Center website: http://www.dmc.org/.
11. Leapfrog Group website: http://www.leapfroggroup.org/cp.
12. Devon M. Herrick, "Medical Tourism: Global Competition in Healthcare," National Center for Policy Analysis, Policy Report No. 304, November 2007.
13. Ashish K. Jha, Zhonghe Li, E. John Orav and Arnold M. Epstein, "Care in US Hospitals—The Hospital Quality Alliance Program," *New England Journal of Medicine* 353 (2005): 265–274.
14. Lauren H. Nicholas, Nicholas H. Osborne, John D. Birkmeyer, and Justin B. Dimick, "Hospital Process Compliance and Surgical Outcomes in Medicare Beneficiaries," *Archives of Surgery* 145 (2010): 999–1004. doi:10.1001/archsurg.2010.191.
15. David M. Shahian, Robert E. Wolf, Lisa I. Iezzoni, Leslie Kirle, and Sharon-Lise T. Normand, "Variability in the Measurement of Hospital-wide Mortality Rates," *New England Journal of Medicine* 363 (2010): 2530–2539.
16. Harris Meyer, "Collaborating Reduces Costs of Healthcare," *USA Today*, January 6, 2012, http://www.usatoday.com/money/industries/health/story/2012-01-05/health-care-collaboratives/52394918/1.
17. Dana Goldman and John A. Romley, "Hospitals as Hotels: The Role of Patient Amenities in Hospital Demand," National Bureau of Economic Research, NBER Working Paper No. 14619, December 2008.
18. Kurt D. Grote, John R. S. Newman, and Saumya S. Sutaria, "A Better Hospital Experience: Hospitals Must Learn What Commercially Insured Patients and Their Physicians Look for When Choosing Facilities—And How to Deliver it," *McKinsey Quarterly*, November 2007.
19. Myung Oak Kim, "Steak or Scallops? Hospitals Add Luxuries to Attract the Well-heeled," *Solutions*, July 13, 2011, http://www.healthpolicysolutions.org/2011/07/13/steak-or-scallops-hospitals-add-luxuries-to-attract-the-well-heeled/.

20. Phil Galewitz (Kaiser Health News), "Hospitals mine patient records in search of customers," *USA Today*, February 5, 2012. http://www.usatoday.com/money/industries/health/story/2012-01-18/hospital-marketing/52974858/1.
21. Nina Bernstein, "Chefs, Butlers, Marble Baths: Hospitals Vie for the Affluent," *New York Times*, January 21, 2012, http://www.nytimes.com/2012/01/22/nyregion/chefs-butlers-and-marble-baths-not-your-average-hospital-room.html.
22. Liz Segre and Marilyn Haddrill, "Other Corrective Procedures," AllAboutVision.com, October 13, 2011, http://www.allaboutvision.com/visionsurgery/cost.htm.
23. J. Russell Teagarden et al., "Dispensing Error Rate in a Highly Automated Mail-Service Pharmacy Practice," *Pharmacotherapy* 25 (2005): 1629–1635.
24. Minnesota HealthScores website: http://www.mnhealthscores.org/.
25. Devon M. Herrick, Linda Gorman, and John C. Goodman, "Information Technology: Benefits and Problems," National Center for Policy Analysis, Policy Report No. 327, April 2010.
26. Herrick et al., "Information Technology: Benefits and Problems."
27. Devon M. Herrick, "Healthcare Entrepreneurs: The Changing Nature of Providers," National Center for Policy Analysis, Policy Report No. 318, December 2008.
28. Paul H. Keckley and Howard R. Underwood, "Medical Tourism: Consumers in Search of Value," Deloitte Center for Health Solutions, 2008.
29. Correspondence with BridgeHealth and North American Surgery. See Devon M. Herrick, "Medical Tourism: Have Insurance Card, Will Travel," National Center for Policy Analysis, Brief Analysis No. 724, September 22, 2010.
30. Patricia Anstett, "Search for World's Best Healthcare is Leading More People to Michigan," *Detroit Free Press*, December 21, 2010.

Chapter 7

1. John C. Goodman, Gerald L. Musgrave, and Devon M. Herrick, *Lives at Risk: Single-Payer National Health Insurance Around the World* (Lanham, MD: Rowman & Littlefield Publishers, Inc., 2004).
2. Ellyn R. Boukus and Peter J. Cunningham, "Mixed Signals: Trends in Americans' Access to Medical Care, 2007–2010," Center for Studying Health System Change, Tracking Report, Results from the Health Tracking Household Survey, No. 25, August 2011.
3. John C. Goodman, "How We Ration Care," *The Healthcare Blog*, September 08, 2011, http://www.ncpa.org/commentaries/how-we-ration-care.
4. Marisa Elena Domino et al., "Increasing Time Costs and Copayments for Prescription Drugs An Analysis of Policy Changes in a Complex Environment," *Health Services Research* 46 (2011): 900–919.
5. Committee on the Consequences of Uninsurance, Board on Healthcare Services, Institute of Medicine, *Care Without Coverage: Too Little, Too Late* (consensus report, Washington DC: National Academy Press, 2002), http://books.nap.edu/openbook.php?record_id=10367.
6. Andrew Wilper et al., "Health Insurance and Mortality in US Adults," *American Journal of Public Health* 99, (2009), http://www.pnhp.org/excessdeaths/health-insurance-and-mortality-in-US-adults.pdf.

7. "Dying for Coverage," Families USA, April 2008, http://www.familiesusa.org/issues/uninsured/publications/dying-for-coverage.html.
8. "New Report Shows How Many People Are Likely to Die in California Due to Lack of Health Coverage," Families USA, Press Release, April 3, 2008, http://www.familiesusa.org/resources/newsroom/press-releases/2008-press-releases/dying-for-coverage-ca.html.
9. June E. O'Neill and Dave M. O'Neill, "Who Are the Uninsured?" Employment Policies Institute, June, 2009. http://www.epionline.org/studies/oneill_06-2009.pdf.
10. Linda Gorman, "Dying for (Media) Coverage," *John Goodman's Health Policy Blog*, May 2, 2008, http://healthblog.ncpa.org/dying-for-media-coverage/; Linda Gorman and John C. Goodman, "Does Lack of Insurance Cause Premature Death? Probably Not," *John Goodman's Health Policy Blog*, November 2, 2009, http://healthblog.ncpa.org/does-lack-of-insurance-cause-premature-death-probably-not/.
11. Helen Levy and David Meltzer, "The Impact of Health Insurance on Health," *Annual Review of Public Health* 29 (2008): 399–409.
12. Richard Kronick, "Health Insurance Coverage and Mortality Revisited," *Health Services Research* 44, No. 4 (2009): 1,211–1,231.
13. Michael F. Cannon, "Perspectives on an Individual Mandate," Cato Institute, October 17, 2008, http://www.cato.org/pub_display.php?pub_id=9722.
14. Steven M. Aschet et al., "Who Is at Greatest Risk for Receiving Poor-Quality Healthcare?" *New England Journal of Medicine* 354 (2006): 1147–1156.
15. Chapin White, "A Comparison of Two Approaches to Increasing Access to Care: Expanding Coverage versus Increasing Physicians Fees," *Health Services Research*, February 2, 2012. Published online doi: 10.1111/j.1475-6773.2011.01378.x.
16. "The Uninsured in America," BlueCross BlueShield Association, Publication W20-04-035, January 2005, http://www.coverageforall.org/pdf/BC-BS_Uninsured-America.pdf.
17. Alain C. Enthoven and Leonard Schaeffer, "Public Coverage Programs: Solving the Enrollment Dilemma," *Health Affairs Blog*, May 9, 2011, http://healthaffairs.org/blog/2011/05/09/public-coverage-programs-solving-the-enrollment-dilemma/.
18. Enthoven and Schaeffer, "Public Coverage Programs: Solving the Enrollment Dilemma."
19. Enthoven and Schaeffer, "Public Coverage Programs: Solving the Enrollment Dilemma."
20. Richard Pérez-Peña, "Trying to Get, and Keep, Care Under Medicaid," *New York Times*, October 18, 2005.
21. Jennifer Brown, "Two University Hospital Clinics Balk at Government Insurance," *Denver Post*, August 27, 2010; Allison Sherry, "Doctors say CU Hospital is Refusing Poor Patients: Medicaid, Medicare Users Can Face 6- to 8-month Waits," *Denver Post*, October 22, 2003.
22. Heath Foster, "Low-Income Patients Left Waiting for Care," *Seattle Post-Intelligencer*, January 26, 2004.
23. Anna S. Sommers et al., "Dynamics In Medicaid and SCHIP Eligibility Among Children In SCHIP's Early Years: Implications For Reauthorization," *Health Affairs* 26 (2007): w598–w607, doi: 10.1377/hlthaff.26.5.w598.
24. Anna S. Sommers et al., "Dynamics in Medicaid and SCHIP Eligibility Among Children in SCHIP's Early Years: Implications for Reauthorization."

25. Lynn M. Olson, Suk-Fong S. Tang, and Paul W. Newacheck, "Children in the United States with Discontinuous Health Insurance Coverage," *New England Journal of Medicine* 353 (2005): 382–391.
26. Benjamin D. Sommers and Sara Rosenbaum, "Issues In Health Reform: How Changes In Eligibility May Move Millions Back And Forth Between Medicaid and Insurance Exchanges," *Health Affairs* 30 (2011): 228–236.
27. Sherry Jacobson, "Parkland Will Treat All Moms-to-be," *Dallas Morning News*, June 12, 2006.
28. Sherry Jacobson, "Parkland Is Brimming with Babies," *Dallas Morning News*, June 11, 2006.
29. Sherry Jacobson, "Parkland Is Brimming with Babies."
30. Minnesota HealthScores Website: http://www.mnhealthscores.org/.
31. "2011 Patient Access to Healthcare Study: A Survey of Massachusetts Physicians' Offices," Massachusetts Medical Society, May 2011.
32. Jack Hadley and John Holahan, "Covering the Uninsured: How Much Would It Cost?" *Health Affairs* Web Exclusive W3.250 (2003): doi: 10.1377/hlthaff.w3.250.
33. Robin DaSilva, "Access to Health Care in Massachusetts: The Implications for Health Care Reform," Massachusetts Medical Society, December 5, 2011, http://www.massmed.org/AM/Template.cfm?Section=Research_Reports_and_Studies2&TEMPLATE=/CM/ContentDisplay.cfm&CONTENTID=65474.
34. *Inequalities in Health*, Black Report (London: UK Department of Health and Social Security, 1980).
35. *Independent Inquiry into Inequalities in Health*, Acheson Report (London: Stationery Office, 1998). See also "Geographic Variations in Health," UK Office for National Statistics, Decennial Supplement 16, 2001.
36. See, for example, "Postcode Lottery in Social Services," *BBC News,* October 13, 2000, http://news.bbc.co.uk/2/hi/health/969110.stm; Sophie Borland, "Laid Bare, Scandal of the Postcode Lottery for Dementia Care," *MailOnline,* December 13, 2011, http://www.dailymail.co.uk/health/article-2073393/Laid-bare-scandal-postcode-lottery-dementia-care.html and; John-Paul Ford Rojas, "Study Reveals Postcode Lottery," *The Telegraph,* December 10, 2011, http://www.telegraph.co.uk/health/8947415/Study-reveals-postcode-lottery.html.
37. Patrick Butler, "Q&A: Postcode Lottery," *The Guardian* (Manchester), November 9, 2000, http://www.guardian.co.uk/society/2000/nov/09/NHS.
38. Dr. Richard Mitchell and Dr. Mary Shaw, "Reducing Health Inequalities in Britain," Joseph Rowntree Foundation, September 2000.
39. "Cancer Trends in England and Wales, 1950–1999," *Health Statistics Quarterly*, 8 (Winter 2000): 18.
40. "Coronary Heart Disease Statistics," British Heart Foundation, Statistics Database, 1998.
41. Sir Charles George, "Coronary Heart Disease Statistics," British Heart Foundation, 1999.
42. A. S. Basinski and C. D. Naylor, "A Survey of Provider Experiences and Perceptions of Preferential Access to Cardiovascular Care in Ontario, Canada," *Annals of Internal Medicine* 129, No. 7, 1998.

43. David A. Alter et al., "Effects of Socioeconomic Status on Access to Invasive Cardiac Procedures and on Mortality after Acute Myocardial Infarction," *New England Journal of Medicine* 341, No. 18 (October 28, 1999): 1359–1367.
44. Sheryl Dunlop, Peter C. Coyte and Warren McIsaac, "Socio-Economic Status and the Utilisation of Physicians' Services: Results from the Canadian National Population Health Survey," *Social Science and Medicine* 51, No. 1 (July 2000): 1–11.
45. June E. O'Neill and Dave M. O'Neill, "Who Are the Uninsured? An Analysis of America's Uninsured Population, Their Characteristics and Their Health," Employment Policy Institute, June 2009.
46. John C. Goodman, Gerald L. Musgrave, and Devon M. Herrick, *Lives at Risk: Single-Payer National Health Insurance Around the World* (Lanham, MD: Rowman & Littlefield Publishers, 2004).
47. John C. Goodman, Gerald L. Musgrave and Devon M. Herrick, *Lives at Risk: Single-Payer National Health Insurance Around the World.*
48. OECD Health Data 2008, Organisation for Co-operation and Development, 2009.
49. John C. Goodman, Gerald L. Musgrave, and Devon M. Herrick, *Lives at Risk: Single-Payer National Health Insurance Around the World.*
50. Linda Gorman, "Community Health Centers: The Rest of the Story," *John Goodman's Health Policy Blog*, December 29, 2010, http://healthblog.ncpa.org/the-rest-of-the-story-3/.

Chapter 8

1. "Medical Education in the United States and Canada: A Report to the Carnegie Foundation for the Advancement of Teaching," Carnegie Foundation, Bulletin No. 4, 1910, http://www.carnegiefoundation.org/sites/default/files/elibrary/Carnegie_Flexner_Report.pdf.
2. For a discussion of the cost-plus system, see John C. Goodman and Gerald L. Musgrave, *Patient Power: Solving America's Healthcare Crisis* (Washington, DC: Cato Institute, 1992), Chapters 5–9.
3. Carl F. Ameringer, "Organized Medicine on Trial: The Federal Trade Commission vs. the American Medical Association," *Journal of Policy History* 12 (2000): 445–472.
4. This section is largely based on John C. Goodman and Gerald L. Musgrave, "A Primer on Managed Competition," National Center for Policy Analysis, Policy Report No. 183, April 1994.
5. The Federal Employees Health Benefits Program (FEHBP) has four main features: (1) federal employees in most places can choose among eight to twelve competing health insurance plans, including BlueCross and a number of HMOs; (2) the government contributes a fixed amount that can be as much as 75 percent of each employee's premium; (3) the extra cost of more expensive plans must be paid by the employee with after-tax dollars; and (4) the plans are forced to community rate, charging the same premium for every enrollee. Public employee health benefit options in the state of Minnesota are similarly organized, as is the California Public Employees' Retirement System (CalPERS).

6. Bryan Dowd and Roger D. Feldman, "Employer Premium Contributions and Health Insurance Costs," in *Managed Care and Changing Healthcare Markets*, ed. Michael Morrisey (Washington, DC: American Enterprise Institute, 1998), 24–54.
7. James Maxwell et al., "Managed Competition in Practice: 'Value Purchasing' by Fourteen Employers," *Health Affairs* 17 (1998): 216–227, doi: 10.1377.
8. The case for managed competition was forcefully argued in Alain Enthoven, *Health Plan: The Only Practical Solution to the Soaring Cost of Medical Care* (Reading, MA: Addison-Wesley, 1980). For an update on Enthoven's views on the advantages and disadvantages of the FEHBP, see Enthoven, "Effective Management of Competition in the FEHBP," *Health Affairs* 8 (1989): 33–50.
9. Congress initially exempted itself and other government employees from Medicare coverage, which meant that younger federal employees had to directly subsidize the premiums of 80- and 90-year-old retirees. The policy was changed for new employees in the early 1980s so that 80 to 85 percent of federal employees now have Medicare coverage—and Medicare is the payer of first resort.
10. Alain Enthoven, "The History and Principles of Managed Competition," *Health Affairs* (1993 Supplement): 35, doi: 10.1377. On the practice of encouraging high-cost patients to "disenroll," see Jonathan E. Fielding and Thomas Rice, "Can Managed Competition Solve the Problems of Market Failure?" *Health Affairs* (1993 Supplement) 222; Joseph Newhouse, "Is Competition the Answer?" *Journal of Health Economics* 1 (1982): 109–116.
11. The HMO would receive premiums only from people who were about to undergo expensive medical procedures. Thus, the average premium would have to equal the average cost of the procedures. It is precisely because most people cannot easily bear such a financial burden that health insurance is desirable in the first place.
12. Reported in Natalie Hopkinson, "Study Finds Medicare HMOs Target Active Seniors but Not Disabled in Ads," *Wall Street Journal*, July 14, 1998.
13. David Hilzenrath, "Showing the Sickest Patients the Door," *Washington Post*, National Weekly Edition, February 2, 1998.
14. David Hilzenrath, "Showing the Sickest."
15. Mark W. Stanton, "The High Concentration of US Healthcare Expenditures," Agency for Healthcare Research & Quality, *Research in Action* No. 19, June 2006, http://www.ahrq.gov/research/ria19/expendria.pdf.
16. Note that the premium does not have to be the same for all plans, but it must be the same for all members of a given plan.
17. More formally, an equilibrium is said to exist when no participant in the market—including all buyers and sellers—can improve his or her position by any unilateral move.
18. Other analysts have recognized this problem, noting that the tendency is one of "the free market pitfalls of managed competition" (p. 118), that "one of managed competition's greatest challenges is to safeguard quality of care without robbing the system of free-market efficiencies" (p. 110) and that "managed competition carries an inherent risk of discrimination against enrollees who incur high healthcare costs" (p. 120). See Alan L. Hillman, William R. Greer and Neil Goldfarb, "Safeguarding Quality in Managed Competition," *Health Affairs* (1993 Supplement): 110–122, doi: 10.1377.

19. Edwin S. Dolan and John C. Goodman, "Flying the Deregulated Skies: Competition, Price Discrimination, Congestion," in *Economics of Public Policy,* 5th ed. (St. Paul, MN: West Publishing Co., 1995), 143–159.
20. Vernon L. Smith and Stephen Rassenti, "Turning on the Lights: Deregulating the Market for Electricity," National Center for Policy Analysis, NCPA Policy Report No. 228, October 1999.
21. See William Tucker, *The Excluded Americans: Homelessness and Housing Policies* (Washington, DC: Regnery Gateway, 1990).
22. Linda Gorman, "Risk Adjustment Doesn't Work in Medicare Advantage," *John Goodman's Health Policy Blog*, September 6, 2011, http://healthblog.ncpa.org/risk-adjustment-doesn%E2%80%99t-work-in-medicare-advantage/.
23. See Joseph P. Newhouse, "Rate Adjusters for Medicare under Capitation," *Healthcare Financing Review* (1986 Annual Supplement), 45–56, cited in Alain Enthoven, "The History and Principles of Managed Competition," *Health Affairs* (Supplement 1993): 24–48, doi: 10.1377.
24. Joseph P. Newhouse, Melinda Beeuwkes Buntin, and John D. Chapman, "Risk Adjustment and Medicare: Taking a Closer Look," *Health Affairs* 16 (1997): 26–43, doi: 10.1377.
25. "Risk Assessment and Risk Adjustment," American Academy of Actuaries, Issue Brief, May 2010,: http://www.actuary.org/pdf/health/Risk_Adjustment_Issue_Brief_Final_5-26-10.pdf.
26. See Harold S. Luft, "Compensating for Biased Selection in Health Insurance," *Milbank Quarterly* 64 (1986): 580; and Alain Enthoven, *Theory and Practice of Managed Competition in Healthcare Finance* (New York: Elsevier Science Publishing Co., 1988), 86; and Newhouse, Buntin, and Chapman, "Risk Adjustment and Medicare," 34–35.
27. Daeho Kim, "Medicare Payment Reform and Hospital Costs: Evidence from the Prospective Payment System and the Treatment of Cardiac Disease," Brown University, Working Paper, November 20, 2011, http://www.econ.brown.edu/students/Daeho_Kim/JMP_Kim.pdf.
28. Kim, "Medicare Payment Reform and Hospital Costs: Evidence from the Prospective Payment System and the Treatment of Cardiac Disease." Under the Prospective Payment System (PPS), there are 503 diagnostic-related groups (DRGs), and physicians and hospitals receive a predetermined amount from the federal government for whatever services they perform. See John C. Goodman and Gerald L. Musgrave, *Patient Power: Solving America's Healthcare Crisis* (Washington, DC: Cato Institute, 1992), 303–306. Also see John Goodman, "Medicare's PPS Made Costs Higher, Not Lower," *John Goodman's Health Policy Blog*, December 16, 2011, http://healthblog.ncpa.org/medicare%E2%80%99s-pps-made-costs-higher-not-lower/.
29. Len Nichols and Linda Blumberg, "A Different Kind of 'New Federalism'? The Health Insurance Portability and Accountability Act of 1996," *Health Affairs*, Vol. 17 No. 3, May/June 1998.
30. HIPAA also requires states to enable certain eligible individuals leaving group coverage to join an individual plan without new underwriting.
31. Departing employees must accept and sign up for COBRA within sixty days or lose that option completely. See "FAQs For Employers About COBRA Continuation Health Coverage," US Department of Labor, undated, http://www.dol.gov/ebsa/faqs/faq_compliance_cobra.html.

PART III

Chapter 9

1. Emmett B. Keeler, Joseph P. Newhouse and Robert H. Brook, "Selective Memories for 25 Years, the RAND Health Insurance Experiment Has Stoked Competing Claims," *RAND Review* 31 (2007): 26–29.
2. See Andrew J. Rettenmaier and Thomas R. Saving, "A Medicare Reform Proposal Everyone Can Love: Finding Common Ground among Medicare Reformers," National Center for Policy Analysis, Policy Report No. 306, December 2007, http://www.ncpa.org/pub/st306; Robin Hanson, "RAND Health Insurance Experiment," *Overcoming Bias* (blog), May 8, 2007, http://www.overcomingbias.com/2007/05/rand_health_ins.html.
3. Thomas A. Massaro and Yu-Ning Wong, "Medical Savings Accounts: The Singapore Experience," National Center for Policy Analysis, Policy Report No. 203, April 1996, http://www.ncpa.org/pub/st203.
4. Shaun Matisonn, "Medical Savings Accounts in South Africa," National Center for Policy Analysis, Policy Report No. 234, June 2000, http://www.ncpa.org/pub/st234.
5. Greg Scandlen, "Medical Savings Accounts Obstacles to Their Growth and Ways to Improve Them," National Center for Policy Analysis, Policy Report No. 216, July 1998.
6. John C. Goodman, "Health Savings Accounts Will Revolutionize American Healthcare," National Center for Policy Analysis, Policy Report No. 464, January 2004, http://www.ncpa.org/pub/ba464/.
7. Devon Herrick, "Health Reimbursement Arrangements: Making a Good Deal Better," National Center for Policy Analysis, Policy Report No. 438, May 2003, http://www.ncpa.org/pub/ba438.
8. "Choosing Independence: An Overview of the Cash & Counseling Model of Self-Directed Personal Assistance Services," Robert Wood Johnson Foundation, 2006.
9. Amelia M. Haviland, Neeraj Sood, Roland McDevitt, and M. Susan Marquis "How Do Consumer-Directed Health Plans Affect Vulnerable Populations?" *Forum for Health Economics & Policy* 14, No. 2, 2011, article 3, http://www.bepress.com/fhep/14/2/3.
10. Jenny Ivy, "2012 HSA and FSA Cheat Sheet," BenefitsPro.com, November 17, 2011, http://www.benefitspro.com/2011/11/17/2012-hsa-and-fsa-cheat-sheet?ref=hp.
11. Amelia Haviland et al., "How Do Consumer-Directed Health Plans Affect Vulnerable Populations?" *Forum for Health Economics & Policy* 14 (2011).
12. Paul Fronstin, "Health Savings Accounts and Health Reimbursement Arrangements: Assets, Account Balances, and Rollovers, 2006–2009," Employee Benefit Research Institute, EBRI Issue Brief No. 343 June 2010.
13. "A Brief History of Health Savings Accounts," National Center for Policy Analysis, Brief Analysis No. 481, August 13, 2004, http://www.ncpa.org/pub/ba481.
14. John C. Goodman and Gerald L. Musgrave, *Patient Power* (Washington, DC: Cato Institute, 1992), 241–261.
15. The annual family plan deductible is twice the annual deductible per individual.
16. Mark V. Pauly and John C. Goodman, "Tax Credits for Health Insurance and Medical Savings Accounts," *Health Affairs* 14 (1995): 125–139.

17. John C. Goodman, "The John McCain Health Plan," National Center for Policy Analysis, Brief Analysis No. 629, September 5, 2008, http://www.ncpa.org/pub/ba629/.
18. Tom Coburn et al., "The Impact of the 2009 The Patient's Choice Act" (Independent assessment by HSI Network LLC, 2009), http://www.hsinetwork.com/HSI_Report_on_PCHOICE_07-21-2009.pdf.
19. Michael F. Cannon, "Flexible Spending Accounts: The Case for Reform," National Center for Policy Analysis, Brief Analyses No. 439, May 13, 2003.
20. John C. Goodman, Gerald L. Musgrave and Devon M. Herrick, "Designing Ideal Health Insurance," in *Lives at Risk: Single-Payer National Health Insurance Around the World* (Lanham, MD: Rowman & Littlefield Publishers, 2004), 235.
21. John C. Goodman, "Ten Small-Scale Reforms for Pre-Existing (Chronic) Conditions," *Health Affairs Blog*, January 27, 2010, http://healthaffairs.org/blog/2010/01/27/ten-small-scale-reforms-for-pre-existing-chronic-conditions/.
22. John Goodman, "Patients Managing Their Own Healthcare Budgets," *John Goodman's Health Policy Blog*, April 19, 2010, http://healthblog.ncpa.org/patients-managing-their-own-health-care-budgets/.
23. Jack A. Meyer, Lise S. Rybowski and Rena Eichler, "Theory and Reality of Value-Based Purchasing: Lessons from the Pioneers," Agency for Healthcare Policy and Research, AHCPR Publication No. 98-0004, November 1997, http://www.ahrq.gov/qual/meyerrpt.htm.
24. Goodman, Musgrave, and Herrick, "Designing Ideal Health Insurance," 235.
25. Vidhya Alakeson, "International Developments in Self-Directed Care," Commonwealth Fund, *Issues in International Health Policy*, February 2010.
26. John C. Goodman, "Patient Power for Chronic Illness," *Health Affairs Blog*, February 12, 2009, http://healthaffairs.org/blog/2009/02/12/patient-power-for-chronic-illness/. An update of these ideas appears in this book as Chapter 12.
27. John C. Goodman, "Designing Ideal Health Insurance for the Information Age," in *Consumer-Driven Healthcare: Implications for Providers, Payers, and Policymakers*, ed. Regina E. Herzlinger (San Francisco: Jossey-Bass, 2004).

Chapter 10

1. John C. Goodman, "What's Wrong with the Way We Pay Doctors?" *John Goodman's Health Policy Blog*, December, 2009, http://healthblog.ncpa.org/what%E2%80%99s-wrong-with-the-way-we-pay-doctors/.
2. About 34 percent of physicians email their patients. *Wall Street Journal* Staff, "Vote: Should Physicians Use Email to Communicate With Patients?" *Wall Street Journal Health Blog*, January 10, 2012, http://blogs.wsj.com/health/2012/01/10/vote-should-physicians-use-email-to-communicate-with-patients/. These are usually messages alerting the patient about an appointment or other notification. Email consultations are rare.
3. John C. Goodman, "Time, Money, and the Market for Drugs," in *Innovation and the Pharmaceutical Industry: Critical Reflections on the Values of Profit*, eds. H. Tristram Engelhardt, Jr. and Jeremy Garrett (Salem, MA: M & M Scrivener Press, 2008), 153–183.
4. Devon M. Herrick, "Why Health Costs Are Still Rising," National Center for Policy Analysis, Brief Analysis No. 731, November 2010.

5. "LASIK Lessons," *Wall Street Journal*, March 10, 2006, A18. Also see Ha T. Tu and Jessica H. May, "Self-Pay Markets in Health Care: Consumer Nirvana Or Caveat Emptor?" *Health Affairs*, 26, No. 2 (2007): w217–w226. doi: 10.1377/hlthaff.26.2.w217.
6. Devon M. Herrick, "Consumer Driven Healthcare: The Changing Role of the Patient," National Center For Policy Analysis, Policy Report No. 276, May 2005.
7. Herrick, "Consumer Driven Healthcare: The Changing Role of the Patient."
8. Devon M. Herrick, "Shopping for Drugs: 2007," National Center for Policy Analysis, Policy Report No. 293, November 2006.
9. Herrick, "Shopping for Drugs: 2007."
10. Devon M. Herrick, "Retail Clinics: Convenient and Affordable Care," National Center for Policy Analysis, Brief Analysis No. 686, January 2010.
11. Minnesota HealthScores website: http://www.mnhealthcare.org/.
12. Devon M. Herrick, "Convenient Care and Telemedicine," National Center for Policy Analysis, Brief Analysis No. 305, November 2007.
13. Devon M. Herrick, "Concierge Medicine: Convenient and Affordable Care," National Center for Policy Analysis, Brief Analysis No. 687, January 2010.
14. "Dallas-based Compass Turns Patients into Smart Consumers," *Dallas Morning News*, September 10, 2011.
15. John C. Goodman, "Ten Small-Scale Reforms For Pre-existing (Chronic) Conditions," *Health Affairs Blog*, January 27, 2010, http://healthaffairs.org/blog/2010/01/27/ten-small-scale-reforms-for-pre-existing-chronic-conditions/.
16. John C. Goodman, "Employer-Sponsored, Personal, and Portable Health Insurance," *Health Affairs* 25, No. 6 (November 2006): 1556–1566.
17. Randall Brown et al., "Cash and Counseling Evaluation Changes Policymakers' Approach to Consumer Directed Care," AcademyHealth, 2009, http://www.academyhealth.org/files/publications/cashandcounseling.pdf.
18. John C. Goodman, "Patient Power for Chronic Illness," *Health Affairs Blog*, February 12, 2009, http://healthaffairs.org/blog/2009/02/12/patient-power-for-chronic-illness/.
19. John H. Cochrane, "Health-Status Insurance: How Markets Can Provide Health Security," Cato Insitute, Policy Analysis No. 633, February 19, 2009, http://www.cato.org/pub_display.php?pub_id=9986.
20. Gail A. Jensen and Michael A. Morrisey, "Employer-Sponsored Health Insurance and Mandated Benefit Laws," *Milbank Quarterly* 77, No. 4 (1999).
21. Terry Neese and John C. Goodman, "Five Family Friendly Policies," National Center for Policy Analysis, Brief Analysis No. 620, July 2008.
22. Noelia Duchovny and Lyle Nelson, "The State Children's Health Insurance Program," Congressional Budget Office, Congress Of The United States, May 2007, http://www.cbo.gov/sites/default/files/cbofiles/ftpdocs/80xx/doc8092/05-10-schip.pdf.
23. Craig L. Garthwaite, "The Doctor Might See You Now: The Supply Side Effects Of Public Health Insurance Expansions," National Bureau of Economic Research, Working Paper No. 17070, May 2011.
24. Institute of Medicine, *Living Well with Chronic Illness: A Call for Public Health Action* (Washington, DC: National Academies Press, 2012).
25. William H. Shrank et al., "The Use of Generic Drugs in Prevention of Chronic Disease Is Far More Cost-Effective Than Thought, and May Save Money," *Health Affairs* 30, No. 7 (2011): 1351–1357.

26. In one study, less than half of those surveyed with a chronic disease had it under control. See Jonathan R. Javors and Judith E. Bramble, "Uncontrolled Chronic Disease: Patient Non-Compliance or Clinical Mismanagement?" *Disease Management* 6, No. 3, (2003): 169–178. doi:10.1089/109350703322425518.
27. Randall Brown et al., "Cash and Counseling: Improving the Lives of Medicaid Beneficiaries Who Need Personal Care or Home- and Community-Based Services," Final Report, Contract No.: Q14690, MPR Reference No.: 8349-110 Mathematica Policy Research, Inc., August 2007, http://www.mathematica-mpr.com/publications/pdfs/CCpersonalcare.pdf.
28. Pamela Villarreal and Devon M. Herrick, "Healthcare Costs During Retirement," National Center for Policy Analysis, Brief Analysis No. 660, May 2009.

Chapter 11

1. The remainder of this chapter is based on John C. Goodman, "Designing Health Insurance for the Information Age," in *Consumer Driven Healthcare: Implications for Providers, Payers, and Policymakers,* Regina E. Herzlinger, ed. (San Francisco: Jossey-Bass, 2004).
2. Although we confine our analysis to health insurance, people in an ideal world would probably be inclined to combine health insurance with other forms of insurance. That is, in an ideal insurance world, coverage probably would include health insurance, disability insurance, long-term care and life insurance.
3. I am ignoring the variance around the expected expenditure amount for ease of presentation.
4. The market would collapse to a market for one-year term insurance; people with terminal illnesses would essentially become uninsurable.
5. Gina Kolata, "Considering When It Might Be Best Not to Know About Cancer," *New York Times*, October 29, 2011.
6. Tammy O. Tengs et al., "Five Hundred Lifesaving Interventions and Their Cost-Effectiveness," *Risk Analysis* 15 (1995); David M. Eddy, ed., *Common Screening Tests* (Philadelphia: American College of Physicians, 1991), 379.
7. Of course, the plan could then require a second opinion, retesting, and so forth.
8. Prior to 2004, such deposits were subject to payroll taxes and income taxes. The exceptions were tax-free MSAs allowed under a federal pilot program for the self-employed and employees of small businesses. However, under the pilot program, year-end withdrawals used for nonmedical purposes faced regular income taxes and a 15 percent penalty. As of 2004, HSAs in principle became available to all nonelderly Americans, and withdrawals for nonmedical purposes prior to age sixty-five face income taxes plus a 20 percent penalty. Withdrawals after age sixty-five face no penalty.
9. The law requires an across-the-board deductible for all covered services with the exception of preventive care.
10. Letter from Alain Enthoven to Gov. Pete Wilson et al., January 6, 1998.
11. Shaun Matisonn, "Medical Savings Accounts in South Africa," National Center for Policy Analysis, Policy Report No. 234, June 2000.
12. Of course, without some oversight, this reimbursement formula encourages discretionary procedures to relocate to a hospital setting.

13. Shaun Matisonn, "Medical Savings Accounts and Prescription Drugs: Evidence from South Africa," National Center for Policy Analysis, Policy Report No. 254, August 2002.
14. A mandatory point of service option when combined with a requirement to reimburse at the same rates in and out of network can raise the cost of health insurance by as much as 11.3 percent. Estimates of M&R for the National Center for Policy Analysis. Cited in Merrill Matthews, "Can We Afford Consumer Protection? An Analysis of the PARCA Bill," National Center for Policy Analysis, Brief Analysis No. 249, November 24, 1997.
15. Niteesh K. Choudhry, Meredith B. Rosenthal, and Arnold Milstein, "Assessing the Evidence for Value-Based Insurance Design," *Health Affairs* 29 (2010): 1988–1994.
16. See A. Faas, F. G. Schellevis, and J. T. Van Eijk, "The Efficacy of Self-Monitoring of Blood Glucose in NIDDM Subjects: A Criteria-Based Literature Review," *Diabetes Care* 20, No. 9: 1482–1486.
17. Shaun Matisonn, "Medical Savings Accounts in South Africa," National Center for Policy Analysis, Policy Report No. 234, June 2000; and Shaun Matisonn, "Medical Savings Accounts and Prescription Drugs: Evidence from South Africa," National Center for Policy Analysis, Policy Report No. 254, August 2002.
18. See John C. Goodman, *Regulation of Medical Care: Is the Price Too High?* (Cato Institute public policy research monograph), 1980.
19. Although for the terminally ill, this is an idea worth considering.
20. Gail A. Jensen and Michael A. Morrisey, "Mandated Benefit Laws and Employer-Sponsored Health Insurance," *Health Insurance Association of America,* January 1999.
21. There is a growing literature on how to design such arrangements. See John H. Cochrane, "Time-Consistent Health Insurance," *Journal of Political Economy* 103 (1995): 445–473; Mark V. Pauly, Howard Kunreuther and Richard Hirth, "Guaranteed Renewability in Insurance," *Journal of Risk and Uncertainty* 10 (1995): 143–156. See also Bradley Herrick and Mark Pauly, "Incentive-Compatible Guaranteed Renewable Health Insurance," National Bureau of Economic Research, NBER Working Paper 9888, July 2003; and Vip Patel and Mark V. Pauly, "Guaranteed Renewability and the Problem of Risk Variation in Individual Health Insurance Markets," *Health Affairs* Web exclusive (2002).
22. What is envisioned here is a market for individual patients. For those who doubt that such a market could develop, recall that the same objection was once raised against a reinsurance market for residential housing.
23. The reason is that sellers have an incentive to charge marginal cost when no third party is involved.
24. Regina E. Herzlinger, *Market Driven Healthcare: Who Wins, Who Loses in the Transformation of America's Largest Service Industry* (Arizona: Basic Books, 1997), 173.
25. Pediatrix Medical Group website. http://www.pediatrix.com/body cfm?id=48&oTop ID=517.
26. Harris Meyer, "Are You Ready for the Competition?" *Hospitals and Health Networks* 72 (1998): 25–30.
27. Cancer Treatment Centers of America Web site. Video available at: http://www.cancercenter.com/pancreatic-cancer/survivors/roger-stump.cfm.

28. One well-known case was profiled in the movie *Sicko*. See Linda Peeno, "Managed Care Ethics: The Close View," Prepared for US House Of Representatives Committee on Commerce, Subcommittee on Health and Environment, May 30, 1996.
29. Mark V. Pauly and John C. Goodman, "Tax Credits for Health Insurance and Medical Savings Accounts," *Health Affairs* 14 (1995), http://content.healthaffairs.org/content/14/1/125.full.pdf.

Chapter 12

1. A. Russell Localio et al., "Relation between Malpractice and Adverse Medical Events Due to Negligence," *New England Journal of Medicine* 325 (1991): 245–251.
2. David M. Studdert et al., "Claims, Errors, and Compensation Payments in Medical Malpractice Litigation," *New England Journal of Medicine* 354 (2006): 2024–2033.
3. Studdert et al., "Claims, Errors, and Compensation Payments in Medical Malpractice Litigation."
4. Estimate based on Brandon Roberts and Irving Hoch, "Malpractice Litigation and Medical Costs in the United States," *Health Economics* 18, No. 12 (2009): 1394–1419.
5. John C. Goodman, Pamela Villarreal and Biff Jones, "The Social Cost of Adverse Medical Events, and What We Can Do About It," *Health Affairs* 30 (2011): 590–595, doi: 10.1377; See also John C. Goodman, "How Safe Is Your Hospital?" *John Goodman's Health Blog* (blog), April 20, 2011, http://healthblog.ncpa.org/how-safe-is-your-hospital/.
6. Richard Epstein, "Medical Malpractice, Imperfect Information, and the Contractual Foundation for Medical Services," *Law and Contemporary Problems* 49, No. 2 (1986): 201–212.
7. For more details, see John C. Goodman et al., "Malpractice Reform: Five Steps to Liability by Contract," in *Handbook on State Healthcare Reform* (Dallas, Texas: National Center for Policy Analysis, 2007), 167–178.
8. John C. Goodman et al., "Malpractice Reform: Ten Principles of a Rational Tort System," in *Handbook on State Healthcare Reform* (Dallas, Texas: National Center for Policy Analysis, 2007), 153–165.
9. John C. Goodman et al., "Malpractice Reform: Five Steps to Liability by Contract," in *Handbook on State Healthcare Reform* (Dallas, Texas: National Center for Policy Analysis, 2007), 167–178.
10. National Vaccine Injury Compensation Program, http://www.hrsa.gov/vaccine compensation/index.html.

Chapter 13

1. This chapter is based on John C. Goodman, "Applying the 'Do No Harm' Approach to Health Policy," *Journal of Legal Medicine* 28 (2007): 37–52. doi: 10.1080/019476406 01180273.
2. Personal correspondence from John Sheils of the Lewin Group. The Lewin Group estimates that in 2011 the federal tax expenditure for employee health coverage was about $274 billion annually.

3. Personal correspondence from John Sheils of the LewinGroup. For a discussion, also see John Sheils and Randall Haught, "The Cost of Tax-Exempt Health Benefits in 2004," *Health Affairs*, Web Exclusive W4 (2004): 106–112, doi: 10.1377.
4. John C. Goodman, "S-CHIP Fiasco," *John Goodman's Health Policy Blog*, October 15, 2007, http://healthblog.ncpa.org/s-chip-fiasco/.
5. David Cutler and Jonathan Gruber, "Does Public Insurance Crowd out Private Insurance?" *Quarterly Journal of Economics* 111, No. 2 (1996): 391–430.
6. Jonathan Gruber and Kosali Simon, "Crowd-Out Ten Years Later: Have Recent Public Insurance Expansions Crowded Out Private Health Insurance?" National Bureau of Economic Research, Working Paper No. 12858, 2007.
7. Mark V. Pauly and John C. Goodman, "Tax credits for health insurance and medical savings accounts," *Health Affairs* 14, no.1 (1995):125-139.

PART III

Chapter 14

1. Andrew J. Rettenmaier and Thomas R. Saving, "Medicare Trustees Reports 2010 and 2009: What a Difference a Year Makes," National Center for Policy Analysis, Policy Report No. 330, November 18, 2010.
2. The Board of Trustees, Federal Old-Age and Survivors Insurance and Federal Disability Insurance Trust Funds, "The 2008 Annual Report of the Board of Trustees of the Federal Old-Age and Survivors Insurance and Federal Disability Insurance Trust Funds," US Government Printing Office, April 10, 2008; John C. Goodman, "A Framework for Medicare Reform," National Center for Policy Analysis, Policy Report No. 315, September 2008, http://www.ncpa.org/pdfs/st315.pdf.
3. Noah Meyerson et al., "The Long-Term Outlook for Health Care Spending," Congressional Budget Office, November 2007. http://www.cbo.gov/ftpdocs/87xx/doc8758/11-13-LT-Health.pdf.
4. CBO, "Selected CBO Publications Related to Health Care Legislation," 2009–2010, Congressional Budget Office, Congress of the United States, Publication No. 4228, December 2010, http://www.cbo.gov/sites/default/files/cbofiles/ftpdocs/120xx/doc12033/12-23-selectedhealthcarepublications.pdf.
5. "2010 Annual Report of the Boards of Trustees of the Federal Hospital Insurance and Federal Supplementary Medical Insurance Trust Funds," Boards of Trustees of the Federal Hospital Insurance and Federal Supplementary Medical Insurance Trust Funds, August 2010, http://www.cms.gov/ReportsTrustFunds/downloads/tr2010.pdf.
6. Alice Rivlin and Paul Ryan, "A Long-Term Plan for Medicare and Medicaid," November 2010, http://paulryan.house.gov/UploadedFiles/rivlinryan.pdf.
7. Paul Krugman, "The Flimflam Man," *New York Times, The Conscience of a Liberal* (blog), August 5, 2010.
8. Ezra Klein, "Creator of Premium Support Says Ryan Has Vouchers, Not Premium Support," *Washington Post Wonkblog* (blog), April 2011, http://www.washingtonpost.com/blogs/ezra-klein/post/creator-of-premium-support-says-ryan-has-vouchers-not-premium-support/2011/04/08/AFAVslLD_blog.html.

9. Austin Frakt, "And, Quietly, We Slip Down the Wonk Hole," *The Incidental Economist* (blog), April 2011, http://theincidentaleconomist.com/wordpress/and-quietly-we-slip-down-the-wonk-hole/.
10. John C. Goodman, "A Framework for Medicare Reform," National Center for Policy Analysis, Policy Report No. 315, September 2008, http://www.ncpa.org/pdfs/st315.pdf.
11. Goodman, "A Framework for Medicare Reform."
12. See the discussion in Chapter 11.
13. Leslie Foster, Randall Brown, Barbara Phillips, Jennifer Schore and Barbara Lepidus Carlson, "Improving The Quality Of Medicaid Personal Assistance Through Consumer Direction," *Health Affairs* Web Exclusive (2003). doi: 10.1377/hlthaff.w3.162.
14. Jason Shafrin, "Why Doctors Don't Like Medicare," *Healthcare Economist* (blog), January 3, 2012, http://healthcare-economist.com/2012/01/03/why-doctors-dont-like-medicare/.
15. John E. Wennberg et al., "The Care of Patients with Severe Chronic Illness: An Online Report on the Medicare Program the Dartmouth Atlas Project," The Dartmouth Atlas of Healthcare 2006, The Center for the Evaluative Clinical Sciences, Dartmouth Medical School, 2006, http://www.dartmouthatlas.org/downloads/atlases/2006_Chronic_Care_Atlas.pdf.
16. Wennberg et al., "The Care of Patients with Severe Chronic Illness: An Online Report on the Medicare Program the Dartmouth Atlas Project."
17. Wennberg et al., "The Care of Patients with Severe Chronic Illness: An Online Report on the Medicare Program the Dartmouth Atlas Project."
18. Amy Hopson and Andrew J. Rettenmaier, "Medicare Spending Across the Map," National Center For Policy Analysis, Policy Report No. 313, July 2008.
19. Reed Abelson, "In Bid for Better Care, Surgery With a Warranty," *New York Times*, May 17, 2007.
20. Vanessa Fuhrmans, "A Novel Plan Helps Hospital Wean Itself Off Pricey Tests," *Wall Street Journal*, January 12, 2007.
21. "The Asheville Project," Supplement to the *Pharmacy Times*, October 1998, http://www.pharmacytimes.com/files/articlefiles/TheAshevilleProject.pdf.
22. American Physician Housecalls website: http://www.aphousecalls.com/.
23. "ICD-10 Code Set to Replace ICD-9," American Medical Association, Transaction Code Set Standards, undated, http://www.ama-assn.org/ama/pub/physician-resources/solutions-managing-your-practice/coding-billing-insurance/hipaahealth-insurance-portability-accountability-act/transaction-code-set-standards/icd10-code-set.page.
24. "ICD-10 Code Set to Replace ICD-9," American Medical Association, Transaction Code Set Standards, undated, http://www.ama-assn.org/ama/pub/physician-resources/solutions-managing-your-practice/coding-billing-insurance/hipaahealth-insurance-portability-accountability-act/transaction-code-set-standards/icd10-code-set.page.
25. Anna Wilde Matthews, "Walked into a Lamppost? Hurt While Crocheting? Help Is on the Way," *Wall Street Journal*, September 13, 2011, http://online.wsj.com/article/SB10001424053111904103404576560742746021106.html.
26. Thomas R. Saving and John C. Goodman, "A Better Way to Approach Medicare's Impossible Task," *Health Affairs Blog*, November 15, 2011, http://healthaffairs.org/blog/2011/11/15/a-better-way-to-approach-medicares-impossible-task/.

27. Devon M. Herrick, "Retail Clinics: Convenient and Affordable Care," National Center for Policy Analysis, Brief Analysis No. 686, January 2010, http://www.ncpa.org/pub/ba686.
28. Devon M. Herrick, "Convenient Care and Telemedicine," National Center for Policy Analysis, Policy Report No. 305, November 2007, http://www.ncpa.org/pub/st305.
29. Devon M. Herrick, "Concierge Medicine: Convenient and Affordable Care," National Center for Policy Analysis, Brief Analysis No. 687, January 19, 2010.
30. Maura Lerner, "Park Nicollet gets sobering lesson in Medicare," *StarTribune*, May 2, 2011.
31. "STARK LAW—Information on penalties, legal practices, latest news and advice," Stark Law, undated, http://starklaw.org.
32. Paul H. Keckley and Howard R. Underwood, "Medical Tourism: Consumers in Search of Value," Deloitte Center for Health Solutions, Item #8174, 2008, http://www.deloitte.com/assets/Dcom-UnitedStates/Local%20Assets/Documents/us_chs_MedicalTourismStudy(3).pdf.
33. BridgeHealth, http://www.bridgehealthmedical.com/.
34. Devon M. Herrick, "Medical Tourism: Global Competition in Health Care," National Center for Policy Analysis, Policy Report No. 304, November 2007
35. Stan Dorn and Baoping Shang, "Spurring Enrollment In Medicare Savings Programs Through a Substitute for the Asset Test Focused on Investment Income," *Health Affairs* 31 No. 2: 367–375, February 2012. doi: 10.1377/hlthaff.2011.0443
36. IntegraNet, http://www.integranettx.com/.
37. "Reductions in Hospital Days, Re-Admissions, and Potentially Avoidable Admissions Among Medicare Advantage Enrollees in California and Nevada, 2006," AHIP Center for Policy and Research, America's Health Insurance Plans, October 2009.

Chapter 15

1. Robert Steinbrook, "Healthcare Reform in Massachusetts—Expanding Coverage, Escalating Costs," *New England Journal of Medicine* 358 (2008): 2757–2760, http://www.nejm.org/doi/full/10.1056/NEJMp0804277. Ben Storrow, "State's Health-Care Coverage Gets Mixed Grades, Daily Hampshire Gazette, February 8, 2010.
2. Kevin Sack, "As Medicaid Payments Shrink, Patients Are Abandoned," *New York Times*, March 15, 2010, http://www.nytimes.com/2010/03/16/health/policy/16medicaid.html.
3. Joanna Bisgaier and Karen V. Rhodes, "Auditing Access to Specialty Care for Children with Public Insurance," *New England Journal of Medicine* 364 (2011): 2324–2333.
4. Brent R. Asplin et al., "Insurance Status and Access to Urgent Ambulatory Care Follow-up Appointments," *Journal of the American Medical Association* 294 (2005): 1248–1254, doi: 10.1001.
5. John C. Goodman et al., "Medicaid Empire: Why New York Spends So Much on Healthcare for the Poor and Near Poor and How the System Can Be Reformed," National Center for Policy Analysis, Policy Report No. 284 (2006): 27, http://www.ncpa.org/pdfs/st284.pdf#page=27.

6. Brent R. Asplin et al., "Insurance Status and Access to Urgent Ambulatory Care Follow-up Appointments," *Journal of the American Medical Association* 294 (2005): 1248–1254. doi: 10.1001/jama.294.10.1248.
7. Merritt Hawkins & Associates, "2009 Survey of Physician Appointment Wait Times."
8. Ron Shinkman, "Kids in Medicaid, CHIP Have Trouble Accessing Specialty Care," *Fierce Healthcare*, April 6, 2011, http://www.fiercehealthcare.com/story/gao-medicaid-chip-shortchanging-children/2011-04-07.
9. "Medicaid and CHIP Information on Children's Access to Care," Government Accountability Office, GAO-10-293R, April 5, 2011, http://www.gao.gov/new.items/d11293r.pdf.
10. Merritt Hawkins & Associates, "2009 Survey of Physician Appointment Wait Times."
11. Ning Tang, John Stein, Renee Y. Hsia, Judith H Maselli and Ralph Gonzales, "Trends and Characteristics of US Emergency Department Visits, 1997–2007," *Journal of the American Medical Association* 304 (2010): 664–670. doi: 10.1001/jama.2010.1112.
12. Linda Gorman, "Medicaid Block Grants and Consumer-Directed Healthcare," National Center for Policy Analysis, Issue Brief No. 102, September 15, 2011.
13. Scott Gottlieb, "Medicaid Is Worse Than No Coverage at All," *Wall Street Journal*, March 10, 2011, http://online.wsj.com/article/SB10001424052748704758904576188280858303612.html?mod=djemITP_h.
14. Joseph Kwok et al., "The Impact of Health Insurance Status on the Survival of Patients with Head and Neck Cancer," *Cancer* 116, No. 2, (2010): 476–485.
15. Damien J. LaPar et al., "Primary Payer Status Affects Mortality for Major Surgical Operations," *Annals of Surgery* 252 (2010): 544–555. doi: 10.1097/SLA.0b013e3181e8fd75.
16. Michael A. Gaglia et al., "Effect of Insurance Type on Adverse Cardiac Events After Percutaneous Coronary Intervention," *American Journal of Cardiology* 107 (2011): 675–680, http://www.ajconline.org/article/S0002-9149(10)02234-4/abstract.
17. Jeremiah C. Allen et al., "Insurance status is an independent predictor of long-term survival after lung transplantation in the United States," *Journal of Heart and Lung Transplantation* 30 (2011): 45–53, http://www.jhltonline.org/article/S1053-2498%2810%2900442-0/fulltext.
18. Avik Roy, "Re: The UVa Surgical Outcomes Study," *The Agenda* (blog) July 18, 2010, http://www.nationalreview.com/agenda/231148/re-uva-surgical-outcomes-study/avik-roy.
19. Damien J. LaPar, "Primary Payer Status Affects Mortality for Major Surgical Operations," *Annals of Surgery* 252 (2010): 544–551, doi: 10.1097.
20. Richard G. Roetzheim, "Effects of Health Insurance and Race on Early Detection of Cancer," *Journal of the National Cancer Institute* 91 (1999): 1409–1415, doi: 10.1093.
21. Rachel R. Kelz, "Morbidity and Mortality of Colorectal Carcinoma Surgery Differs by Insurance Status," *Cancer* 101 (2004): 2187–2194.
22. Jeannine K. Giacovelli et al., "Insurance Status Predicts Access to Care and Outcomes of Vascular Disease," *Journal of Vascular Surgery* 48 (2008): 905–911, doi: 10.1016.
23. Michael T. Halpern et al., "Association of insurance status and ethnicity with cancer stage at diagnosis for 12 cancer sites: a retrospective analysis," *Lancet Oncology* 9 (2008): 222–231. doi:10.1016/S1470-2045(08)70032-9.

24. Avik Roy, "Re: The UVa Surgical Outcome Study," *National Review* (Online), July 18, 2010, http://www.nationalreview.com/agenda/231148/re-uva-surgical-outcomes-study/avik-roy.
25. Austin Frakt, "Medicaid-IV Summary," *The Incidental Economist* (blog), October 14, 2010, http://theincidentaleconomist.com/wordpress/medicaid-iv-summary/.
26. Benjamin D. Sommers and Sara Rosenbaum, "Issues In Health Reform: How Changes In Eligibility May Move Millions Back And Forth Between Medicaid And Insurance Exchanges," *Health Affairs* 30 (2010): 228–236. doi: 10.1377/hlthaff.2010.1000.
27. Austin Frakt, "Medicaid and Health Outcomes Again," *The Incidental Economist* (blog), March 2, 2011, http://theincidentaleconomist.com/wordpress/medicaid-and-health-outcomes-again/.
28. Devon Herrick, "Report: Uninsured Emergency Room Use Greatly Exaggerated," *Healthcare News*, July 2010, http://news.heartland.org/newspaper-article/report-uninsured-emergency-room-use-greatly-exaggerated.
29. Amy Finkelstein et al., "The Oregon Health Insurance Experiment: Evidence from the First Year," NBER Working Paper No. 17190 (2011), http://www.rwjf.org/files/research/72577.5294.oregon.nber.pdf.
30. Robin Hanson, "The Oregon Health Insurance Experiment," *Overcoming Bias* (blog), June 19, 2011, http://www.overcomingbias.com/2011/07/the-oregon-health-insurance-experiment.html.
31. "Medicaid Fraud and Abuse: Stronger Action Needed to Remove Excluded Providers From Federal Health Programs," Government Accountability Office, 1997, http://www.gao.gov/products/HEHS-97-63.
32. Clifford J. Levy and Michael Luo, "New York Medicaid Fraud May Reach Into Billions," *New York Times*, July 18, 2005.
33. Clifford J. Levy and Michael Luo, "New York Medicaid Fraud May Reach Into Billions."
34. Pamela Villarreal and Michael Barba, "Update on Federal Medicaid Funding," National Center for Policy Analysis, Brief Analysis No. 744, May 10, 2011.
35. Villarreal and Barba, "Update on Federal Medicaid Funding."
36. Linda Gorman, "Medicaid Block Grants and Consumer-directed Healthcare," National Center for Policy Analysis, Issue Brief No. 102, September 2011.
37. "Rhode Island's Medicaid Lesson," *Wall Street Journal*, March 28, 2011, http://online.wsj.com/article/SB10001424052748704893604576198710204114624.html#articleTabs%3Darticle.
38. "Medicaid Managed Care Enrollment Report," Centers for Medicare and Medicaid Services, US Department of Health and Human Services, undated, https://www.cms.gov/MedicaidDataSourcesGenInfo/downloads/2010Trends.pdf.
39. Tarren Bragdon, "Florida's Medicaid Reform Shows the Way to Improve Health, Increase Satisfaction, and Control Costs," Heritage Foundation, Backgrounder No. 2620, November 9, 2011.
40. "Healthy Indiana Plan" website: http://www.in.gov/fssa/hip/.
41. Avik Roy, "Obama Administration Denies Waiver for Indiana's Popular Medicaid Program," *The Apothecary* (blog), November 11, 2011. http://www.*Forbes*.com/sites/aroy/2011/11/11/obama-administration-denies-waiver-for-indianas-popular-medicaid-reform/

42. Timothy K. Lake, Vivian L. H. Byrd, and Seema Verma, "Healthy Indiana Plan: Lessons for Health Reform," Mathmatica Policy Research, No. 1, January 2011. http://www.mathematica-mpr.com/publications/PDFs/health/healthyindianaplan_ib1.pdf.
43. Kenneth Artz, "Obama Administration May Wipe Out Daniels' Healthy Indiana Plan," *Healthcare News*, November 11, 2011. http://news.heartland.org/newspaper-article/2011/11/11/obama-administration-may-wipe-out-daniels-healthy-indiana-plan.
44. Avik Roy, "Obama Administration Denies Waiver for Indiana's Popular Medicaid Program," *The Apothecary* (blog), November 11, 2011. http://www.Forbes.com/sites/aroy/2011/11/11/obama-administration-denies-waiver-for-indianas-popular-medicaid-reform/
45. Conversations with Foundation for Health Coverage Education President, Ankeny Minoux, and Executive Director, Phil Lebherz.

Chapter 16

1. Patient Protection and Affordable Care Act of 2009, HR 3962, 111th Congress, 1st session.
2. Laura Landro, "Unexpected Limits of New, Free Preventive Care," *Wall Street Journal*, January 18, 2011.
3. Congressional Budget Office, "Estimate of Changes in Direct Spending and Revenue Effects of the Reconciliation Proposal Combined with HR 3590 as Passed by the Senate," March 20, 2010, http://www.cbo.gov/ftpdocs/113xx/doc11379/AmendReconProp.pdf.
4. Centers for Medicare and Medicaid Service, "Estimated Financial Effects of the 'Patient Protection and Affordable Care Act,' as Amended," April 22, 2010, http://republicans.waysandmeans.house.gov/UploadedFiles/OACT_Memorandum_on_Financial_Impact_of_PPACA_as_Enacted.pdf.
5. Robert Book believes the proportion of Americans without health coverage will rise under the Affordable Care Act. Microsimulation analysis by Book finds that previously insured Americans will forgo coverage for a variety of reasons: many employers may drop employee health coverage, some individuals will not qualify for an exchange subsidy, and individuals can always enroll in the event they become sick. See Robert A. Book, "Who will be Insured, and Uninsured, Under the 2010 Health Reform Law?" *American Action Forum*, forthcoming 2012.
6. Congressional Budget Office, "Estimate of Changes in Direct Spending and Revenue Effects of the Reconciliation Proposal Combined with HR 3590 as Passed by the Senate."
7. Centers for Medicare and Medicaid Service, "Estimated Financial Effects of the 'Patient Protection and Affordable Care Act,' as Amended."
8. Boards of Trustees of the Federal Hospital Insurance and Federal Supplementary Medical Insurance Trust Funds, "2010 Annual Report of the Boards of Trustees of the Federal Hospital Insurance and Federal Supplementary Medical Insurance Trust Funds," August 5, 2010, https://www.cms.gov/ReportsTrustFunds/downloads/tr2010.pdf.
9. "Five Unaffordable Facts About the New Healthcare Law: The Patient Protection and Affordable Care Act," National Federation of Independent Businesses, April 2010,

http://www.nfib.com/Portals/0/PDF/AllUsers/IssuesElections/healthcare/April%2010%20Five%20Unaffordable%20Facts%20about%20the%20New%20Healthcare%20Law.pdf.

10. "The WellPoint Revelation: Private Insurance Premiums Could Triple under ACA," *Wall Street Journal*, October 28, 2009, A22; and "Healthcare Reform Premium Impact in California—December 2009 Addendum," Wellpoint, December 2009, http://www.wellpoint.com/prodcontrib/groups/wellpoint/@wp_news_research/documents/wlp_assets/pw_d014969.pdf.
11. "The Budget and Economic Outlook: An Update," Congressional Budget Office, Congress of the United States, August 1, 2010, http://cbo.gov/publication/21670.
12. "Health Costs and the Federal Budget," *Congressional Budget Office Director's Blog* (blog), May 28, 2010, http://cboblog.cbo.gov/?p=1034.
13. Centers for Medicare and Medicaid Service, "Estimated Financial Effects of the 'Patient Protection and Affordable Care Act,' as Amended."
14. "Analysis of the Patient Protection and Affordable Care Act (HR 3590)," RAND Corporation, 2010, http://www.rand.org/pubs/research_briefs/2010/RAND_RB9514.pdf.
15. Nadeem Esmail, "Waiting Your Turn: Hospital Waiting Lists in Canada 2009 Report," Fraser Institute, October 2009. David C Dugdale, Ronald Epstein and Steven Z Pantilat, "Time and the Patient-Physician Relationship," *Journal of General Internal Medicine* 14 (1999): S34–S40, doi: 10.1046/j.1525-1497.1999.00263.x.
16. Centers for Medicare and Medicaid Service, "Estimated Financial Effects of the 'Patient Protection and Affordable Care Act,' as Amended." Carla K. Johnson, "Health Overhaul May Mean Longer ER Waits, Crowding," *USA Today*, July 2, 2010, http://www.usatoday.com/news/health/2010-07-02-emergency-room_N.htm.
17. Atul Gawande, "The Velluvial Matrix," *New Yorker*, June 16, 2010, http://www.newyorker.com/online/blogs/newsdesk/2010/06/gawande-stanford-speech.html.
18. Karen Davis, "How Will the Healthcare System Change Under Health Reform?" *The Commonwealth Fund Blog* (blog), June 29, 2010, http://www.commonwealthfund.org/Blog/How-Will-the-Health-Care-System-Change.aspx.
19. Peter Orszag, "Reforming Medicare's Payment System," *The Opinionator* (blog), October 21, 2010, http://opinionator.blogs.nytimes.com/2010/10/21/reforming-medicares-payment-system/.
20. Peter Orszag, "Malpractice Methodology," *New York Times*, October 20, 2010, http://www.nytimes.com/2010/10/21/opinion/21orszag.html?_r=1.
21. Ryan Lizza, "Obama Memos: The Verdict on Malpractice," *New Yorker News Desk* (Blog), January 27, 2012, http://www.newyorker.com/online/blogs/newsdesk/2012/01/obama-memos-malpractice.html.
22. For a discussion, see Anna Wilde Mathews, "Can Accountable-Care Organizations Improve Health Care While Reducing Costs?" *Wall Street Journal*, January 23, 2012.
23. Jeff Goldsmith, "The Accountable Care Organization: Not Ready for Prime Time." Amy Goldstein, "Experiment to Lower Medicare Costs did not Save Much Money," *Washington Post*, June 1, 2011.
24. David Dranove, "Quality Disclosure and Certification: Theory and Practice," *Journal of Economic Literature*, 48 (2010): 935–963, doi: 10.1257/jel.48.4.935.

25. Ashley D. Black et al., "The Impact of eHealth on the Quality and Safety of Healthcare: A Systematic Overview," *PloS Medicine* (2011), http://www.plosmedicine.org/article/info%3Adoi%2F10.1371%2Fjournal.pmed.1000387
26. Brian Serumaga et al., "Effect of Pay for Performance on the Management and Outcomes of Hypertension in the United Kingdom: Interrupted Time Series Study," British Journal of Medicine (2011), doi: 10.1136/bmj.d108.
27. Scott Gottlieb, "Accountable Care Organizations: The End of Innovation in Medicine?" American Enterprise Institute for Public Policy Research, No. 3, February 2011, http://www.aei.org/files/2011/02/16/HPO-2011-03-g.pdf.
28. Gottlieb, "Accountable Care Organizations: The End of Innovation in Medicine?"
29. Reed Abelson, "Insurers Push Plans That Limit Choice of Doctor," *New York Times*, July 18, 2010.
30. "Fact Sheet: Keeping the Health Plan You Have: The Affordable Care Act and 'Grandfathered' Health Plans," HealthCare.gov, http://www.healthreform.gov/newsroom/keeping_the_health_plan_you_have.html.
31. "Employer Reaction to Healthcare Reform: Grandfathered Status Survey," Aon Hewitt, August 2011, http://www.aon.com/attachments/Employer_Reaction_HC_Reform_GF_SC.pdf.
32. Kay Lazar, "Firms Cancel Health Coverage," *Boston Globe*, July 18, 2010, http://www.boston.com/news/health/articles/2010/07/18/firms_cancel_health_coverage/.
33. Congressional Budget Office, "Summary of Preliminary Analysis of Health and Revenue Provisions of Reconciliation Legislation Combined with H.R. 3590 as Passed by the Senate," March 18, 2010, http://www.politico.com/static/PPM110_100318_cbo_score.html.
34. Centers for Medicare and Medicaid Service, "Estimated Financial Effects of the 'Patient Protection and Affordable Care Act,' as Amended."
35. Douglas Holtz-Eakin, "Labor Markets and Healthcare Reform: New Results," American Action Forum, May 2010, http://americanactionforum.org/files/LaborMkts HCRAAF5-27-10.pdf.
36. McKinsey & Company, "Employer Survey on US Healthcare Reform," June 20, 2011, http://www.mckinsey.com/Features/US_employer_healthcare_survey.aspx.
37. Centers for Medicare and Medicaid Service, "Estimated Financial Effects of the 'Patient Protection and Affordable Care Act,' as Amended."
38. Avery Johnson, "Private Medicare Plans Are Retrenching," *Wall Street Journal*, November 19, 2010.
39. Janet Adamy, "3M to Change Health-Plan Options for Workers," *Wall Street Journal*, October 4, 2010.
40. Jack Hoadley et al., "Medicare Part D: A First Look at Part D Plan Offerings in 2012," Kaiser Family Foundation, October 2011, http://www.kff.org/medicare/upload/8245.pdf.
41. Chris Jacobs (Republican Policy Committee) review of waiver requests granted by the US Department of Health and Human Services, January 6, 2012.
42. Many individuals may choose health plans that are less comprehensive than the average plans sold in the exchange. The CBO estimates the minimum (bronze) plan sold

in the exchange will cost individuals between $4,500 and $5,000 (family plans from $12,000 to $12,500). See "Premiums for Bronze Plan—Letter to Honorable Olympia Snowe," Congressional Budget Office, January 11, 2010, http://www.cbo.gov/ftpdocs/108xx/doc10884/01-11-Premiums_for_Bronze_Plan.pdf. The actual cost will vary by plan design, region, and age of applicant.

43. Committee on Ways and Means Republican Report, "The Wrong Prescription: Democrats' Health Overhaul Dangerously Expands IRS Authority," March 18, 2010, http://republicans.waysandmeans.house.gov/News/DocumentSingle.aspx?DocumentID=176997.
44. Douglas W. Elmendorf, "Analysis of the Major Health Care Legislation, Enacted in March 2010," Testimony before the Subcommittee on Health, Committee on Energy and Commerce, U.S. House of Representatives, March 30, 2011, http://www.cbo.gov/sites/default/files/cbofiles/ftpdocs/121xx/doc12119/03-30-healthcarelegislation.pdf.
45. Keith Hennessey, "How Would the Reid Bill Affect the Middle Class?" December 10, 2009, http://keithhennessey.com/2009/12/10/reid-bill-middle-class/.
46. Joint Economic Committee, "Unwinding ACA," April 22, 2010, http://jec.senate.gov/republicans/public/?a=Files.Serve&File_id=1d63d12d-0e1b-45ee-8633-e3624a8ddcd4.
47. Duff Wilson, "Drug Makers Raise Prices in Face of Healthcare Reform," *New York Times*, November 15, 2009, http://www.nytimes.com/2009/11/16/business/16drugprices.html?_r=2&adxnnl=1&adxnnlx=1323872339-vjJx4koVTRgysY/ce+JDAA.
48. Kelly Phillips Erb, "Deduct This: The History of the Medical Expenses Deduction," *Forbes*, June 20, 2011, http://www.Forbes.com/sites/kellyphillipserb/2011/06/20/deduct-this-the-history-of-the-medical-expenses-deduction/.
49. Thomas R. Saving, "How Will the Affordable Care Act Affect the Elderly and Disabled on Medicare?" National Center for Policy Analysis, http://www.ncpa.org/pdfs/NCPA-Social-Security-Trustees-Briefing-2010.pdf.
50. Robert A. Book and James C. Capretta, "Reductions in Medicare Advantage Payments: The Impact on Seniors by Region," Heritage Foundation, September 14, 2010, http://www.heritage.org/research/reports/2010/09/reductions-in-medicare-advantage-payments-the-impact-on-seniors-by-region.
51. John D. Shatto and M. Kent Clemens, "Projected Medicare Expenditures under an Illustrative Scenario with Alternative Payment Updates to Medicare Providers," Office of the Actuary, Centers for Medicare & Medicaid Services, U.S. Department of Health & Human Services, August 5, 2010, http://www.cms.gov/Research-Statistics-Data-and-Systems/Statistics-Trends-and-Reports/ReportsTrustFunds/downloads//2010TRAlternativeScenario.pdf
52. Kris Maher, Ellen E. Schultz, and Bob Tita, "Companies Take Health-Care Charges," *Wall Street Journal*, March 26, 2010; David Reilly, Ellen E. Schultz and Ron Winslow, "AT&T Joins in Health Charges," *Wall Street Journal*, March 27, 2010.
53. Congressional Budget Office, "Comparison of Projected Medicare Part D Premiums under Current Law and under Reconciliation Legislation Combined with H.R. 3590 as Passed by the Senate," March 19, 2010, http://www.cbo.gov/ftpdocs/113xx/doc11355/Comparison.pdf.
54. Todd Ackerman, "Texas Doctors Fleeing Medicare in Droves," Houston Chronicle, May 18, 2010, http://www.chron.com/news/houston-texas/article/Texas-doctors-fleeing-Medicare-in-droves-1718866.php. "Medicare and the Mayo Clinic," *Wall*

Street Journal, January 8, 2010, http://online.wsj.com/article/SB10001424052748703436504574640711655886136.html.

55. Kathleen Sebelius, "Securing Medicare's Future," *Yahoo! News*, July 29, 2010, http://old.news.yahoo.com/s/ynews_excl/ynews_excl_pl3287.
56. Congressional Budget Office, "Letter to the Honorable Jeff Sessions," January 22, 2010, http://www.cbo.gov/ftpdocs/110xx/doc11005/01-22-HI_Fund.pdf.
57. Centers for Medicare and Medicaid Service, "Estimated Financial Effects of the 'Patient Protection and Affordable Care Act,' as Amended."
58. "Mayberry Misleads on Medicare," FactCheck.org, Annenberg Public Policy Center, July 31, 2010, http://factcheck.org/2010/07/mayberry-misleads-on-medicare/.
59. Chris Jacobs, "AARP's Healthcare Bailouts," Republican Policy Committee, April 19, 2010, http://www.ncpa.org/pdfs/E-mail-from-Chris-Jacobs-RPC.pdf.
60. Paul Fronstin, "Findings from the 2010 EBRI/MGA Consumer Engagement in Healthcare Survey," Employee Benefit Research Institute, EBRI Issue Brief No. 352, December 2010.
61. Ron Bachman, "Congress Declares War on HSAs," National Center for Policy Analysis, Brief Analyses No. 698, March 5, 2010.
62. "Actuarial Value and Cost-Sharing Reductions Bulletin," US Department of Health and Human Services, February 24, 2012, http://www.ncpa.org/pdfs/HHS-EHB-Actuarial-Equivalence-Bulletin-022412.pdf. Also see Mark E. Litow et al., "Impact of Medical Loss Ratio Requirements Under PPACA on High Deductible Plans / HSAs in Individual and Small Group Markets," Milliman Inc., January 6, 2012.
63. "The WellPoint Revelation," *Wall Street Journal*, October 28, 2009; "Healthcare Reform Premium Impact in California—December 2009 Addendum," Wellpoint, December 2009, http://www.wellpoint.com/prodcontrib/groups/wellpoint/@wp_news_research/documents/wlp_assets/pw_d014969.pdf.
64. Eric Johnson, "IRS announces new HSA limits for 2012," BenefitsPro.com, May 23, 2011, http://www.benefitspro.com/2011/05/23/irs-announces-new-hsa-limits-for-2012.
65. "Employer Mandate Penalties: Calculations," National Federation of Independent Business, undated, http://www.nfib.com/LinkClick.aspx?fileticket=8lmj3UFCpy0%3D&tabid=1083.
66. "Interim Final Rules for Group Health Plans and Health Insurance Coverage Relating to Status as a Grandfathered Health Plan under the Patient Protection and Affordable Care Act," *Federal Register*, June 17, 2010, http://www.ncpa.org/pdfs/employees-not-grandfathered-in.pdf#page=54.
67. Chris Jacobs, "Did Unions Just Obtain Another Backroom Healthcare Deal?" Republican Policy Committee, June 14, 2010.
68. Many individuals may choose health plans that are less comprehensive than the average plans sold in the exchange. The CBO estimated the minimum (bronze) plan sold in the exchange will cost individuals between $4,500 and $5,000 (families $12,000–$12,500). See Douglas W. Elmendorf, "Letter to Honorable Olympia Snowe," Congressional Budget Office, January 11, 2010, http://www.cbo.gov/ftpdocs/108xx/doc10884/01-11-Premiums_for_Bronze_Plan.pdf.
69. The Henry Kaiser Family Foundation, "Health Reform Subsidy Calculator," June 22, 2010, http://healthreform.kff.org/SubsidyCalculator.aspx.

70. Dan Danner, "ACA vs. Small Business," *Wall Street Journal*, May 27, 2010.
71. Douglas W. Elmendorf, "Letter to the Honorable Harry Reid," Congressional Budget Office, December 19, 2009, http://www.cbo.gov/ftpdocs/108xx/doc10868/12-19-Reid_Letter_Managers_Correction_Noted.pdf; Greg Scandlen, "Whatever Happened to the Small Business Tax Credit?" *John Goodman's Health Policy Blog*, December 28, 2011, http://healthblog.ncpa.org/whatever-happened-to-the-small-business-tax-credit/.
72. The Honorable J. Russell George, "Implementation and Effectiveness of the Small Business Healthcare Tax Credit," (Hearing Before the Committee on Ways and Means Subcommittee on Oversight, US House of Representatives, November 15, 2011), http://waysandmeans.house.gov/UploadedFiles/GeorgeTestimonyOS911.pdf.
73. Patricia Thompson, American Institute of Certified Public Accountants (Testimony Before the Committee on Ways and Means Subcommittee on Oversight, US House of Representatives, November 15, 2011), http://waysandmeans.house.gov/Uploaded Files/ThompsonTestimonyOS1115.pdf.
74. "White House Unveils Subsidies to Preserve Early-Retiree Coverage," *Kaiser Health News*, May 5, 2010, http://www.kaiserhealthnews.org/Daily-Reports/2010/May/05/early-retirees-wednes.aspx.
75. "Comparison of Projected Medicare Part D Premiums Under Current Law and Under Reconciliation Legislation Combined with HR 3590 as Passed by the Senate," Congressional Budget Office, Congress of the United States, March 19, 2010, http://www.cbo.gov/ftpdocs/113xx/doc11355/Comparison.pdf.
76. "Preventive Services Covered under the Affordable Care Act," HealthCare.gov, July 2010, http://www.healthcare.gov/news/factsheets/2010/07/preventive-services-list.html.
77. "Designated Health Professional Shortage Areas (HPSA) Statistics," Office of Shortage Designation, Bureau of Health Professions, Health Resources and Services Administration (HRSA), US Department of Health & Human Services, December 12, 2011, http://ersrs.hrsa.gov/ReportServer?/HGDW_Reports/BCD_HPSA/BCD_HPSA_SCR50_Smry&rs:Format=HTML3.2.
78. David Brown, "In the Balance: Some Candidates Disagree, but Studies Show It's Often Cheaper to Let People Get Sick," *Washington Post*, April 8, 2008.
79. Louise B. Russell, "Preventing Chronic Disease: An Important Investment, But Don't Count On Cost Savings," *Health Affairs* 28, No. 1 (2009): 42–45. doi: 10.1377.
80. Louise B. Russell, "Preventing Chronic Disease: An Important Investment, But Don't Count On Cost Savings," *Health Affairs* 28 (2009): 42–45, doi: 10.1377.
81. "Breast Cancer Screening Recommendations for Women at Higher Risk," Susan G. Komen for the Cure, http://ww5.komen.org/BreastCancer/Recommendationsfor WomenwithHigherRisk.html
82. Michelle Andrews. "Preventing Pregnancy: Should Patients Get Contraceptives from Health Plans At No Cost?" *Kaiser Health News*, July 6, 2010.

Chapter 17

1. Conversation with Republican Senate staff; compilation based on pages of Federal Register regulations and notices.
2. Uwe E. Reinhardt, Peter S. Hussey, and Gerard F. Anderson, "US Healthcare Spending in an International Context," *Health Affairs* 23, No. 3 (May 2004): 10–25.

3. Many people will opt for more comprehensive plans. See Douglas W. Elmendorf, "Letter to Honorable Olympia Snowe," Congressional Budget Office, January 11, 2010, http://www.cbo.gov/ftpdocs/108xx/doc10884/01-11-Premiums_for_Bronze_Plan.pdf.
4. Katherine Baicker and Helen Levy, "Employer Health Insurance Mandates and the Risk of Unemployment," *Risk Management and Insurance Review* 11 (2008): 109–132. doi: 10.1111/j.1540-6296.2008.00133.x.
5. Victoria C. Bunce and J. P. Wieske, "Health Insurance Mandates in the States, 2010," Council for Affordable Health Insurance, http://www.cahi.org/cahi_contents/resources/pdf/MandatesintheStates2010.pdf.
6. John C. Goodman and Gerald L. Musgrave, "Freedom of Choice in Health Insurance," National Center for Policy Analysis, NCPA Policy Report No. 134, 1988; Gail A. Jensen and Michael A. Morrisey, "Mandated Benefit Laws and Employer-Sponsored Health Insurance," Health Insurance Association of America, January 25, 1999; and Stephen T. Parente, et al., "Consumer Response to a National Marketplace for Individual Insurance," Office of the Assistant Secretary for Planning and Evaluation, US Department of Health and Human Services, Final Report, June 28, 2008, http://aspe.hhs.gov/health/reports/08/consumerresponse/report.html.
7. The Henry Kaiser Family Foundation, "Health Reform Subsidy Calculator," June 22, 2010, http://healthreform.kff.org/SubsidyCalculator.aspx.
8. Daniel P. Kessler, "How Health Reform Punishes Work," *Wall Street Journal*, April 25, 2011, http://www.hoover.org/news/daily-report/76401.
9. Jason Brown et al., "How Does Risk Selection Respond to Risk Adjustment? Evidence from the Medicare Advantage Program," National Bureau of Economic Research, NBER Working Paper 16977, April 18, 2011, http://www.nber.org/papers/w16977.pdf.
10. Robert O. Morgan et al., "The Medicare-HMO Revolving Door—The Healthy Go in and the Sick Go Out," *New England Journal of Medicine* 337 (1997): 169–175, http://www.nejm.org/doi/full/10.1056/NEJM199707173370306?ck=nck.
11. Kay Lazar, "Short-term Insurance Buyers Drive Up Cost in Mass.," *Boston Globe*, June 30, 2010, http://www.boston.com/news/local/massachusetts/articles/2010/06/30/short_term_insurance_buyers_drive_up_cost_in_mass/.
12. Jay Hancock, "IRS to Enforce Health Coverage with 'Honor System'," *The Baltimore Sun, Jay Hancock's Blog*, March 30, 2010, http://weblogs.baltimoresun.com/business/hancock/blog/2010/03/irs_enforcement_for_health_cov.html.
13. Timothy Jost, "Implementing Health Reform: Preventive Services," *Health Affairs Blog*, July 15, 2010, http://healthaffairs.org/blog/2010/07/15/implementing-health-reform-preventive-services/.
14. Damon Adams, "Who has 7-Plus Hours a Day to Put Toward Preventive Care?" *American Medical News*, April 21, 2003, http://www.ama-assn.org/amednews/2003/04/21/prsc0421.htm.
15. Louise B. Russell, "Preventing Chronic Disease: An Important Investment, but Don't Count on Cost Savings," *Health Affairs* 28 (2009): 42–45. doi: 10.1377/hlthaff.28.1.42.
16. John C. Goodman, "For the Vulnerable, Expect Less Access to Care," John Goodman Health Policy Blog, November 16, 2011, http://healthblog.ncpa.org/for-the-vulnerable-expect-less-access-to-care/.

17. Devon M. Herrick, "Concierge Medicine: Convenient and Affordable Care," National Center for Policy Analysis, Brief Analysis No. 687, January 19, 2010.
18. Julian Pecquet, "Investment in Healthcare Workforce Announced as Doctor Shortage Looms," *Healthwatch, The Hill's Healthcare Blog*, June 16, 2010, http://thehill.com/blogs/healthwatch/health-reform-implementation/103575-invetment-in-healthcare-workforce-announced-as-doctor-shortage-looms.
19. Doug Trapp, "Primary Care Gets Boost with $250 Million in HHS Grants," *American Medical News*, July 1, 2010, http://www.ama-assn.org/amednews/2010/06/28/gvsf0701.htm.
20. "Fact Sheet: Creating Jobs and Increasing the Number of Primary Care Providers," Health Reform.Gov, December 12, 2010, http://www.healthreform.gov/newsroom/primarycareworkforce.html/.
21. The Henry Kaiser Family Foundation, "Total Nurse Practitioners, 2010," State Health Facts, http://www.statehealthfacts.org/comparemaptable.jsp?typ=1&ind=773&cat=8&sub=103&sortc=1&o=a.
22. Virginia Traweek and John C. Goodman, "The Doctor's Out, Where is the Nurse?" National Center for Policy Analysis, Brief Analysis No. 757, November 10, 2011.
23. "2010 County-Level Poverty Rates for Texas," US Department of Agriculture Economic Research Services, December 2, 2011, http://www.ers.usda.gov/Data/povertyrates/PovListpct.asp?st=TX&longname=Texas.
24. Anna Gorman, "Free Clinic Plagued by Red Tape," *Los Angeles Times*, October 12, 2011, http://www.latimes.com/news/local/la-me-freeclinic-20111012,0,1784326.story.
25. John C. Goodman, "Emergency Room Visits Likely to Increase under ACA," National Center for Policy Analysis, Brief Analysis No. 709, June 18, 2010, http://www.ncpa.org/pdfs/ba709.pdf.
26. Douglas W. Elmendorf, "Letter to Speaker Nancy Pelosi," Congressional Budget Office, March 20, 2010, http://www.ncpa.org/pdfs/Managers-Amendment-to-Reconciliation-Proposal.pdf.
27. John D. Shatto and M. Kent Clements, "Projected Medicare Expenditures under an Illustrative Scenario with Alternative Payment Updates to Medicare Providers," Center for Medicaid &Medicare Services, August 5, 2010, https://www.cms.gov/ReportsTrustFunds/downloads/2010TRAlternativeScenario.pdf.
28. Joseph P. Newhouse, "Assessing Health Reform's Impact on Four Key Groups of Americans," *Health Affairs* 29 (2010): 1714–1724, doi: 10.1377/hlthaff.2010.0595.
29. For example see: Robert A. Berenson, "From Politics To Policy: A New Payment Approach In Medicare Advantage," *Health Affairs* 27, No. 2 (2008): w156–w164. doi: 10.1377/hlthaff.27.2.w156.
30. Robert A. Berenson, "From Politics To Policy: A New Payment Approach In Medicare Advantage," Health Affairs 27, No. 2 (2008): w156–w164 (Published online) doi: 10.1377/hlthaff.27.2.w156. Also see Lisa Wangsness, "Democrats Seek Cuts in Medicare Advantage: Citing Perks, GOP says Obama Misled," *Boston Globe*, September 24, 2009.
31. John C. Goodman, "The Puzzling War on the Elderly," *John Goodman's Health Policy Blog*, August 24, 2009, http://healthblog.ncpa.org/the-puzzling-war-on-the-elderly/.
32. David Cutler and Jonathan Gruber, "Does Public Insurance Crowd out Private Insurance?" *Quarterly Journal of Economics* 111, No. 2 (1996): 391–430.

33. Thomas M. Suehs, "Federal Health Care Reform — Impact to Texas Health and Human Services Commission," Presentation to Texas House Select Committee on Federal Legislation, April 22, 2010. http://www.hhsc.state.tx.us/news/presentations/2010/HouseSelectFedHlthReform.pdf.
34. Author calculations based on estimates of the ratio of Medicare to private insurers' physicians fees and data from Kaiser State Health Facts. Also see Devon Herrick, "Medicaid Expansion will Bankrupt the States," National Center for Policy Analysis, Brief Analysis No. 729, October 25, 2010, http://www.ncpa.org/pdfs/ba729.pdf.
35. Katherine Hobson, "HHS Releases Final Medical Loss Ratio Regulations," *Wall Street Journal Health Blog*, November 22, 2010, http://blogs.wsj.com/health/2010/11/22/hhs-releases-final-medical-loss-ratio-regulations/.
36. Grace Marie-Turner, "A Radical Restructuring of Health Insurance: Millions to Lose the Health Coverage They Have Now," Galen Institute, December 2011, http://www.galen.org/fileuploads/RadicalRestructuring.pdf.
37. David W. Emmons, José R. Guardado and Carol K. Kane, *Competition in Health Insurance: A Comprehensive Study of US Markets, 2011 Update,* American Medical Association, https://catalog.ama-assn.org/Catalog/product/product_detail.jsp?productId=prod1940016.
38. "Actuarial Value and Cost-Sharing Reductions Bulletin," US Department of Health and Human Services, February 24, 2012. http://www.ncpa.org/pdfs/HHS-EHB-Actuarial-Equivalence-Bulletin-022412.pdf. Also see Mark E. Litow et al., "Impact of Medical Loss Ratio Requirements Under PPACA on High Deductible Plans / HSAs in Individual and Small Group Markets," Milliman Inc., January 6, 2012.
39. Greg Scandlen, "New Regulation Threatens Agents, HSA Plans," *John Goodman's Health Policy Blog*, December 12, 2011, http://healthblog.ncpa.org/new-regulation-threatens-agents-hsa-plans/.

Chapter 18: Conclusion

1. John Rawls, *A Theory of Justice* (Cambridge, MA: Belknap Press of Harvard University Press, 1971).
2. "High Blood Pressure and Cholesterol," *Vital Signs*, Centers for Disease Control and Prevention, US Department of Health and Human Services, February 2012, http://www.cdc.gov/vitalsigns/CardiovascularDisease/.
3. J.D. Kleinke, "Access Versus Excess: Value-Based Cost Sharing for Prescription Drugs," *Health Affairs* 23, No. 1 (2004): 34–47.

Index

About the Author

JOHN C. GOODMAN is Research Fellow at the Independent Institute and President and Kellye Wright Fellow in Health Care at the National Center for Policy Analysis. The *Wall Street Journal* and the *National Journal*, among other media, have called him the "Father of Health Savings Accounts."

John Goodman's *Health Policy Blog* is a premier healthcare blog where solutions to healthcare problems are routinely examined and debated by top health policy experts throughout the country. He is frequently invited to testify before Congress on healthcare reform, and he is the author of more than fifty studies on health policy, retirement reform, and tax issues plus nine books, including *Lives at Risk: Single Payer National Health Insurance Around the World*; *Leaving Women Behind: Modern Families, Outdated Laws*; and the trailblazing *Patient Power: Solving America's Health Care Crisis*, which has sold more than 300,000 copies.

Dr. Goodman regularly appears on television and radio news programs on Fox News Channel, CNN, PBS, Fox Business Network and CNBC, and his articles appear in *The Wall Street Journal*, *Investor's Business Daily*, *National Review*, *Health Affairs*, *Kaiser Health News* and other national publications. Goodman was also the pivotal lead expert in the grassroots public policy campaign, "Free Our Health Care Now," an unsurpassed national education effort to communicate patient-centered alternatives to a government-run health care system. The initiative resulted in the largest online petition ever delivered on Capitol Hill.

Dr. Goodman holds a Ph.D. in economics from Columbia University, and he has taught and completed research at Columbia University, Stanford University, Dartmouth College, Southern Methodist University, and the University of Dallas.

Independent Studies in Political Economy

THE ACADEMY IN CRISIS | *Ed. by John W. Sommer*
AGAINST LEVIATHAN | *Robert Higgs*
ALIENATION AND THE SOVIET ECONOMY | *Paul Craig Roberts*
AMERICAN HEALTH CARE | *Ed. by Roger D. Feldman*
ANARCHY AND THE LAW | *Ed. by Edward P. Stringham*
AQUANOMICS | *Ed. by B. Delworth Gardner & Randy T. Simmons*
ANTITRUST AND MONOPOLY | *D. T. Armentano*
AQUANOMICS | *Ed. by B. Delworth Gardner and Randy T. Simmons*
ARMS, POLITICS, AND THE ECONOMY | *Ed. by Robert Higgs*
BEYOND POLITICS | *Randy T. Simmons*
BOOM AND BUST BANKING | *Ed. by David Beckworth*
CAN TEACHERS OWN THEIR OWN SCHOOLS? | *Richard K. Vedder*
THE CAPITALIST REVOLUTION IN LATIN AMERICA | *Paul Craig Roberts & Karen Araujo*
THE CHALLENGE OF LIBERTY | *Ed. by Robert Higgs & Carl P. Close*
CHANGING THE GUARD | *Ed. by Alexander Tabarrok*
THE CHE GUEVARA MYTH AND THE FUTURE OF LIBERTY | *Alvaro Vargas Llosa*
THE CIVILIAN AND THE MILITARY | *Arthur A. Ekirch, Jr.*
CUTTING GREEN TAPE | *Ed. by Richard L. Stroup & Roger E. Meiners*
THE DECLINE OF AMERICAN LIBERALISM | *Arthur A. Ekirch, Jr.*
DELUSIONS OF POWER | *Robert Higgs*
DEPRESSION, WAR, AND COLD WAR | *Robert Higgs*
THE DIVERSITY MYTH | *David O. Sacks & Peter A. Thiel*
DRUG WAR CRIMES | *Jeffrey A. Miron*
ELECTRIC CHOICES | *Ed. by Andrew N. Kleit*
THE EMPIRE HAS NO CLOTHES | *Ivan Eland*
ENTREPRENEURIAL ECONOMICS | *Ed. by Alexander Tabarrok*
THE ENTERPRISE OF LAW | *Bruce L. Benson*
FAULTY TOWERS | *Ryan C. Amacher & Roger E. Meiners*
FINANCING FAILURE | *Vern McKinley*
FIRE & SMOKE | *Michael I. Krauss*
THE FOUNDERS' SECOND AMENDMENT | *Stephen P. Halbrook*
FREEDOM, FEMINISM, AND THE STATE | *Ed. by Wendy McElroy*
GOOD MONEY | *George Selgin*
HAZARDOUS TO OUR HEALTH? | *Ed. by Robert Higgs*
HOT TALK, COLD SCIENCE | *S. Fred Singer*
HOUSING AMERICA | *Ed. by Randall G. Holcombe & Benjamin Powell*
JUDGE AND JURY | *Eric Helland & Alexander Tabarrok*
LESSONS FROM THE POOR | *Ed. by Alvaro Vargas Llosa*
LIBERTY FOR LATIN AMERICA | *Alvaro Vargas Llosa*
LIBERTY FOR WOMEN | *Ed. by Wendy McElroy*
LIVING ECONOMICS | *Peter J. Boettke*
MAKING POOR NATIONS RICH | *Ed. by Benjamin Powell*
MARKET FAILURE OR SUCCESS | *Ed. by Tyler Cowen & Eric Crampton*
MONEY AND THE NATION STATE | *Ed. by Kevin Dowd & Richard H. Timberlake, Jr.*
NEITHER LIBERTY NOR SAFETY | *Robert Higgs*
THE NEW HOLY WARS | *Robert H. Nelson*
NO WAR FOR OIL | *Ivan Eland*
OPPOSING THE CRUSADER STATE | *Ed. by Robert Higgs & Carl P. Close*
OUT OF WORK | *Richard K. Vedder & Lowell E. Gallaway*
PARTITIONING FOR PEACE | *Ivan Eland*
PLOWSHARES AND PORK BARRELS | *E. C. Pasour, Jr. & Randal R. Rucker*
A POVERTY OF REASON | *Wilfred Beckerman*
PRICELESS | *John C. Goodman*
PRIVATE RIGHTS & PUBLIC ILLUSIONS | *Tibor R. Machan*
PROPERTY RIGHTS | *Ed. by Bruce L. Benson*
THE PURSUIT OF JUSTICE | *Ed. by Edward J. López*
RACE & LIBERTY IN AMERICA | *Ed. by Jonathan Bean*
RECARVING RUSHMORE | *Ivan Eland*
RECLAIMING THE AMERICAN REVOLUTION | *William J. Watkins, Jr.*
REGULATION AND THE REAGAN ERA | *Ed. by Roger E. Meiners & Bruce Yandle*
RESTORING FREE SPEECH AND LIBERTY ON CAMPUS | *Donald A. Downs*
RESURGENCE OF THE WARFARE STATE | *Robert Higgs*
RE-THINKING GREEN | *Ed. by Robert Higgs & Carl P. Close*
SCHOOL CHOICES | *John Merrifield*
SECURING CIVIL RIGHTS | *Stephen P. Halbrook*
STRANGE BREW | *Douglas Glen Whitman*
STREET SMART | *Ed. by Gabriel Roth*
TAXING CHOICE | *Ed. by William F. Shughart, II*
TAXING ENERGY | *Robert Deacon, Stephen DeCanio, H. E. Frech, III, & M. Bruce Johnson*
THAT EVERY MAN BE ARMED | *Stephen P. Halbrook*
TO SERVE AND PROTECT | *Bruce L. Benson*
TWILIGHT WAR | *Mike Moore*
VIETNAM RISING | *William Ratliff*
THE VOLUNTARY CITY | *Ed. by David T. Beito, Peter Gordon, & Alexander Tabarrok*
WINNERS, LOSERS & MICROSOFT | *Stan J. Liebowitz & Stephen E. Margolis*
WRITING OFF IDEAS | *Randall G. Holcombe*